Mental Health of Children and Adolescents in the 21st Century

Edited by Marco Carotenuto

Published in London, United Kingdom

Mental Health of Children and Adolescents in the 21st Century
http://dx.doi.org/10.5772/intechopen.111275
Edited by Marco Carotenuto

Contributors
Ambreen Tharani, Andrea Landini, Anneliese Dörr, Ann Hemingway, Blanca Mas, Helen Johnson, Henry Drasiku, Ioana Darjan, Joel Masete, Jolyon Grimwade, Jonathan Glazzard, Juan M. Guiote, Katrina Robson, Magdalen Akia, Marco Carotenuto, Miguel Ángel Vallejo, Mihai Predescu, Milton Anguyo, Monica Oxford, Patricia Crittenden, Paulina Chávez, Razia Bano Momin, S. Kezia Sullivan, Sharifa Lalani, Shireen Shehzad Bhamani, Siw Karlsen, Steve Farnfield, Susana Roque López, Susan Spieker, Vicki Ellis, Yasodha Rohanachandra, Zahra Tharani, Zoe Ash

First published in London, United Kingdom, 2024 by IntechOpen
IntechOpen is the global imprint of INTECHOPEN LIMITED, registered in England and Wales, registration number: 11086078, 167-169 Great Portland Street, London, W1W 5PF, United Kingdom

British Library Cataloguing-in-Publication Data
A catalogue record for this book is available from the British Library

Additional hard and PDF copies can be obtained from orders@intechopen.com

Mental Health of Children and Adolescents in the 21st Century
Edited by Marco Carotenuto
p. cm.
Print ISBN 978-0-85466-518-1
Online ISBN 978-0-85466-517-4
eBook (PDF) ISBN 978-0-85466-519-8

For EU product safety concerns:
IN TECH d.o.o., Prolaz Marije Krucifikse Kozulić 3, 51000 Rijeka, Croatia,
info@intechopen.com or visit our website at intechopen.com.

Meet the editor

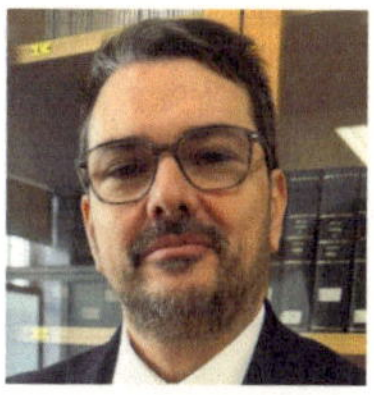

Dr. Marco Carotenuto is a distinguished expert in child neuropsychiatry, with an impressive educational and professional background. Graduating with a master's degree in medicine and surgery from the University of Campania "Luigi Vanvitelli," Italy, in 2000, he went on to specialize in child neuropsychiatry in 2005 after extensive training in the United Kingdom. His pursuit of knowledge led him to obtain a Ph.D. in Behavioral Sciences and Learning Disorders in 2008. Dr. Carotenuto's dedication to advancing his expertise continued as he undertook further training at prestigious Italian research centers, culminating in his appointment as Professor of Child Neuropsychiatry and Director of the Child Neuropsychiatry Unit in 2018. With a portfolio of more than 200 scientific journal articles, Dr. Carotenuto's research focuses on the diagnostic evaluation and therapeutic management of neurodevelopmental disorders, emphasizing childhood autism, sleep disorders, pediatric headaches and epilepsies, as well as neurocognitive and behavioral rehabilitation in children.

Contents

Preface

The surge in mental health problems has reached epidemic proportions, evolving into a silent and invisible pandemic that affects individuals across all stages of life, particularly during childhood, adolescence, and the transition to adulthood. The COVID-19/SARS-2 pandemic has significantly altered this landscape, bringing the magnitude of the problem into sharp focus.

Dedicating an entire book to the mental health problems of children and adolescents is no longer unusual or strange; rather, it is necessary. It is now evident that many psychiatric pathologies in adults have their roots in childhood. Specialized health workers such as child neuropsychiatrists are called upon every day to deal with these problems, which have grown increasingly complex over time. Mental health challenges develop alongside children, and as the child grows, so does the pathology. The beginnings are subtle and insidious, and the emotional fragility of today's youth has become a problem that is too evident to be ignored.

Adolescents today face unique challenges. The formation of their identity is increasingly fragmented and influenced by social media, where issues such as social withdrawal, once considered isolated, have evolved into well-recognized disorders like *hikikomori*. Additionally, violent and harmful interactions on social platforms have led to the rise of cyberbullying. Although there may be generational differences in the perception of these problems, it is crucial to approach them with empathy, care, and respect.

At the same time, our ability to diagnose and understand these issues has improved dramatically. This is not about pathologizing normal behavior, but rather about recognizing and addressing subthreshold or hidden situations early on, allowing for timely intervention through family support, rehabilitation, and pharmacological therapy, all within an integrated vision.

This book is an updated resource for understanding the mental health challenges faced by children and adolescents. Just as these age groups are constantly evolving, so too is our understanding of the conditions they face. It is our hope that this contribution will shed light on the ever-evolving field of child and adolescent mental health and provide valuable insights for those working in this area.

Marco Carotenuto
Department of Mental and Physical Health and Preventive Medicine,
University of Campania "Luigi Vanvitelli",
Caserta, Italy

Section 1

Conceptualizing Change and Shifts

Chapter 1

Introductory Chapter: Mental Health in Developmental Age

Marco Carotenuto

1. Introduction

The term "mental health" refers to an individual's psychological and emotional well-being, allowing them to utilize their cognitive and emotional abilities, function within society, meet daily needs, build healthy relationships, engage positively with societal changes, and adapt to internal and external challenges. This concept varies depending on culture, subjective assessments, and reference theories related to mental functioning. While many experts consider mental health as the absence of mental illness, normality, social adaptation, and happiness, these factors are not necessarily interchangeable. The World Health Organization's general definition of "health" is "a state of complete physical, mental, and social well-being, rather than just the absence of disease or infirmity." The World Health Organization eloquently describes "health" as not just the lack of disease or infirmity but as a state of complete physical, mental, and social well-being. This comprehensive definition underscores the holistic nature of health, emphasizing the importance of addressing not only physical ailments but also mental and social aspects [1].

Critical attributes of mental health include the ability to establish satisfying social relationships, participate constructively in social changes, develop one's personality through social engagement, resolve conflicts in a balanced manner, adapt to internal and external challenges, possess a positive self-image, and be aware of one's emotions, affections, and relational methods.

Mental health is crucial to overall well-being, particularly during the formative years, as up to 50% of adult psychiatric disorders begin before the age of 14. Economic and employment status, education level, standard of living, physical health, family cohesion, discrimination, human rights violations, and exposure to adverse events can all impact mental health. Integrated multi-sectoral strategies are necessary for health promotion and mental distress prevention.

The given definition marks a significant step forward in distancing mental health from the idea of simply the absence of mental illness. However, it raises a few concerns because it could be misinterpreted as suggesting that positive emotions and positive functioning are the only essential aspects of mental health [2].

2. Epidemiology

Early diagnosis and management actions are crucial in addressing psychiatric disorders in children and adolescents. According to a recent UNICEF report, more than 1 in 7 adolescents aged 10–19 have a diagnosed mental disorder, with anxiety and

IntechOpen

depression accounting for 40% of diagnosed cases. Sadly, almost 46,000 teenagers die from suicide each year, and Western Europe has high rates.

Investments in mental health must align with the significant impact that mental health challenges have on children and young people, especially in the context of the ongoing COVID-19 pandemic. There are still significant gaps between mental health needs and dedicated funding [3].

3. The societal cost

Diagnosed mental health issues, such as ADHD, anxiety, autism, bipolar disorder, conduct disorder, depression, eating disorders, intellectual disability, and schizophrenia, can substantially affect the health, education, achievement, and earning capacity of children and young people.

The report from the London School of Economics highlights that the economic impact of mental health issues causing disability or death among young people is estimated at nearly $390 billion annually. However, the actual impact on children's lives is immeasurable [3].

There is an increasing body of evidence supporting mental health and psychosocial support interventions for children and adolescents in low-resource and humanitarian settings. However, there has been limited research assessing family interventions in these contexts despite solid evidence for the vital role that families play in protecting the mental health of children and adolescents. Evidence also suggests that parent and family interventions are highly effective for various mental health and child protection outcomes in high-income countries and non-humanitarian contexts. Conversely, research on family interventions in these contexts remains scarce despite solid evidence for their crucial role-playing in safeguarding developmental age mental health [4].

It is crucial to remember that half of all mental disorders begin before the age of 14 and often stem from non-specific emotional and social issues. These issues can escalate into significant mental disorders, accounting for 45% of the global disease burden among individuals aged 0–25. Although some strides have been made in providing mental health services for young people, there remains a considerable unmet need for support during this critical period. This underscores the importance of reevaluating preventive strategies using a youth-focused, multidisciplinary approach to identify and address potential mental health issues early on [5].

Moreover, evidence suggests that relying solely on mental health professionals to promote and prevent mental health issues is unrealistic. Integrated and multidisciplinary services are necessary to expand the range of available interventions and reduce the risk of long-term adverse outcomes, potentially leading to cost savings in the healthcare system. At the same time, mental health professionals have a responsibility to guide social, political, and other healthcare entities in meeting the mental health needs of young people [5].

The evidence suggests that placing the sole responsibility for promoting and preventing mental health issues on mental health professionals is not practical. We need integrated and multidisciplinary services to expand the range of possible interventions and reduce the risk of poor long-term outcomes. This approach could also lead to cost benefits for the healthcare system. Nevertheless, mental health professionals have a scientific, ethical, and moral obligation to offer guidance to all social, political, and healthcare entities involved in addressing the mental health needs of young people [6].

4. Cyberbullism

The widespread use of the Internet and Information and Communications Technologies (ICT) has significantly transformed society in recent decades. One of the risks that adolescents face in this new reality is the transition from traditional face-to-face bullying to the virtual environment, known as cyberbullying. This study aimed to investigate the relationship between cyberbullying and behaviors such as internet and mobile usage, as well as other risky online behaviors.

Cyberbullying is also found to be associated with Problematic Internet Use and behaviors such as sexting, gambling, and contacting strangers. Additionally, parental monitoring could play a role in moderating these behaviors and should be considered in the development of prevention strategies [7–9]. While numerous studies have examined cyberbullying among high school students, there is a need for more research in different cultural contexts due to potential variations in prevalence, nature, and consequences across societies. Understanding these cultural nuances is crucial for developing effective, context-specific interventions and policies to combat cyberbullying and its adverse effects.

In the fast-evolving digital landscape of today, cyberbullying has emerged as a prevalent and concerning problem, particularly impacting high school students. With the increased amount of time adolescents spend on various social media and online platforms, they are more vulnerable to experiencing this type of aggressive behavior [7, 9, 10].

Cyberbullying extends beyond traditional bullying by using electronic communication technologies to repeatedly and intentionally engage in hostile behavior toward others. It has the ability to persist without relenting, even encroaching into the daily lives of targets while they are within the confines of their own homes, causing them to feel confined and lacking in power. The widespread occurrence of cyberbullying and its capacity to cause serious psychological harm has sparked considerable worry among educators, mental health experts, and parents, underscoring the pressing necessity for a thorough grasp of this digital issue [7, 9, 11, 12].

5. Conclusion

The term "mental health" refers to an individual's psychological and emotional well-being, allowing them to function within society, build healthy relationships, and adapt to challenges. Key factors include social relationships, personality development, conflict resolution, and self-awareness. Early detection and management of psychiatric disorders in children is crucial. Mental health challenges greatly impact young people, with significant gaps in funding. Diagnosed mental health issues can affect education, achievement, and earning capacity, with an estimated cost of $390 billion annually. There is limited research on family interventions despite their critical role in safeguarding child and adolescent mental health. It is essential to address potential mental health issues early on using a youth-focused, multidisciplinary approach.

Acknowledgements

The authors declare that they used Grammarly AI software only for lexical and linguistic improvement, not for creating the reported content.

Author details

Marco Carotenuto
Department of Mental and Physical Health and Preventive Medicine, Child and Adolescent Neuropsychiatry, University of Campania "Luigi Vanvitelli", Naples, Italy

*Address all correspondence to: marco.carotenuto@unicampania.it

References

[1] Skiadas CH, Skiadas C. Preliminary notes. In: Skiadas CH, Skiadas C, editors. Demography of Population Health, Aging and Health Expenditures, The Springer Series on Demographic Methods and Population Analysis. Vol. 50. Cham: Springer International Publishing; 2020. pp. 1-6. DOI: 10.1007/978-3-030-44695-6_1

[2] Gautam S, Jain A, Chaudhary J, Gautam M, Gaur M, Grover S. Concept of mental health and mental well-being, it's determinants and coping strategies. Indian Journal of Psychiatry. 2024;**66**(Suppl. 2):S231-S244. DOI: 10.4103/indianjpsychiatry.indianjpsychiatry_707_23

[3] UNICEF. The State of the World's Children 2023: For Every Child, Health [Internet]. New York: United Nations Children's Fund; 2023 [cited 2024 June 30]. Available from: https://www.unicef.org/reports/state-of-worlds-children

[4] Bosqui T et al. Parenting and family interventions in lower and middle-income countries for child and adolescent mental health: A systematic review. Comprehensive Psychiatry. 2024;**132**:152483. DOI: 10.1016/j.comppsych.2024.152483

[5] Colizzi M, Lasalvia A, Ruggeri M. Prevention and early intervention in youth mental health: Is it time for a multidisciplinary and trans-diagnostic model for care? International Journal of Mental Health Systems. 2020;**14**(Suppl. 1):23. DOI: 10.1186/s13033-020-00356-9

[6] McElvaney R, Tatlow-Golden M. A traumatised and traumatising system: Professionals' experiences in meeting the mental health needs of young people in the care and youth justice systems in Ireland. Children and Youth Services Review. 2016;**65**:62-69. DOI: 10.1016/j.childyouth.2016.03.017

[7] Catone G et al. Epidemiological pattern of bullying using a multi-assessment approach: Results from the bullying and youth mental health Naples study (BYMHNS). Child Abuse and Neglect. 2019;**89**:18-28. DOI: 10.1016/j.chiabu.2018.12.018

[8] Feijóo S, Foody M, O'Higgins Norman J, Pichel R, Rial A. Cyberbullies, the cyberbullied, and problematic internet use: Some reasonable similarities. Psicothema. 2021;**33**(2):198-205. DOI: 10.7334/psicothema2020.209

[9] Ramadan OME et al. Digital dilemma of cyberbullying victimization among high school students: Prevalence, risk factors, and associations with stress and mental well-being. Children. 2024;**11**(6):634. DOI: 10.3390/children11060634

[10] Miraglia Del Giudice M et al. Behavioral and sleep disorders in children and adolescents following COVID-19 disease: A case-control study. Children (Basel). 2023;**10**(7):1189. DOI: 10.3390/children10071189

[11] Catone G et al. Psychotic-like experiences in help-seeking adolescents: Dimensional exploration and association with different forms of bullying victimization—A developmental social psychiatry perspective. The International Journal of Social Psychiatry. 2017;**63**(8):752-762. DOI: 10.1177/0020764017733765

[12] Cavallo ND et al. Neuropsychiatric manifestations, reduced self-esteem and poor quality of life in children and adolescents with neurofibromatosis type 1 (NF1): The impact of symptom visibility and bullying behavior. Children (Basel). 2023;**10**(2):330. DOI: 10.3390/children10020330

Chapter 2

Lessons from the Twentieth Century for Child and Adolescent Mental Health Practice in the Twenty-First Century

Jolyon Grimwade

Abstract

A review of the past one hundred and fifty years of child and adolescent mental health practice, in five three-decade periods, is presented to background the upcoming developments in this century, while also documenting what has been of value as the field moves forward. There has been much loss of corporate memory as we have moved into the Twenty-First Century. Professional amnesia is a condition with grave consequences. The final list of twenty lessons provide a view as to how these lessons can be absorbed into clinical training and into clinical practice. This summary is necessarily brief, but the references will provoke enquiry and the learning of old ideas.

Keywords: child mental health, twentieth century history, social changes, diagnostic changes, lessons for practice

1. Introduction

Over the past fifteen decades, the knowledge base for child and adolescent mental health practice has been built by various actors and through various social processes in the Western world. As we explore the opportunities for expanding this knowledge in this century, we need to retain the best parts of what we already know. This is a paper that documents how the knowledge was acquired and what needs to be retained, by breaking the one hundred and fifty years into five thirty-year periods. This phasing is not meant to be veridical; rather it allows for an overview of the emerging field and places new developments in wider social and historical contexts, while demonstrating how understanding has built across time. The intention is not to chide or criticize beginning professionals for a lack of understanding of the history, but rather to celebrate the achievements of those who innovated and to communicate the special joy that comes with elucidating a puzzling presentation. Hopefully teachers will review their practices, as well.

Along the way, there has always been a tension between the nomothetic and idiopathic. Social agents have wanted to implement policies that effect change in a systematic way across populations. But, clinicians have usually been working with unique presentations that require tailored responses. This remains an active tension today and will be the final point of this paper as I try to elucidate how my learning of the following lessons has affected my practice.

Briefly, we can describe the period from 1870 on as a time of social response to social changes that arose from the American Civil War. The next period, from the turn of the century is the time of establishment of the professions and their practices with the emergence of Western style democracy determining the need to help the disadvantaged. The third period, from 1930, begins the processes of specialization and the fallout from the Second World War. From 1960, there is much development with respect to families and to the research base of interventions and vulnerability. The final period, from 1990, has seen emphasis upon the brain, trauma, and technology.

Wardle [1] summarized his view of the twentieth century, by looking to an Austrian American innovator: Leo Kanner, who, in his third edition of *Child Psychiatry*, divided the growth of child psychiatry, from 1900, into four decades, to which Wardle added explanatory examples:

> *"first decade: thinking about children (e.g., child studies, psychodynamic theories);*
>
> *second decade: doing things to children (e.g., sending them to special institutions);*
>
> *third decade: doing things for children (e.g., making changes in family and school);*
>
> *fourth decade: working with children (e.g., individual treatment of children, and play therapy).*
>
> *It is a neat simplification; if we continued Kanner's model up to the end of the century, it might read:*
>
> *fifth decade: working with mothers;*
>
> *sixth decade: working with fathers, marriages, and groups;*
>
> *seventh decade: working with whole families, and institutions for children;*
>
> *eighth decade: working within an interactional model and with protective positive factors in child and family;*
>
> *ninth decade: promoting resilience in the child and protective factors in the school;*
>
> *tenth decade: promoting protective factors for children in society, preventive child psychiatry" (p. 65).*

Wardle's [1] summary using Kanner's [2] ideas captured some of that which will be documented here but does not address why the field came into existence and does not provide for the complexity of what has unfolded. Overlapping the period-by-period description of acquired knowledge, thirteen themes (Social change, Domestic violence, Prevention, Philanthropy, Juvenile Justice, Social Welfare, Discovery of childhood, Individualization, the Freudian turn, Family intervention, Cognitivism, Consumerism, and Diversity) in this history can be identified. As we develop our understanding of neurology, we need also to integrate that knowledge with understanding of social, interpersonal, and cultural processes. There will be separate sections covering psychoanalytic practice, diagnosis (DSM), CBT, and trauma.

Further, across the period from 1870 to 2020, there have been mass movements of people across the globe that has often been associated with war, but always concerned with safe housing. Sociology and anthropology have provided some hints about how people and nations have been affected by such factors, as housing, poverty, war, trauma, emigration, family violence, and disease. The assumption of the Western economic man as modal citizen has often obscured clinical responses to a variety of human tragedies.

Prior to 1870 there were a few contributions to the field of child and adolescent mental health. Aristotle (~270 BC) believed children to be "pathologically weak, physically disproportionate, and above all irrational" ([3], p. 659). Erasmus [4], in 1530 published *A handbook on good manners for children*, was keen to have raised well-behaved children. A book from 1545 contained tips for child rearing (Thomas Phaire *The Boke of Chyldren.* Section titles cited by Howells and Osborn [5] included: Terrible Dreames and Feare in the Slepe, and of pissing in the Bedde). Jean-Jacques Rousseau, in 1776 [6] had revolutionary ideas on child rearing and learning. In 1860, a young Scottish doctor, James Crichton-Browne [7], presented the first medical text on childhood mental health [6]. There may have been other systematically developed models of response, but these do not compare with those which began post-Civil War in the United States.

Prior to this were several welfare changes in the United Kingdom with the funding of asylums at the municipal level in 1808 and the Poor Law Amendment Act of 1834 [8] which was designed to reduce the costs of looking after the poor and to take beggars off the streets, among other reforms, defined what a child is by age and stipulated hours of work in the poor houses [9]. This was not a wholly successful enterprise, but began a rethinking of welfare services in the UK and the USA [8, 10].

2. 1870

The platform for many social changes over the past century and a half, was the aftermath of the American Civil War. But there was also another civil war, which went by the name of closing the frontier [11]. While the American Civil War united the states and the edges of the continent, there were vast tracts of land to be brought under central control by subduing the indigenous peoples and then by traversing the continent with railways. Other minorities were also subject to the effects of colonization and domination by Europeans: African Americans (former slaves) and Latin Americans who migrated from the south.

With the movement north of southern African-American communities and the dislocation of families due to war deaths, there was a great load upon voluntary assistance organizations, especially churches. A conference in 1870 (National Conference of Charities, which later became the National Conference of Charities and Corrections in 1884) [8], brought together thoughts about the provision of social services. Over the course of thirty years, social research was developed, further conferences held, and the modern profession of Social Work (1892) was born, along with the pioneering initiatives of Jane Addams at Hull House in Chicago [8].

Women's rights were a central part of Addams' intentions. The first case of domestic violence was prosecuted in 1876 in the United States. Earlier, in 1868, Elizabeth Packard [12] wrote *The prisoner's life* in which she described the enforced removal of her from her children through her placement in an asylum by her pastor husband. By 1873, laws were changed to prevent such incarceration and to allow overview of asylum residency. Mental health consumerism began in this American decade.

Addams [13] established, in 1890, a many faceted community called Hull House, which provided housing for single mothers, employment in various service occupations (child care, catering, washing, and cleaning) provided income for the resident families. Hull House was the starting place of many important persons, including Julia Lathrop, who became head of the Children's Bureau (established out of the first Presidential Conference on Childhood in 1909). Addams [14] was energetic in the founding of the Illinois Psychopathic Institute (which became Healy's Institute for Juvenile Research).

One of the achievements of the eighteenth century was the development of techniques and technologies for the measurement of all sorts of variables: quantity, time, temperature, and weight. In the nineteenth century this was extended to measurement of human bodies and human capacities. This was given impetus by Charles Darwin's [15] 1859 publication of *On the origin of species by means of natural selection*. One of his cousins, Francis Galton took to measuring intelligence based on the discredited pseudo-sciences of phrenology and of eugenics, which laboratory work he pursued through his role as head of anthropology at the British Association for the Advancement of Science [12]. In 1890 the Vineland Hospital for feeble-minded children was opened and, subsequently, Goddard [16] produced the first test of functionality in 1919; a test that has been revised many times but is still in use. In 1891, Stanley Hall at Clark University started a twenty-year program of child study where a range of attributes were documented. The first test of intelligence was devised by Frenchman, Alfred Binet, in 1905: this test was renewed at Stanford University with many subsequent revisions and remains in professional use. Psychology entered the twentieth century with a firm base in measurement of attributes [12]. A new conception of childhood was being formed.

One history of child guidance was entitled, *The century of the child* [12], another was entitled, *Before it's too late* [17] and was followed by [14] *Science in the service of the child*; each gave reference to a change in philosophy about children and childhood.

Philanthropy was brought forward as a major force at about the same time. The opening up of oilfields in West Virginia and in Philadelphia enabled expansion of many industries and the generation of hitherto unthought of wealth among a lucky few citizens [12]. Some industrialists and miners have donated huge sums of money ever since. It is difficult to know which of the benefactors were the most influential; but the Carnegies, the Rockefellers, and the Harkness' family's Commonwealth Fund were very important, as was Johns Hopkins in his formation of a university around a hospital complex.

American philanthropy's professional genealogy within health had begun in 1879 when Johns Hopkins' bequest established a place of learning and a place of treatment in Boston [12]. Graduates of the medical and psychology schools appear throughout the story of the National Committee on Mental Hygiene (NCMH) and of child guidance, especially through the influence of scholars Adolf Meyer and William James, in the formation of the Rockefeller and Harkness philanthropic funds [12] and through the other training facilities spawned by Johns Hopkins University at Yale and in Philadelphia.

Nineteenth century medicine was much about sitting with suffering and making note of observations of the patient during the course of disease. This was the foundation of evidence-based practice [18]. Psychiatric diagnosis was no exception with

Kraepelin having defined dementia praecox in the 1890s, and later Bleuler, in 1911, calling the syndrome schizophrenia, with autism as one of the symptoms [19]. This is what mental health innovators of the late 1800s would do and what Breuer encouraged in his neurology colleague, Freud [20] (*Studies on hysteria*, 1895). In the "sitting with" came an understanding of symptoms and release from suffering, that Freud's patient, Anna O., called the talking cure.

By the end of the nineteenth century, the professions of social work, psychology, and psychiatry were forming, a new conception of the child was emerging, women's mental health rights were being legislated, and philanthropy was a driven activity of successful business people. An optimism pervaded much of the Western world as the new century began, but the next thirty years ended in economic collapse following a disastrous world war.

3. 1900

Smuts [14] noted three different sorts of interest that promoted the founding of child guidance clinics after the First World War: Child Study (Stanley Hall, and then *Iowa Child Welfare Research Station*), Mental Hygiene (and Healy's studies of delinquency), and government policy (Presidential conferences on childhood in 1909, 1919, and 1930; and the Children's Bureau). In the background was the interest of philanthropy, especially those with female backers (Laura Spelman Rockefeller, Anne E Harkness, Lizzie Merrill-Palmer, Cora Bussey Hillis, and Ethel Dummer; the last being particularly influential in the establishment of the *Judge Baker Clinic*) [14].

Mental Hygiene came from direct experience within the dreary history of asylums. In 1841, asylums in Britain had undergone a major change [19, 21] with the foundation of the Medico-Psychological Association whose membership was the medical directors of the asylums in England. This allowed for medical oversight and the accumulation of knowledge about mental illnesses and the development of treatments. Progress was rapid, but the old philosophy of incarceration and occupation within minimal, prison-like facilities took over a hundred years to overturn. The Boston Asylum of 1874 [19] was seen as a great step forward with much sunlight entering through windows and more focus on healthy exercise, but this facility reverted under the strain of admission rates to substandard accommodation by the turn of the century.

One admission in 1901 would prove very important [22]. A young man, Clifford Beers, was suicidal following the death by suicide of his brother and he endured a terrible internment in an asylum and left determined to document his experience of admission. The book [23] was published 1908 (re-released 2004), entitled, *The mind that found itself*, and soon after he launched the Connecticut Committee on Mental Hygiene and the National Committee on Mental Hygiene the following year, with a brief to prevent disorders and to treat patients humanely [17].

Mental Hygiene was proposed to mirror the great social effects achieved with the provision of physical hygiene systems in the previous two decades [17]. Clifford Beers was supported in the activity by the most senior psychiatrist Adolf Meyer, and the most senior psychologist, William James. Funding was provided by philanthropists. Meyer envisaged interventions with youth to prevent ill adolescents entering adulthood in a poor state of wellbeing [12]. This was not the preferred path for Beers, but money could be raised for Meyer's purpose.

Earlier, in 1906, Judge Harvey Humphrey Baker founded a children's court in Boston where the aim was to deter juveniles from a life of crime. Orders were made by

Baker that amounted to rudimentary rehabilitation programs. In time, William Healy, a medical doctor, was commissioned in 1909 to study the lives of the children referred to the court and to design interventions of rehabilitation. Thus, was established the *Judge Baker Clinic*. The research was reported by Healy [23] in 1915: *The individual delinquent* [12, 14, 17]. This research was one outcome of the first Presidential Conference on Childhood.

Originally, the central research question was whether criminality was constitutional or situational [12]. Healy's research [23] demonstrated that commission of crimes was an effect of the living circumstances of the children, not their genetic make-up. The basic methodology was the collection of information from the child by the medical doctor, on the child's academic potential by a psychologist, and information on the family's social position by a social researcher.

Healy and his psychologist collaborator, Augusta Fox Bronner, moved to Chicago in 1917 and proceeded to provide social treatments of juvenile criminality [17]. Using the professional model developed in the Boston study, the roles of psychologist and social worker were expanded to assess and better treat children who were attending the juvenile court. This professional profile endured into the 1990s in Australia and other Western countries. Intervention in cases in need of child protection and of juvenile crime have remained an abiding challenge for Western governments.

Each professional would gather information and bring it to a three-hour meeting of all the professionals to formulate what the cause of the trouble was and then to suggest interventions that were designed to help the child and family recover [17]. In the last hour the parent or parents would attend to receive the recommendation for action. Frequently, the suggestion was made to the mother to move house: away from the father and away from the cohort of juvenile criminals.

The success of this work was soon to be measured on a grand scale with the launch of Demonstration Projects in child mental hygiene. Horn [17] described three phases in the pre-Second World War history of child guidance. The Commonwealth Fund supported the seven demonstration clinics of 1922 to 1927 (St Louis, Missouri; Norfolk, Virginia; Dallas, Texas; Los Angeles, California; Twin Cities, St Paul and Minneapolis, Minnesota; Cleveland, Ohio; Philadelphia, Pennsylvania). Movement building occurred between 1927 and 1933, with the establishment of the Institute of Child Guidance and the operation of some sixty clinics throughout the United States and Canada and the Islington Clinic in London in 1928 [24]. Thereafter, the Commonwealth Fund withdrew, and clinics became state or local authority funded. Professionals then ran the clinics autonomously.

The first British child guidance clinic was the Institute of Medical Psychology opened in Tavistock Square, London in 1918, whose first client was a child [25]. The Commonwealth Fund opened the Islington clinic in 1928. Australia's first child guidance clinic opened in 1929 under John Francis Williams at the (now Royal) Children's Hospital in Melbourne [26].

It should be noted that the effect of the First World War (WWI) upon the development of child guidance is rarely commented upon. For Americans, WWI was a 1917 to 1918 event. The Second World War (WWII) had a very different set of effects on child mental health. 1917 might have seen the Russian revolution but in the welfare world of the USA, it was the year that Richmond released her book on psychiatric social work entitled: *Social Diagnosis* [27] along with the move of Healy and Fox Bronner to Chicago. Yet, Freud [28] had commented that the effects of war upon returned soldiers confirmed many of the hypotheses of underlying pathology expressed in terrifying nightmares and memories that distorted daily living.

4. An overview: psychoanalytic thought applied to children's disorders

Freud's [29] famous case of childhood therapy was more like the supervision of Little Hans' father, rather than in person therapy. Hermine Hug-Helmuth published several short papers upon play therapy from 1912 [30]. Melanie Klein [31, 32] did much to pioneer such treatments. Anna Freud [33] was also very influential and particularly through her work with Dorothy Burlingham [34] with whom she started a pre-school in Vienna and then took this to Hampstead Heath in London in 1936.

A central focus of Freud was upon childhood development: The three essays on sexuality [35] and child abuse (The etiology of hysteria [36]; A child is being beaten [37]). The case most reported is his study of the autobiography of Judge Daniel Schreber who developed a paranoid psychosis [38] which was further elucidated by Schatzman [39] in *Soul murder*, where the athletic disciplines of the father were enacted against the son's body with devastating effect.

Earlier than this was the work of Alfred Adler who was expelled from the Viennese psychoanalytic circle by Freud over his views regarding the education of children. Adler thought the best approach was to work with the parents. This was not so different in essence to the case of Little Hans [29] but the focus was upon the moral education of children not upon treatment of disorder. This work continued with Adler as part of what he called Individual Psychology and was most famously pursued in the work of Rudolf Dreikurs [40]. In contemporary times, work with parents has continued and in Australia there is the TripleP parenting program [41] (a CBT based model) and the Tuning into Kids [42] program (one based in emotion coaching).

As the Child Guidance Demonstration Projects progressed, the attention of the professionals moved from juvenile delinquents to neurotic children, who were more amenable to in clinic therapy, rather than the environmental adjustment approach of Healy and Fox Bronner. The third generation of Child Guidance clinics in the early 1930s were much about Child Psychoanalytic Play Therapy: this became known as the "Freudian Turn" [43]. In fact, many mental hygiene programs were taking such a turn with practitioners seeking psychoanalytic treatment for themselves, as well as supervision in their work with children.

But there was another change afoot in psychoanalytic circles as the second generation of theorists and practitioners emerged. Klein developed Object-Relations theory from the work of her mentor Karl Abraham [44] and in competition and collaboration with Protestant Scot, Ronald Fairbairn, and grounded in the firm belief that interpretation was the basis of child psychoanalytic work, except the language was that of play. Anna Freud [33] took an alternate view that not until later in childhood were children able to develop transference responses with their therapist and that a supportive, psychoeducational approach was needed for the younger child (this was also the position of Hug-Helmuth) [30]. Therein lay a feud that was never resolved and still exists in British psychoanalytic circles, today.

But two other psychoanalytic traditions were emerging in the Western world. In France, Jacques Lacan produced his thesis on the mirror stage (1936, but not published until 1949, and translated into English in 1968) [45]. Meanwhile, the exodus of Jewish analysts to the United States and elsewhere in the 1930s, saw the development of psychoanalysis in major American cities, especially New York and in the medical profession. Not long after, in 1936, Anna Freud [46] produced *The ego and the mechanisms of defense* which was adopted by a series of New York emigres and the school of Ego Psychology developed. Underpinning this development was a focus upon rationality and upon the developmental theory of Erik Erikson [47] and a change in focus to adolescent mental health [48].

Lacan was fierce in his critique of Ego Psychology as he developed his return to Freud and a focus on the Unconscious [49]. He put the focus on language and how it obscures and reveals. The differences between schools of thought are cultural as well as theoretical (Grimwade) [50] the second generation. Lacan's technical innovations caused problems within the International Psychoanalytic Association and led to an enquiry headed by Donald Winnicott, who was otherwise a supporter of Lacan [49].

The next generation saw the adoption of object-relations theory by many American practitioners and a combination of Lacanian and Object-Relations thought in the work of French analyst Andre Green (Kohon) [51]. In the next generation this has been found in Relational Psychoanalysis. The move within the discipline from internalist, biological, and mechanical descriptions to relational ones is significant over the course of a century.

Among child psychodynamic practitioners the relevance of interpersonal and relational factors was always relevant. One could not work with a child without the consent and cooperation of the child's parent. This is one reason that family therapy became a development in the 1950s. The development of attachment theory by John Bowlby [52, 53] was another major relational redevelopment within psychoanalytic thought. But we are now getting well beyond the parameters of the second three decades in this presentation.

Whereas the first three decades of the Twentieth Century began with hope and ended with despair, the next three decades began with despair, involved a terrible world war, but ended with much optimism. Within child mental health the work moved away from juvenile justice to neurosis, from social treatment to psychoanalytic treatment, and then to drug, behavioral, and family treatment. The war changed many aspects of social and community life and psychosocial theory.

5. 1930

As knowledge grew about child mental health, the focus of the clinicians also changed. The capacity to influence juvenile offending proved very difficult, but neurotic children could be helped. The Demonstration Projects were intended to develop broad templates for action across all sorts of childhood presentations, but the accumulating knowledge among the treating professionals was about the differences between children. Treatment became individualized and the clinicians used technique derived from psychoanalytic practice, in what became called the "Freudian turn" [27, 43].

After WWII, there were many changes to the way psychiatric services were provided. The Mental Hygiene movement became the Mental Health movement in 1948 [22]. Efforts began to formalize psychiatric diagnosis with the publication of the Diagnostic and Statistical Manual of the American Psychiatric Association (DSM) [54].

Freud, who died in 1938, conceded that there was a problem with the rate of change in *Analysis: terminable and interminable* [55]. The focus on a passive individual patient was challenged on many fronts. Action methods focusing on the body were developed such as Moreno [56] with his Psychodrama. After WWII, a number of physicalist mental health treatments were developed with injured soldiers. Psychopharmacology and psychosurgery were popular treatments at the Palo Alto Naval Veterans' hospital. But, on other wards, Bateson, Jackson, Haley, and

Weakland [57] were considering how relational factors within families were causing mental distress. The ideas of cybernetics and ecology developed in the sciences of war machines and of environmental degradation were applied to studying families by these pioneers [58].

The second research group that developed from these pioneers under Watzlawick [59, 60] focused specifically on communicational patterns within families. They were all anti-Freudian, except for anthropologist and cetacean researcher, Bateson. As a family therapist, Bateson was a conversationalist, not a technical adjuster of communication patterns. In the talk with families, relational movement occurred.

There are other versions of the exchange between psychoanalytic thought and family therapy practice during this period. Harry Goolishian moved from individual psychoanalytic psychotherapy practice to psychodynamic couple therapy, and then to his version for family therapy practice [61] during the same period of time as the Palo Alto group were establishing themselves in the early 1950s. Nathan Ackerman [62] established his New York family therapy clinic as an extension of his group analytic work, but the Ackerman Institute was anti-psychodynamic for many years after his death. In the 1960s, Ivan Boszormenyi-Nagy developed his Contextual Family Therapy [63]. Gurman and Kniskern [64] observed that in family work the thinking was psychodynamic, but the intervention was something else. Deborah Luepnitz's [65] *The family interpreted* was very much in this domain, but she moved from family work to psychoanalytic practice. The recent spate of works linking family interventions with attachment theory [66–68] seems bizarre given a misreading of Bowlby back in 1949 [69], inspired a number of anti-psychoanalytic family therapy practitioners in the 1950s, especially those in Palo Alto.

Other models of psychological practice were appearing in the 1950s, based on the behavioral theories of Skinner [70], Eysenck [71], Wolpe [72], and Pavlov [73]. Applied Behavioral Analysis [74] was used to settle children in classrooms. Elsewhere, the theories of Piaget [75] were being used to understand how children learn. By 1955, the use of stimulant medication for the treatment of hyperactive children (now, Attention Deficit Hyperactivity Disorder; ADHD) had become common [76].

While American child guidance had become child psychiatry, with the three professions providing input to cases, in Britain [24], Child Guidance was the province of school and municipal psychologists and social workers, with child psychiatry part of hospital clinics. Australia still had child guidance clinics and the relevant Victorian department still had the name of Mental Hygiene Branch, although that changed with the World Mental Health conference of 1960 [22, 77].

Broader still, WWII with its atomic ending changed international relations and the Western view. Many ascribe to the bombing a recognition that expansion through material and mechanical innovation had reached a moral limit. The Modern world became the Post-Modern world [78], although this was not really apparent until the 1980s, and Modernism still exists in many relationships to scientific experimentation, despite the contemporary climate crisis.

The impact of the atomic bombs had at least two other consequences: the mass movement of homeless, scared, and stateless people and the problems of social reconstruction in Japan. The soldiers who were assigned the tasks of helping Japanese people rebuild lives and homes were frustrated by the lack of cooperation from the Japanese. The Marshall plan was failing, and an anthropologist was asked to find a way to allow for assistance. Benedict [79] published *The chrysanthemum and the sword* in 1946, in which she described two different moral codes. The Western way concerned Truth and Guilt. The Eastern way was Honor and Shame.

By offering the Japanese help, the Americans were demonstrating the truth that the Japanese had lost which caused the Japanese shame and dishonor. Not accepting help avoided the loss of honor [78]. This distinction was taken up by Christian missionaries [80, 81] in various parts of the world and was seen to apply across Asian and Pacific communities, including Australian Aboriginal communities [82]. But in sub-Saharan Africa a different moral parameter was described and was also evident in African American and Caribbean communities: Power and Fear. The African Big Man could maintain his power by having the shaman confront fears. This is a finding that might have affected cross-cultural counseling practice, but seems to be little known in the mental health world.

Another effect of WWII was the development of attachment theory by John Bowlby. He noticed that children who had been removed from London during the blitz and placed in safe keeping in northern parts of Britain, had particular troubles when returned to the care of their parents. This led to the paper that sparked interest in family therapy in the United states, even though Bowlby [69] in his very English way, had spoken of working with the family to re-establish connections between children and parents. In his paper "family" actually meant "parents", not the child, or other children, or other generations.

Attachment theory developed across four decades with its final rendering as *A secure base* in 1988. It had been taken up by USA based researcher, Mary Ainsworth [83] using an experimental method called the "strange situation" which led to description of four types of attachment style; a style that would be present for many children throughout their childhood and sometimes throughout their lives. The work has been used to establish grounds for removal of children and placement in out-of-home care, worldwide. I am not attached to attachment theory as it does not allow for hate and anger to be considered primary emotions. But without the development of attachment theory, it may have been more difficult to have generated the far more compelling description of "adventures in companionship" [84], Stern's [85] *Interpersonal world of the infant* and Infant Mental Health as a specific discipline, along with Panksepp's [86] description of the primary emotions of mammals (both discussed later). But attachment is a basis for considering the effects of mass migration post-WWII.

The mass movement of people from wars is ongoing and, in Australia, we have had waves of immigration from different ethnic groups across time and there is a discernible pattern of transgenerational trauma associated with the migration [87]. Many Jewish people arrived in Melbourne between the two World Wars [87, 88] After the way came many southern (Italian, Greek, Yugoslavian) and central European (Czechoslovak, Hungarian, Baltic states). In the 1970s came Vietnamese fleeing the war and Lebanese fleeing civil war. In the 1990s came people from the breakup of the former Yugoslavia [86]. In the 2000s came people from China. In the 2010s many people arrived from India. These waves had effects upon the second and third generations [88] with mental health problems prominent in some families and among youth who were torn between the culture of origin and the Australian community.

It is possible to describe the new arrivals as principally coming from their culture, coming to Australia, or coming with their culture. Many families traveled together to Australia, while some families arrived in parts and gradually rebuilt over some years. Often these migrations were successful as there was family support, and three generations were in place. If the migrating family had the attitude of coming to Australia for wellbeing gains, they have done rather better than those who fled.

Fleeing a country has a different psychological meaning to the other forms of migration. Only some people fled. Those who remained behind did so to be with family and friends in the familiar generational structure. The fleeing migrants may not have felt they had a choice, but were probably not so connected to families and communities. Because they had not been culturally attached, they lacked these skills when coming to the new country and these families were consequently subject to mental health challenges [88].

Another feature was that these families tended to be two generation families. Whereas in the country of origin, the elderly were venerated and played important roles in the acculturation of the grandchildren; no such elders existed in the new country [88]. Children were attracted to the culture of the new. However, having no other relatives, the migrant parents valued their children as the only family, in a way that was not present in the country of origin. This gave the children a power over their parents that led to dominance of the parents in some families and unsettled family lives, with domestic violence and alienation of the children, leading to mental health difficulties for both generations, and especially, in the next generation. This pattern can be identified in the many waves of migrants that have arrived in Australia [87].

But before the arrival of people from wars, the colonization war of Australia involved forced migration from land of indigenous people and the breaking up of cultural knowledge through attacks on language and family structures, especially removal of children from their parents, which is called the stolen generations. This knowledge needs to be taken into account when doing cross-cultural family work. The assimilation of this knowledge about the traumatic impact of war and colonization is still being absorbed into usual practice in Australia.

In 1959, Jerome Frank published his first edition of *On persuasion and healing* [89] where it was proposed that much of the effect of psychotropic drugs and of psychotherapies of many different sorts was a placebo effect. Frank estimated the size of the effect to be about thirty percent. As far as can be ascertained, Fish (1972, cited in Pentony) [90] deliberately embraced the placebo effect in his Placebo Therapy, a behavioral intervention. The rationale was simple: the placebo effect applies, so just let the momentum that such an effect has upon the beginnings of the work take place. The task of the therapist is to appear credible while getting out of the way of the healing effect of seeking healing. This remains an issue of contention [91], but it could be a form of encouragement to any beginning therapist who can be confident that when a person presents they have come for change and will be accepting of whatever the prescriptions, direct or implied.

6. 1960

The next three decades were periods of prosperity across much of the Western world. There was a major war in Vietnam that caused mass migrations in the 1970s and 1980s, and there was also a war on drugs. Substance misuse was a problem throughout the Twentieth Century and before, but was much more commonplace during this period as disposable income was higher and production of such drugs became more practical, with new concoctions developed in laboratories.

This was a period of innovation and research in mental health. New theories and practices emerged. Cognitive-behavioral therapies had been pioneered by Beck [92] and by Ellis [93] from the early 1960s, but these became a unified set of interventions in the 1980s. The publication by Watzlawick et al. [60] of *Change: principles of problem formation and problem resolution* placed family therapy squarely in the domain of child guidance clinics and child psychiatry.

The 1960s had two further social changes: black rights' movements and consumer rights. The emancipation of African Americans across these decades was very important for the mental health of millions of people who were able to achieve economic goals and have racism markedly reduced, although it is still evident in many social forums, as the contemporary Black Lives Matter movement has underlined. Emancipation of non-Western peoples remains a challenge for practitioners who try to reconcile social circumstances with states of psychological distress.

In 1962, US President Kennedy introduced laws to protect the rights of consumers [94] the right to safety, the right to be informed, the right to choose, and the right to be heard. This legislation was taken up by those in asylums and other mental health services to tear down the asylums within the decade and to liberate the patients. The notion was slow in application to the field of child and adolescent mental health, but most public services have consumer advocates. Child advocates are often affected teenagers and, when they achieve adulthood, may not continue in mental health advocacy as they seek to live lives outside of the shadow of mental ill health. Parent advocates tend to stay involved for much longer, wanting to help families avoid the troubles that they endured. In Australia this has been formalized within a government policy: *Mental health statement of rights and responsibilities* [95].

Family therapies and cross-cultural counseling practices highlighted the need for practitioners to take context into account. For instance, Ivan Boszormenyi-Nagy [63], a Hungarian American, developed a model of practice he entitled Contextual Family Therapy. In the 1980s, contextual approaches received a new impetus from White's Narrative therapy [96]. By placing life experience within narratives of adaptation and change rather than narratives of stasis and destructiveness, language was used to facilitate change by choice. New contexts for living could be fashioned through questioning. This work continues and is persuasive. Most therapies, in contemporary times, are described in terms of narratives and contexts.

As will be seen shortly, context has been absorbed into diagnostic systems over the last sixty years. But the way to work with overlapping contexts remains a work in progress. In my work, and as a result of learning from writings from diverse therapeutic approaches and settings, supervision, and in work with people, I aim to disentangle contexts in therapy with lone persons, couples, and families. Such fluid work with persons in therapy lies in contrast to the efforts to systematize diagnosis and treatments that is embedded in the DSM and its years of revision.

7. A second overview: DSM

In 1952, the Diagnostic and Statistical Manual, Mental Disorders (DSM) was published by the American Psychiatric Association [54]. This was another effect of the WWII as this diagnostic system was based on the psychiatric diagnosis system of the Veterans' Administration. It primarily focused upon classification of adult disorders and was underpinned by psychodynamic principles. DSM II arrived in 1968 [97]. There were now 182 disorders, and the manual had 134 pages.

Again, DSM-II reflected the predominant psychodynamic psychiatry, with also included concepts from Kraepelin's system of classification. Sociological and biological factors were included, with the boundary between normality and abnormality not severe and symptoms not specified in detail for any specific disorders. A sharp distinction was made between neurosis, based on anxiety and depressive symptoms and psychosis, which required hallucinations and delusions. The diagnostic art was to elucidate broad underlying conflicts or maladaptive reactions to life problems.

Dissatisfaction with the system was articulated by Rutter, Shaffer, and Shepherd [98] who suggested a multi-axial approach to diagnosis that included psychosocial effects of the disorder, functionality of the person, and other medical conditions. DSM-III [99] listed 265 diagnostic categories and had 494 pages. The scheme transformed mental health diagnosis. Data on the reliability of diagnosis was assessed by a panel of experts that included several factors, not just prevalence of the specified conditions. Diagnosis of child and adolescent disorders was much expanded.

DSM-III-R [100] published as a revision of the DSM-III, was 567 pages with 292 diagnoses. Further efforts had been made for the diagnoses to be descriptive rather than inferential, but diagnosis of the Personality Disorders, still required diagnostic inference. Childhood disorders were further expanded with particular focus on Attention Deficit Disorder, Autism, and Asperger's Syndrome.

DSM-IV [101] featured further changes to the definition of Asperger's syndrome. In 1991, Frith [102] published a translation of Asperger's [103] paper which described, unlike Kanner's [104] paper, a population of intellectually normal children with autistic features. This has changed the way autism has been seen ever since. It is unclear why the paper took so long to be translated, but Asperger had been involved in Nazi human [105]. Another reason was that it had emerged that two of Asperger's collaborators had gone to work with Kanner as early as 1938 and assisted with the research, which questioned the originality of the preeminent child psychiatrist of the time.

DSM-IV [101] was very important for the definition of Autism and of Attention-Deficit Hyperactivity Disorder (ADHD). Finally, the diagnosis of one of these did not exclude the diagnosis of the other. We have come to know that thirty per cent of autistic children also have ADHD and that autistic children can have other disorders, as well, including Post-Traumatic Stress Disorder (PTSD). This is another disorder finally described in DSM-IV.

The ADHD criteria had the subsequent effect of adults being able to be diagnosed as ADHD and able to receive the stimulant treatment that was allowed for children but had been banned for adults from 1971 to 2009 [75, 106]. But it was some time before psychiatrists were comfortable to diagnose ADHD and treat with stimulant medication. Diagnosed children still lost their medication when they turned eighteen years, until recently in Australia.

DSM-IV-TR in 2000 [107] was a text revision of DSM IV with only nine diagnoses changed: the majority of the text was unchanged. Two childhood disorders were dramatically changed: Pervasive Developmental Disorder NOS (not otherwise specified) was returned to its DSM-III-R wording, and Asperger's disorder was almost completely rewritten.

DSM-5 in 2013 [108] involved the deletion of the subtypes of schizophrenia (paranoid, disorganized, catatonic, undifferentiated, and residual). There was combination of the subsets of autism (Asperger's syndrome, classic autism, Rett syndrome, childhood disintegrative disorder and pervasive developmental disorder not otherwise specified) under a new class represented as a spectrum of intensity (mild, moderate, and severe) and called Autism Spectrum Disorder.

The major change for DSM-5 [108] was the dropping of multi-axial diagnosis as a general approach, to incorporation of these sorts of factors, when relevant, within each diagnosis with estimates of severity, chronicity, and functional disturbance.

There had been no specific scientific merit of the multi-axial approach. The DSM, fifth edition, text revision, published in 2022 [109], expanded the range of relevant psychosocial factors requiring specification within a diagnosis to include issues of gender, sex and sexuality, culture, suicidality, ethnicity, and social inclusion.

DSM-5-TR [109] has 1120 pages and had revised criteria for a further 70 disorders. The DSM-5-TR also included the addition of three new diagnoses: Prolonged Grief Disorder, Unspecified Mood Disorder and Stimulant-induced Mild Neurocognitive Disorder. The last reflected the widespread abuse of the illicitly manufactured drug known as "ice". The DSM journey has been a long one driven by data collection. We can use the changes to map our advancement in understanding mental health and its variations. Most of the changes are about context.

As reflected in the revisions of the DSM, this period of thirty years from 1960 to 1990 saw the proliferation and diversification of research programs: prominent endeavors were attachment theory, stress and psychopharmacology, psychotherapy theory, process, and outcome research, and much expansion of studies of neurology as new techniques of imaging were developed. All such programs were expanded further in the three decades that followed into 2020. This book will contain much about such work.

8. Another overview: CBT

Cognitive-behavioral practice (CBT) is into its fourth wave. This very recent: process-oriented CBT [110]. These waves reflect a battle between the nomothetic prescription of set technique for diagnosed conditions and the idiopathic response to variations from standard presentation, including multiple diagnoses, and the need to treat in a way that is acceptable to the patient.

The first wave (~1960) was Ellis [93] and Beck [92] postulating that thinking about anxieties can relieve anxieties and promote more adaptive behavior. The second wave (~1980) included the contributions of Meichenbaum [111], Lazarus [112], and Mahoney [113] and the new version of Ellis' [114] formulation as Rational Emotive Behavioral Therapy (REBT). These approaches like those of the subsequent waves, have tried to provide strategies for overcoming any reluctance to engage with the cognitive work.

The mid-1990s were a period of great triumphalism among CBT researchers who would claim that therapies had to be Empirically Validated (EVT) or Empirically Supported (EST) [115]. The nomothetic dominated and was seen as a scientific repudiation of inter-personal and psychodynamic therapies.

But by the end of the decade three new CBTs emerged: Acceptance and Commitment Therapy (ACT) [116], Dialectical Behavior Therapy (DBT) [117], and Schema Therapy (ST) [118]. Each had absorbed a developmental view of presentation and recovery, and each had a moral/philosophical framework. Within certain well-controlled therapeutic environments these methods were shown to be successful, but the behavioral side of the work was almost replaced by other strategies, other than as criterion for outcome as behavioral change. Each has as a starting point the emotional status of the consumer and how this emotional status must be used to secure treatment and to resolve difficulties.

The fourth wave has arrived with an emphasis on process, as previously described [110]. The new CBT is relationship based, developmentally understood, emotionally mapped, and includes in another variation an understanding of death anxiety [119].

Sexuality is the only part missing in contemporary CBT of the Freudian paradigm of one hundred and twenty years earlier.

Throughout this history of technical development, there have been practitioners applying techniques for the special cognitive and emotional needs of children. Just as interpretation of play activities became the basis of child psychoanalysis, the use of games, visual prompts, and images of facial expressions have been the mainstays for application of CBT to children. The homework exercises on recording frequency of events and thought diaries used with adults have become worksheets and card games for children. All of which are designed to bring anxiety under cognitive control through emotion regulation. The problem is that such technique can work well away from distressing events, but is often unavailable when under threat. Helping people think clearly when under threat and in trauma has a long history in mental health work. Halder and Mahato, in 2019 [120], have provided an interesting cross-cultural view of the challenges and gaps in practice that have emerged across time and for the Indian cross-cultural context.

There is one other problem with CBT: it has no theory of language and how language influences therapeutic outcome. The body of work is technical, often mechanical, and not narrativist, although process-oriented therapists are concerned with the story of the patient [121].

9. A further overview: trauma and grief

Along with changing waves of CBT, there have been development of sets of techniques for specific disorders: for instance, CBT-E for eating disorders [122]. There has also been the development of Trauma-focused CBT (TF-CBT) for children and families [123].

But trauma is one of the defining themes for the development of mental health services in the twentieth century. Several of Freud's early cases involved child sexual abuse [36]. War trauma confirmed in clinical cases many of the postulates of psychoanalysis [124]. The Vietnam war led to systematic observation of the effects of trauma, as did motor vehicle collisions. The DSM-IV [100] recognized a specific mental health condition associated with trauma: PTSD. The International Classification of Diseases in its most recent iteration (ICD-11) [125] has recognized Complex PTSD as a diagnosis in its own right. The complexity referred to concerns multiple events across time and place, not just a single exposure as would occur with a car crash.

Meanwhile, many practitioners have adapted their practices to working in trauma-focused way. Trauma-focused psychotherapy is a generic name for a variety of practices and techniques. There has been one important new method for treating trauma: Eye Movement Desensitization and Re-training (EMDR).

EMDR was developed by Francine Shapiro [126] following recovery from breast cancer and was dealing with her own trauma issues when she made a discovery about her own eye movements. She became a psychologist and developed her ideas from 1988 onwards and produced her defining book in 2001. EMDR has been subsequently developed and researched by many practitioners and has been applied to children who have suffered trauma [127].

In the background of trauma has been the problem of grief. Much has been written about grief and mourning treatments, but it always surprises me that experienced supervisees do not think automatically of the grief implications of events. Longing has many implications. Many in the eating disorders community do not know of the work of psychiatrist, Christopher Dare, with Social Worker, Lily Pincus [128] in the domain of grief and how this led to the beginning the program now called the Maudsley model of family-based care [129, 130]. So much concern in matters of extreme self-starvation is focused upon lost opportunities and the fear of a child dying. The next three decades have seen considerable focus on adolescent mental health and upon eating disorders.

There are two more parts to this digression for which I have very few references to add other than professional experience: post-natal depression (PND) and sibling rivalry. These have been part of my learning since I began working as a child psychologist. Things have been written about the life enhancing qualities of the continuity of sibling relationships [131] but rarely has the problem of rivalry been adequately addressed. There is an unpublished paper of Lacan (unpublished for copyright reasons, but well translated) from 1938 [132] called Family Complexes and the murderous dislike of the new arrival is well described as are impacts in adult life. Winnicott provided a small glimpse of this in *The Piggle* [133] with the little girl having accepted the name given by her sister, which her parents thought was cute, but as the dark thoughts cleared, Winnicott knew that she wished to reclaim her name from the mean label provided by her sibling.

Winnicott is a great source of inspiration and wisdom for me and my practice; I saw *Therapeutic consultations in child psychiatry* [134] on a library shelf and decided this was what I wanted to do. I have really enjoyed his collection of letters [135] where he frequently complained of his lack of facility with "correct" terminology.

I am grateful for the wise, older women who showed me the traumatic effects of PND on families, when I started work at a rural child development centre. The presentation at any age of a woman having trouble managing a child that others can manage is instantly reason to question PND. PND damages mothers, babies, relationships, and siblings. The damage goes in to the next generation and can emerge from the past generation. Much grief is generated. If I could get rid of one mental health condition PND would be it.

10. 1990

Knowledge has expanded across the field across the century, and it is difficult to locate the significance of contemporary developments. The establishment of Infant Mental Health as a practice and as a research focus continues to be significant. But there are some that are important to my practice and have been gladly integrated into my professional activities with all those other past experiences. Commentary upon significant developments in this last period will be covered in other chapters as others as they describe current and emerging research programs.

However, three research programs associated with Colwyn Trevarthen have nurtured my contemporary practice and seem very pertinent to future practice. In 2005, Trevarthen [84] published his "adventures in companionship" as an alternative to attachment theory as the basis for understanding early infantile and maternal experience. One part of that work was his description of pride and shame as the first social emotions. He had come to an Australian Infant Mental health conference in the late 1990s and in a rapidly convened side talk outlined his ideas that had only occurred in the previous month about pride and shame. I understood it intuitively and spent over a decade exploring the application of the ideas to cross-cultural counseling, especially with couples of different ethnic backgrounds, and to the treatment of low level but chronic depression. Unfortunately, I did not see the 2005 paper until 2011.

Pride and shame are opposites and pride is the natural treatment of shame [84]. I began asking depressed patients about whether their parents had expressed pride in what they had done, and whether a central tactic of parenting included shaming. Shaming was common, but more pernicious was the lack of expression of pride. Parents learning how to be proud in themselves can be relieving of chronic depression in their children.

The centrality of pride and shame as the first social emotions also explains to me the cross-cultural difference presented earlier of honor versus shame, truth versus guilt, and power versus fear. In the wider cultural context of the respective communities, shame can be transmuted as guilt or fear; and pride can become honor, or truth, or power. With such early experience being a social given those who seek truth abhor those who seek power or honor. Those who feel shame dislike the misuse of truth against them to cause dishonor.

Trevarthen also introduced me to the work of Panksepp [86] on the basic mammalian emotions and how these are present well before the development of the frontal cortex, which seems like a further de-centring of mankind from importance or centrality, that Freud commented upon referencing Copernicus, Darwin, and his theory of the Unconscious. We are mammals and the brain stem not the cortex is the seat of our humanity. I have begun to use these seven basic emotions as a guide to the relating style of some of my patients. But, perhaps, Panksepp's mammalian emotions are just an extension of the de-centring explicated by Darwin. There is much to be learned about human experience through the study of the early stages of life and of early relationships.

Trevarthen also introduced me to his collaborator, Jonathon Delafield-Butt, and their work on autism. Over the past ten years or so, people with autism have been referred to me for therapeutic work. But my training is psychodynamic and often find people who have been turned into automatons by Applied Behavior Analysis with unusual accents learnt from their speech pathologist. Delafield-Butt and Trevarthen [136] have noted such treatments as problematic and advocate for expressive therapies that engage the body in action to help with the processing of sensory information.

Helping families and couples to understand neurodiversity, rather than displaying anger or shame, requires a subtle mix of psycho-education around reading the signs of difference, and then acknowledging feelings of stigma in the partners and siblings of a neurodiverse adult or child. The differences do constrain the neurodiverse person, but there are often hidden super powers that can be highlighted.

There are two other things that this history of ideas in child and adolescent mental health needs to have incorporated: the primacy of relating and the primacy of language. In fact, relational understanding is well-established in some quarters, but there is a Western notion that is stubbornly resistant to re-formulation: that of the individual. I prefer not to use the term.

The etymology of individual involves two prefixes and an adjectival suffix around the Latin root "videre" to see. It is the same "vid" in evidence and video. "Di" means two parts and "in" is the negation of what follows: that is, not able to be seen in parts, or complete unto itself. This is the Western Rational Economic Man; a concoction of the nineteenth century who Freud [137] promoted, especially through his translation into German of the philosophy of John Stuart Mill [138]. But Freud was not a fan of rationality as the usual human experience, but he did want to assist his patients to think more clearly. But he did like the idea of an independent man acting in the best interests of himself and his family. This version of personhood cannot survive in culturally diverse liberal societies.

I prefer to use "person". Sanders [139] suggested that the prefix and root word of "sonare" can be literally interpreted to be "with sound", but more usefully rendered as "sounding through". The person appears through the conversations with others. Meaning is established through the logos according to Corradi-Fiumara [140].

Logos is the Ancient Greek practice of seeking understanding through exchange [140]. The speaker needs signs from the listener that the listener has understood what has been said. The listener gestures or murmurs understanding, and the speaker responds likewise to indicate that meaning has been transferred. This iterative cycle is completed with both understanding that what was said has been understood.

Language is our medium for living. It is how we sound through in ordinary conversation and when conducting neurological experiments. While an understanding of the mechanisms of signaling and information transfer within neurological systems is very important to the development of new treatments, we need to be able to talk with each other to define terms and methods, to determine what the experiments mean, and to engage patients in treatments. When scientists discover new phenomena, they usually rely on Latin words to label the phenomena. Sometimes acronyms are used to make new words, but each initial letter within the acronym has ancient origins.

Freud [141] claimed the Unconscious was a third de-centring of mankind. I think the third de-centring is the recognition that language speaks us. We may say novel combinations of words, but the words themselves have been used before and in many similar combinations of which we cannot be aware. In reading or listening to narratives, language allows us to connect to other narratives and histories, beyond our immediate attention, yet persuasive to our responses to the primary narrative.

This is why this history of child and adolescent mental health has been written; to show how former practices can continue to enrich current practice, especially through the gentle art of listening. Medications can moderate, modify, and resolve mental health conditions, but not without a careful assessment through listening and then listening to the consumer and carer describe any changes. The talking cure has survived, but not in the context experienced by Bertha Pappenheim (Anna O.) [20].

11. Conclusion

So what might be a summary of the lessons for me (there are eighteen such insights):

- Childhood, like infancy and adolescence, are unique and precious stages of life,
- family relationships and environment is the source of most developmental influence, other than through trauma,
- it is important to consider grief in all presentations,
- juvenile justice and child protection have been demonstrable failures of the development of child and adolescent mental health,
- allow for the possibility of the placebo effect to enhance the starting process,

- treatment can involve internal processes of the child so long as the parents' experience is taken into account and other environmental influences modified,
- specific medicines can be effective in certain presentations,
- understanding the developments in neurology can make sense of childhood disturbance,
- systematic approaches to diagnosis can be helpful, but these have changed considerably across time,
- cross-cultural factors affect the speaking and listening of patients and of practitioners, a range of other factors influence mental health (including sexuality, gender, ethnicity, migration, housing, income, access to services, physical health, stability of the home, stigma),
- mental health consumerism helps deliver more appropriate services through accredited lived experience practitioners,
- the insights of Freud remain relevant even if his practices concerning individual adults do not apply in child and family contexts,
- family based therapy can be the most efficient,
- team based, multi-disciplinary approaches allow for better understanding in complex cases,
- notice the shadows on family life of post-natal depression and sibling rivalry,
- work like a Winnicottian,
- therapy and supervision are oral practices, and
- listening is the key.

This is a rich field for acquiring knowledge, understanding, and wisdom.

Much of my learning has come from patients, from colleagues, from supervision and from supervisees. Without direct experience, the things to be learnt would be ungrounded. Books are valuable sources, but ideas need to be lived in practice.

Listening as a mental health professional is complex, multi-faceted, and multi-leveled. Longing can be simple but obscured. Language can be incisive, or hurtful, or obstructive, but is brought to bear, seemingly from nowhere, within the flow that is therapeutic exchange.

Acknowledgements

I wish to acknowledge the Wurundjeri people of the Kulin nation who are the custodians of the land upon which this manuscript was created. And pay respects to their elders past, present, and emerging. I acknowledge the support of First Peoples' Health and Wellbeing primary care service.

I am grateful to the Committee members of Mental Health for the Young and their Families (Victorian group) (MHYF Vic) for their commentaries upon the text and for similar input from Ms. Marell Lynch.

Conflict of interest

I believe that I have no conflicts of interest as I produced the document on my own with a view to publication, only.

Author details

Jolyon Grimwade
Mental Health for the Young and their Families (Victorian Group),
First Peoples' Health and Wellbeing, Australia

*Address all correspondence to: jolyongrimwade@gmail.com

References

[1] Wardle C. Twentieth-century influences on the development in Britain of services for child and adolescent psychiatry. British Journal of Psychiatry. 1991;**159**:53-68

[2] Kanner L. Child Psychiatry. 3rd ed. Springfield, IL: Charles C. Thomas; 1955

[3] Monteils-Laeng L. Aristotle's perception of childhood. Archives de Philosophie. 2017;**80**(4):659-676

[4] Erasmus of Rotterdam. A Handbook on Good Manners for Children (New Translation). London: Penguin; 1530/2011

[5] Howells J, Osborn M. The history of child psychiatry in the United Kingdom. Acta Paedopsychiatrica. 1980;**46**:193-202

[6] Rousseau J. Emile, or on Education. (Trans. Allan Bloom). New York: Basic Books; 1776/1979

[7] Crichton-Browne J. The psychical diseases of early life. Journal of Mental Science. 1860;**6**:284-320

[8] Goldstein H. Social Work: A Unitary Approach. Columbia, SC: University of South Carolina Press; 1973

[9] Goulding P, Middleton S. Images of Welfare: Press and Public Attitudes to Poverty. Oxford: Martin Robertson; 1982

[10] Winchester S. The Men Who United the States: America's Explorers, Inventors, Eccentrics and Mavericks, and the Creation of One Nation, Indivisible. New York: Harper; 2013

[11] Trattner W. From Poor Law to Welfare State. New York: Free Press; 1974

[12] Richardson T. The Century of the Child: The Mental Hygiene Movement and Social Policy in the United States and Canada. New York: SUNY Press; 1989

[13] Addams J. Twenty Years at Hull House. New York: Macmillan; 1910/1966

[14] Smuts A. Science in the Service of Children, 1893-1935. New Haven, CT: Yale University Press; 2006

[15] Darwin C. On the Origin of Species by Means of Natural Selection. London: John Murray; 1859

[16] Goddard H. Psychology of the Normal and Subnormal. New York: Dodd; 1919

[17] Horn M. Before It's Too Late: The Child Guidance Movement in the United States, 1922-1945. Philadelphia, PA: Temple University Press; 1989

[18] Porter R. The Greatest Benefit to Mankind: A Medical History of Humanity. New York: Norton; 1997

[19] Shorter E. A History of Psychiatry: From the Era of the Asylum to the Age of Prozac. New York: John Wiley and Sons; 1997

[20] Breuer J, Freud S. Studies on Hysteria, Standard Edition of the Complete Psychological Works of Sigmund Freud. Vol. II (Trans J. Strachey). London: Hogarth Press and the Institute of Psychoanalysis; 1895/1955

[21] Foucault M. Madness and Civilisation: A History of Insanity in the Age of Reason. London: Tavistock/Routledge; 1961/1971

[22] Bertolote J. The roots of the concept of mental health. World Psychiatry. 2008;**7**(2):113-116

[23] Beers C. The Mind That Found Itself. Salt Lake City, UT: Guttenberg Project; 1908/2004

[24] Keir G. A history of child guidance. British Journal of Educational Psychology. 1952;**22**:5-29

[25] Healy W. The Individual Delinquent: A Text-Book of Diagnosis and Prognosis for all Concerned in Understanding Offenders. Boston: Little, Brown & Co; 1915

[26] Springthorpe A. John Francis Williams. London: Royal College of Physicians Munk's Roll; 1971

[27] Leighninger L, editor. Creating a New Profession: The Beginnings of Social Work Education in the United States. Alexandria, VA: Council on Social Work Education; 2000

[28] Gertz N. Blood/lust: Freud and the trauma of killing in war. Formations. 2010;**1**:65-79

[29] Freud S. Two case histories ('little Hans' and the 'rat man'). In: Standard Edition of the Complete Psychological Works of Sigmund Freud. Vol. X. London: Hogarth Press and the Institute of Psychoanalysis; 1909/1955

[30] Plastow M. Hermine hug-Hellmuth, the first child psychoanalyst: Legacy and dilemmas. Australasian Psychiatry. 2011;**19**(3):206-210

[31] Klein M. The Psycho-Analysis of Children. London: Hogarth Press; 1932

[32] Klein M. Narrative of a child analysis: The conduct of the psycho-analysis of children as seen in the treatment of a ten-year-old boy. In: The Writings of Melanie Klein, Volume 4. London: Hogarth Press and The Institute of Psychoanalysis; 1975

[33] Freud A. The Psychoanalytic Treatment of Children. London: Imago; 1946

[34] Freud A, Burlingham D. Infants Without Families. London: Allen and Unwin; 1943

[35] Freud S. Three Essays on Sexuality, Standard Edition of the Complete Psychological Works of Sigmund Freud. Vol. VII (Trans J. Strachey). London: Hogarth Press and the Institute of Psychoanalysis; 1905/1953

[36] Freud S. The Aetiology of Hysteria, Standard Edition of the Complete Psychological Works of Sigmund Freud, Vol: III. London: Hogarth Press and the Institute of Psychoanalysis; 1996/1962

[37] Freud S. A child is being beaten. In: Standard Edition of the Complete Psychological Works of Sigmund Freud. Vol. XVII (Trans J. Strachey). London: Hogarth Press and the Institute of Psychoanalysis; 1919/1966

[38] Freud S. The case of Schreber, papers on technique and other works. In: Standard Edition of the Complete Psychological Works of Sigmund Freud. Vol. XVII (Trans J. Strachey). London: Hogarth Press and the Institute of Psychoanalysis; 1913/1958

[39] Schatzman M. Soul Murder: Persecution in the Family. Harmondsworth: Penguin; 1973

[40] Dreikurs R. Happy Children: A Challenge to Parents. Glasgow: William Collins; 1964

[41] Sanders MR. Development, evaluation, and multinational dissemination of the triple p-positive parenting program. Annual Review of Clinical Psychology. 2012;**8**:345-379

[42] Havighurst S, Harley A. Tuning in to Kids: Emotionally Intelligent Parenting: Program Manual. Melbourne: University of Melbourne; 2007

[43] Stevenson GS, Smith G. Child Guidance Clinics; a Quarter Century of Development. New York: Commonwealth Fund; 1934

[44] Hinshelwood R. Clinical Klein. London: Free Association Books; 1993

[45] Lacan J. The Language of the Self: The Function of Language in Psychoanalysis. (Trans A. Wilden). London: Delta; 1949/1968

[46] Freud A. The Ego and the Mechanisms of Defense. London: Hogarth Press and the Institute of Psychoanalysis; 1936

[47] Erikson E. Childhood and Society. New York: Norton; 1950

[48] Erikson E. Identity: Youth and Crisis. New York: Norton; 1968

[49] Schneiderman S. Jacques Lacan: Death of an Intellectual Hero. Cambridge, MA: Harvard University Press; 1983

[50] Grimwade J. Psychoanalysis: A traveller's guide for family therapists. Australian & New Zealand Journal of Family Therapy. 1998;**19**:81-88

[51] Kohon G. The Dead Mother: The Work of André Green. London: Routledge; 1999

[52] Bowlby J. Child Care and the Growth of Love. Harmondsworth: Penguin; 1953

[53] Bowlby J. A Secure Base: Clinical Applications of Attachment Theory. London: Tavistock; 1988

[54] APA. Diagnostic and Statistical Manual of the American Psychiatric Association. Washington, DC: APA; 1952

[55] Freud S. Analysis: Terminable and Interminable, Standard Edition of the Complete Psychological Works of Sigmund Freud. Vol. XXII (Trans J. Strachey). London: Hogarth Press and the Institute of Psychoanalysis; 1937/1964

[56] Moreno JL. Psychodrama Volume One. New York: Beacon House; 1946/1977

[57] Bateson G, Jackson D, Haley J, Weakland J. Toward a theory of schizophrenia. Behavioural Science. 1956;**1**(4):251-264

[58] Bateson G. Steps to an Ecology of Mind: Collected Essays in Anthropology, Psychiatry, Evolution, and Epistemology. Northvale, NJ: Jason Aronson; 1972

[59] Watzlawick P, Beavin Bavelas J, Jackson D. Pragmatics of Human Communication: A Study of Interactional Patterns, Pathologies and Paradoxes. New York: Norton; 1968

[60] Watzlawick P, Weakland J, Fisch P. Change: Principles of Problem Formation and Problem Resolution. New York: Norton; 1974

[61] Anderson H, Goolishian H. Human systems as linguistic systems: Preliminary and evolving ideas about the implications for clinical theory. Family Process. 1988;**27**:371-394

[62] Ackerman N. The Psychodynamics of Family Life. New York: Basic Books; 1958

[63] Boszormenyi-Nagy I, Krasner B. Between Give and Take: A Clinical Guide to Contextual Therapy. New York: Brunner-Mazel; 1986

[64] Gurman A, Kniskern D. Handbook of Family Therapy. 1st ed. New York: Taylor and Francis; 1981

[65] Luepnitz D. The Family Interpreted: Feminist Theory in Clinical Practice. New York: Basic Books; 1988

[66] Dallos R, Vetere A. Systemic Therapy and Attachment Narratives: Applications in a Range of Clinical Settings. New York: Routledge/Taylor; 2009

[67] Diamond GS, Reis B, Diamond GM, Siqueland L, Isaacs L. Attachment-based family therapy for depressed adolescents: A treatment development study. Journal of the American Academy of Child & Adolescent Psychiatry. 2002;**41**:1190-1196

[68] Erdman E, Caffery T. Attachment and Family Systems: Conceptual, Empirical, and Therapeutic Relatedness. New York: Brunner-Routledge; 2003

[69] Bowlby J. The study and reduction of group tensions in the family. Human Relations. 1949;**2**:123-128

[70] Skinner B. About Behaviorism. New York: Alfred A Knopf; 1974

[71] Eysenck H, editor. Behaviour Therapy and the Neuroses. London: Pergamon Press; 1960

[72] Wolpe J. Reciprocal inhibition as the main basis of psychotherapeutic effects. Archives of Neurology and Psychiatry. 1954;**72**(2):205-226

[73] Plaud J, Wolpe J. Pavlov's contributions to behavior therapy: The obvious and the not so obvious. American Psychologist. 1997;**52**(9):966-972

[74] Ayllon T, Michael J. The psychiatric nurse as a behavioral engineer. Journal of the Experimental Analysis of Behavior. 1959;**2**(4):323-334

[75] Piaget J. The theory of stages in cognitive development. In: Green D, editor. Measurement and Piaget. New York: McGraw-Hill; 1971. pp. 1-11

[76] Lange KW, Reichl S, Lange KM, Tucha L, Tucha O. The history of attention deficit hyperactivity disorder. ADHD Attention Deficit Hyperactivity Disorders. 2010;**2**:241-255

[77] Brody E. The World Federation for Mental Health: its origins and contemporary relevance to WHO and WPA policies. World Psychiatry. 2004;**3**(1):54-55

[78] Lyotard J-F. The Postmodern Condition: A Report on Knowledge. Minneapolis, MN: University of Minnesota Press; 1979

[79] Benedict R. The Chrysanthemum and the Sword: Patterns of Japanese Culture. New York: Houghton Mifflin; 1946/1989

[80] Hiebert P. Anthropological Insights for Missionaries. Grand Rapids, MI: Baker Book House; 1985

[81] Nida E. Customs and Cultures: Anthropology for Christian Missions. New York: Harper; 1954

[82] Drahm-Butler T. De-colonising identity stories. In: Wingard B, Johnson C, Drahm-Butler T, editors. Aboriginal Narrative Practice: Honouring Storylines of Pride, Strength and Creativity. Adelaide, South Australia: Dulwich Centre Publications; 2015

[83] Ainsworth MD, Blehar M, Waters E, Wall S. Patterns of Attachment: A Psychological Study of the Strange Situation. Hillsdale, NJ: Lawrence Erlbaum; 1978

[84] Trevarthen C. Stepping away from the mirror: Pride and shame in adventures of companionship: Reflections on the nature and emotional needs of infant intersubjectivity. In: Carter C, Ahnert L, Grossman K, Hardy S, Lamb M, Porges S, Sachser N, editors. Attachment and Bonding: A New Synthesis. Cambridge, MA: MIT Press; 2005

[85] Stern D. The Interpersonal World of the Infant: A View from Psychoanalysis and Developmental Psychology. London: Routledge; 1985

[86] Panksepp J. How primary process emotional systems guide child development: Ancestral regulators of human happiness and suffering. In: Narvaez D, Panksepp J, Schore A, Gleason T, editors. Evolution, Early Experience and Human Development: From Research to Practice and Policy. Oxford: Oxford University Press; 2013

[87] Richards E. Destination Australia: Migration to Australia Since 1901. Sydney: University of New South Wales Press; 2008

[88] Lang M. The long shadow. Generation: A Journal of Australian Jewish Life, Thought & Community. 1994;**4**(1):22-49

[89] Frank J, Frank J. Persuasion and Healing: A Comparative Study of Psychotherapy. 3rd. ed. Baltimore: Johns Hopkins; 1991

[90] Pentony P. Models of Influence in Psychotherapy. New York: The Free Press; 1980

[91] Harrington A. Introduction. In: Harrington A, editor. The Placebo Effect: An Interdisciplinary Exploration. Cambridge, MA: Harvard University Press; 1997

[92] Beck AT. The Diagnosis and Management of Depression. Philadelphia, PA: University of Pennsylvania Press; 1967

[93] Ellis A, Harper R. A Guide to Rational Living. Englewood Cliffs, NJ: Prentice-Hall; 1961

[94] Tomes N. From patients' rights to consumers' rights: Historical reflections on the evolution of a concept. In: Robertson S, Kellehear K, Teeson M, Miller V, editors. Making History: Shaping the Future. Proceedings of the 8th Annual TheMHS Conference. Hobart, TAS: Mental Health Services Conference of Australia and New Zealand; 1999

[95] Commonwealth of Australia. Mental Health Statement of Rights and Responsibilities. Canberra: Commonwealth of Australia; 2012

[96] White M, Epston D. Literate Means to Therapeutic Ends. Adelaide, South Australia: Dulwich Centre Publications; 1989

[97] APA. Diagnostic and Statistical Manual of the American Psychiatric Association. 2nd ed. DSM II). Washington, DC: APA; 1968

[98] Rutter M, Shaffer D, Shepherd M. A Multiaxial Classification of Child Psychiatric Disorders. Geneva: World Health Organization; 1975

[99] APA. Diagnostic and Statistical Manual of the American Psychiatric Association. 3rd ed., DSM III. Washington, DC: APA; 1981

[100] APA. Diagnostic and Statistical Manual of the American Psychiatric Association. 3rd edn., revised ed, DSM IIIR). Washington, DC: APA; 1987

[101] APA. Diagnostic and Statistical Manual of the American Psychiatric Association. 4th ed., DSM IV. Washington, DC: APA; 1994

[102] Frith U, editor. Autism and Asperger Syndrome. Cambridge: Cambridge University Press; 1991

[103] Asperger H. Autistic psychopathy in childhood (U. Frith, Trans.). In: Frith U, editor. Autism and Asperger Syndrome. Cambridge, UK: Cambridge University Press; 1944/1991

[104] Kanner L. Autistic disturbances of affective contact. Nervous Child. 1943;**2**:217-250

[105] Czech H. Hans Asperger, National Socialism, and "race hygiene" in Nazi-era Vienna. Molecular Autism. 2018;**9**:1-43

[106] Geffen J, Forster K. Treatment of adult ADHD: A clinical perspective. Therapeutic Advances in Psychopharmacology. 2018;**8**(1):25-32

[107] APA. Diagnostic and Statistical Manual of the American Psychiatric Association. 4th ed., text revision, DSM IV TR). Washington, DC: APA; 2000

[108] APA. Diagnostic and Statistical Manual of the American Psychiatric Association. 5th ed., DSM 5. Washington, DC: APA; 2013

[109] APA. Diagnostic and Statistical Manual of the American Psychiatric Association. 5th ed., text revision, DSM 5TR). Washington, DC: APA; 2022

[110] Hayes S, Hoffman S, editors. Process-Based CBT: The Science and Core Clinical Competencies of Cognitive Behavioral Therapy. Oakland, CA: New Harbinger; 2018

[111] Meichenbaum D. Cognitive-Behavior Modification: An Integrative Approach. New York: Plenum; 1977

[112] Lazarus R, Folkman S. Stress, Appraisal, and Coping. New York: Springer; 1984

[113] Mahoney MJ, editor. Psychotherapy Process: Current Issues and Future Directions. New York: Plenum; 1980

[114] Ellis A. Rational-emotive therapy and cognitive behavior therapy: Similarities and differences. Cognitive Therapy and Research. 1980;**4**(4):325-340

[115] Chambless DL, Hollon SD. Defining empirically supported therapies. Journal of Consulting & Clinical Psychology. 1998;**66**:7-1810

[116] Hayes SC, Strosahl K, Wilson KG. Acceptance and Commitment Therapy: An Experiential Approach to Behavior Change. New York: Guilford Press; 1999

[117] Dimeff L, Linehan M. Dialectical behavior therapy in a nutshell. The California Psychologist. 2001;**34**(3):10-13

[118] Young JE, Klosko J, Weishaar ME. Schema Therapy: A Practitioner's Guide. New York: Guilford; 2003

[119] Menzies RE, Menzies RG, Iverach L, editors. Curing the Dread of Death: Theory, Research and Practice. Brisbane: Australian Academic Press; 2018

[120] Halder S, Mahato A, K. Cognitive behavior therapy for children and adolescents: Challenges and gaps in practice. Indian Journal of Psychological Medicine. 2019;**41**(3):279-283

[121] Ong C, Hayes S, Hoffman S. A process-based approach to cognitive

behavioral therapy: A theory-based case illustration. Frontiers in Psychology. 2022;**13**:1002849. DOI: 10.3389/fpsyg.2022.1002849

[122] Fursland A, Watson H. Eating disorders: A hidden phenomenon in outpatient mental health? International Journal of Eating Disorders. 2014;**47**(4):422-425

[123] Cohen J, Mannarino A. Trauma-focused cognitive behavioral therapy for traumatized children and families. Child & Adolescent Psychiatric Clinics of North America. 2015;**24**(3):557-570

[124] Freud S. Introduction to psycho-analysis and the war neuroses. In: Standard Edition of the Complete Psychological Works of Sigmund Freud. Vol. XII (Trans J. Strachey). London: Hogarth Press and the Institute of Psychoanalysis; 1919/1966

[125] World Health Organization (WHO). International Classification of Diseases (ICD-11). Geneva: United Nations; 2018

[126] Shapiro F. Eye Movement Desensitization and Reprocessing: Basic Principles, Protocols, and Procedures. New York: Guilford Press; 2001

[127] Civilotti C, Margola D, Zaccagnino M, Cussino M, Callerame C, Vicini A, et al. Eye movement desensitization and reprocessing in child and adolescent psychology: A narrative review. Current Treatment Options in Psychiatry. 2021;**8**:95-109

[128] Pincus L, Dare C. Secrets in the Family. London: Faber & Faber; 1978

[129] Russell G, Szmukler G, Dare C, Eisler I. An evaluation of family therapy in anorexia nervosa and bulimia nervosa. Archives of General Psychiatry. 1987;**44**(12):1047-1056

[130] Szmukler G, Dare C, Treasure J, editors. Handbook of Eating Disorders: Theory, Treatment and Research. Chichester, UK: Wiley; 1995

[131] Sanders R. Sibling Relationships: Theory and Issues for Practice. London: Bloomsbury; 2004

[132] Lacan J. Family Complexes in the Formation of the Individual. Antony Rowe; 1938

[133] Winnicott D. The Piggle: An Account of the Psychoanalytic Treatment of a Little Girl. New York: International Universities Press; 1977

[134] Winnicott D. Therapeutic Consultations in Child Psychiatry. London: Hogarth Press and the Institute of Psychoanalysis; 1971

[135] Rodman FR, editor. The Spontaneous Gesture: Selected Letters of D.W. Winnicott. London: Routledge; 1987

[136] Delafield-Butt J, Trevarthen C. On the brainstem origin of autism: Disruption to movements of the primary self. In: Torres EB, Whyatt C, editors. Autism: The Movement Sensing Perspective. Abingdon: CRC Press; 2017. pp. 119-138

[137] Freud S. The ego and the Id. In: Standard Edition of the Complete Psychological Works of Sigmund Freud. Vol. XIX (Trans J. Strachey). London: Hogarth Press and the Institute of Psychoanalysis; 1923/1961

[138] Molnar M. John Stuart mill translated by Siegmund Freud. Psychoanalysis and History. 1999;**1**(2):195-205

[139] Sanders B. Sudden Glory: Laughter as Subversive History. Boston: Beacon Press; 1996

[140] Corradi-Fiumara G. The Other Side of Language: A Philosophy of Listening. London: Routledge; 1990

[141] Fletcher J. Freud and the Scene of Trauma. New York: Fordham University Press; 2013

Chapter 3

Contemporary Challenges in Adolescent Mental Health

Anneliese Dörr and Paulina Chávez

Abstract

The aim of this chapter is to show the possible relations between the particularities of our time and certain pathologies in mental health that our young people experience today. It is in adolescence that the various mental illnesses begin to manifest themselves and that to understand them properly, it is essential to include the historical, social and cultural particularities dominant at a given time, this chapter sets forth some of the current difficulties observed in young people that would hinder them from entering adulthood. This chapter will focus on the psychopathological manifestations and the concomitant subjective discomfort that would afflict the young person and make it difficult for them to successfully adapt to their environment. Specifically, we will review the most prevalent phenomenon that physicians may face in their clinical work with adolescents will be reviewed, namely, borderline personality disorder (BPD) and three of its most frequent manifestations: addictions, self-harm and eating disorders.

Keywords: adolescence, identity, borderline personality disorders, self-injuries, addictions, eating disorders late modernity

1. Introduction

The different knowledge disciplines are in consensus as to the way in which mental pathologies manifest themselves is related to the historical period and the prevailing culture at a given time. Thus, for example, when going over the studies that deal with the history of mood illness and schizophrenia, we find that the pathology of schizophrenic psychosis, as we know it today, was first described in the year 1800 only, within the framework of a modern rationality that does not allow for arbitrary logic but seeks scientific certainty. Before the enlightenment and rationalism, the "madman" had a place in art and religion, creative and timeless spheres in which such people develop best [1]. Studies on the historical origins of this pathology conclude that before the nineteenth century schizophrenia did not exist and its description would be a consequence of civilization, so, therefore, schizophrenia and civilization would be strongly correlated [2].

Respecting mood disorders, that is, depression, bipolar disorder and mania, we see changes related to their classification and diagnosis. In the twentieth century, cross-cultural studies show differences in the intensity and form of presentation between countries. The first studies on this subject belong to Hoch [3], who found that in India

IntechOpen

depressions were not seen in psychiatric hospitals, but in the general population. In parallel, Yap [4], who researched manic-depressive psychosis, shows us that in certain parts of Africa forms of bipolar disorder type I would be more prevalent, with a very low rate of suicides, while in other parts of that continent, melancholic depressions would be more common. At the same time, there are descriptions that point to how, for example, for the Egyptians, climate was a determinant of mood [5].

All this shows how sensitive diseases are to social and cultural influences and invites us to reflect on how, in our current time, factors such as changes in family structure, the growth in urban population and longer life expectancy may be influencing. Thus, it should be considered that in each era there are people unable to properly adapt to the demands of the new times, so their ways of living are socially unsuitable for that community.

Examples of the importance of social factors in the manifestation of psychopathological conditions would be the relationship between the ideal of thinness prevailing in society and anorexia or between morbid obesity and the philosophy of life of unbridled consumerism or the picture of conversion hysteria described in the nineteenth century and the repression of sexuality at the time [1]. Thus, various cross-cultural studies on the manifestations of mental pathologies throughout history make us see the influence the environment has on the way suffering, illness or subjective discomfort occurs.

Regarding adolescence, as a qualitatively different stage of life, social scientists agree on the importance of social and cultural determinations to understand the experience of the adolescent subject.

In the second half of the last century, adolescence came to be defined as a specific phase of the course of human life and its conceptualization has become increasingly complex. In the West, adolescence is characterized by its long duration, its indeterminacy, its burden of conflicts and the great asynchrony between sexual and social maturity (Salazar in [6]). However, the "from" and "to" adolescence, in terms of its chronological delimitation, is a dynamic criterion, not fixed, subject to the era, cultural context and scientific discoveries. This would be one of the reasons to explain why there is no total coincidence, or rather equivalence, between the socio-legal criteria and the latest discoveries made by neuroscience about the age at which the maturity of brain development is reached to enter adulthood. Notwithstanding the above, it should be noted that in the last 20 years, the criteria for determining the age range for adolescence have not changed much, according to what the World Health Organization established: from 16 to 20 for women and from 17 to 21 for men [7].

On the other hand, neuroscience also contributes to the understanding of adolescence and the period it covers. In recent times, this discipline has shown how the brain develops and learns, being a plastic organ that reaches its maturity between the second and third decades of life. The brain of a newborn is only a quarter of the size of the adult brain and during childhood and adolescence, it will experience an intensive and massive growth of neurons, a biological phenomenon that will be conditioned by the environment. That is, the brain grows and specializes according to a genetic program and with modifications given by environmental influences. But it is in adolescence when the changes that mainly distinguish homo sapiens from other species occur, by which we refer to the most anterior portion of the frontal lobe or prefrontal cortex. This region would be the one that makes us "more human," since it regulates functions of our species, such as logical reasoning (inductive and deductive), decision-making, working memory, the ability to plan an idea and carry it out, the inhibition of impulses and other functions related to the ethical dimension, necessary to live in society. Thus, from adolescence until the third decade of life, the frontal lobes would finish maturing and produce a brain remodeling as a result of neuronal pruning, which would eventually be transformed into more efficient brain circuits. If the development is optimal, the young person will have the ability to control the most impulsive behavior, the possibility of accessing abstract thinking, imagining, planning as well as to consolidate identity, that is, knowing who they are, who they were and who they want to be. Thus, we see how knowing these phenomena of brain maturation is a contribution that can help to illuminate the understanding of the strengths and potentialities of adolescents as well as the age period that comprises this stage [8, 9].

Finally, regarding our current era and its relationship with the way in which certain psychopathological conditions manifest themselves in youth, the contributions of certain philosophers and sociologists to the understanding of these clinical phenomena are very illuminating. Luis Zoja, Byung-Chul Han, Zygmund Bauman and James Côté offer us theoretical keys that shed new light on the understanding of the particularities of our societies as well as the challenges and difficulties they pose to young people.

2. Adolescence in the twenty-first century

Zoja [10], an Italian sociologist, writer, psychoanalyst and economist, argues that in our society there would be a loss of common life and closeness to the others, stating that after the "death of God" announced by Nietzsche, there would be a "death of the other," an essential loneliness that would occur, basically, due to the effects of overpopulation in cities (of people and stimuli) and the irruption of technology that would have an impact by increasing the experience of the other's distance. With regard to the former, he argues that in the context of the exacerbation of the self-indulgence of narcissistic and egocentric values, typical of our time, the experience of encountering the other as an existential companion "on the journey" or "in the destination" would have been damaged, so that the man from the city would be surrounded by strangers so they would need to put distance to protect themselves from this other seen as an invader. In other words, our society would have lost the "shame of narcissism,", which results in an individuality characterized by an autarkic self that demands that its desires be satisfied without others or against others. This distance from others will have the effect of "a deprivation that represents real psychic damage" ([10], p. 23), a psychological fragilization.

As for technology, he argues that, although it enables us to increase the possibility of communication, it entails, at the same time, the so-called "paradox of the internet," which consists of the illusion of being connected, but with a non-real, non-close being, whom one cannot touch, a fact that promotes the experience of emptiness. Thus, because human beings are social beings, this emotional and psychological distance from a real other would generate psychic damage that is experienced as a distressing and threatening emptiness. This predominance "of distance and relationships mediated by technology" means that intimacy is experienced in a tortuous way, "disguised as sexuality or other impulses that are now formally permitted" (p. 14).

Bauman [11], a sociologist and philosopher of Polish-British origin, calls our era "liquid modernity" and states that in this society change would be the only permanent thing in an abundance of uncertainties and unrest. Things become temporary, fleeting, without permanence and their correlation in human relationships is that they are characterized by the fluidity, inconsistency and fragility of bonds, all of which would affect the process of identity formation. Like Zoja, Bauman believes that being part of the liquid society leads young people to experience a sense of emptiness, along with a lack of meaning and try to anesthetize themselves through drug consumption and abuse, self-harm and technology, etc.

In a dizzying and changing sociocultural scenario, where the old references of meaning and identity have fallen, adolescents encounter a series of difficulties on their path to finding themselves and strengthening their convictions, values and self-identity. In this regard, it is worth quoting in extenso the words of Novella [12] as to the impact of post-traditional societies on the construction of identity:

> *the unstable identities of our time and their clinical variants refer us—as it could not be otherwise—to a world that has lost its way and its referents, but which offers all kinds of navigation tools and possibilities of identification; a world that fosters expressive richness, but tends to dissolve it in the incessant search for spectacularity, immediacy and impact; a world, in short, that permanently oscillates between omnipotence and insufficiency, opportunity and despair, abundance and emptiness (p. 134)*

In the same line, the South Korean philosopher Byung-Chul Han [13] in his work "The Fatigue Society," speaks of a "hypertransparency" or existence traversed by overexposure and highlights, like previous authors, a subjective discomfort associated with the experience of emptiness and meaninglessness. This phenomenon is significantly linked to the technical world inhabited by today's young people, in which "the other," constitutive of the formation of a stable self, disappears, and there is a virtual other that applauds or attacks them through the networks. Han [14] also argues that social networks make us live in a kind of "digital swarm," where there are many people, but ultimately no one. These would be new groupings or a new "mass" or "digital swarm," which differs in several ways from a classic mass, in which a leader or a conductor is expected to exist. In the case of the digital swarm, there would be no leaders or voices that manage to integrate this mass, which is why, in the end, we live in a space of solitude, made up of isolated individuals, who lack a "we" capable of guiding a common action. Thus, for the swarm, there are no "places of congregation" as for the traditional mass. In Han's words: "The digital inhabitants of the network do not congregate. They lack the *intimacy of the congregation*, which would produce a *we*. They form a *concentration without congregation*, a multitude without interiority, *a group without soul or spirit*." ([14], p. 17).

At the same time, social networks favor a kind of immediate emptying or unloading: young people have quick experiences and go from one image to another without stopping. It is an immediate and rapid transport of affection, which hinders the achievement of certain tasks involved in the adolescent stage, such as the elaboration of grief, meaning the loss of the child's body, the change in the image we had of our parents and the distance from parental authority. Grief is a spiral of experiences that require a period of processing and elaboration and a time of silence.

Thus, we see that these three authors, Luigi Zoja with his idea of the death of others, Byung-Chul Han and his concept of the society of tiredness, and Zygmut Bauman with his interpretation of liquid modernity, come to the same conclusion: our current Western society would promote feelings of emptiness in young people that would have a negative impact on the possibility of consolidating identity, making it difficult for them to enter adulthood.

Regarding this problem, we need to mention the German philosopher Martin Heidegger, who enlightens us with his reflections. Surprising is Heidegger's [15] visionary way of thinking about the technical world and the difficulties that it could give us in our way of life, a reflection that can be linked to manifestations of subjective discomfort that we observe in our young people. In his words:

> *What is truly disturbing... is not that the world is entirely technified. Much more disturbing is that human beings are not prepared for this universal transformation; that we have not yet been able to meditatively face what is properly coming in this age. (p. 25)*

Han [14], when referring to Heidegger's warning about irrational technological development, speaks of the fragmentation, acceleration, discontinuity and atomization of time, noting that: "when time loses its rhythm, when it flows into the open without stopping aimlessly, any appropriate or good time also disappears" (p. 20).

Another thinker who has profoundly studied the issue of how adolescent identity is configured in different historical moments is Côté [16], an American sociologist who argues that cultures promote certain personality characteristics by fostering "character types."

In pre-modern societies, young men were led by tradition, while in modern societies, they would have been self-made men. In the current or postmodern era, young people would be led by others, and these "others" would be the means of consumption, a sort of being what one has and, at the same time, not knowing who one is. The biggest problem with being directed by the means of consumption is that these incessantly stimulate a greater consumption of ephemeral, obsolescent and transitory objects, which would be detrimental to the construction of a "firm floor" from which young people can situate themselves and face the world, thus remaining at the mercy of a changing internal and external world, a kind of presentist, unanchored and "seismographic" existence [17], which would affect the sense of historical continuity, the sense of belonging to a succession of generations (...), any firm concern for posterity" ([18], p. 5).

According to Côté, this would happen due to the crisis and discredit of traditional socializing institutions (family, parents and school), which fail to constitute a sufficiently solid guide to help young people to shape their identity and thus enter adulthood. This failure of institutional support gives way to excessive consumption (of objects, people, experiences and relationships) that does not offer institutional support and guidance to make the transition to development (Côté in [19]).

This background reaffirms the need for an understanding and a contextualized clinical approach to the main psychopathological manifestations of our current youth, which we will review below.

3. Adolescence and psychopathology

In general, in adolescence, the different mental pathologies begin to manifest themselves. This chapter will not refer to the most serious ones, such as schizophrenia and manic-depressive psychosis, which are diseases for whose diagnosis and treatment there is agreement and common criteria, but it will concentrate on the psychogenic conditions that account for a subjective discomfort that makes it difficult for young people to successfully adapt to their environment. Specifically, the most prevalent phenomenon that physicians may face in their clinical work with adolescents will be reviewed, namely, borderline personality disorder (BPD) and three of its most frequent manifestations: addictions, self-harm and eating disorders.

The essential developmental task of adolescence is the achievement of a new sense of identity that is associated with an experience of internal cohesion: I recognize myself as the same person who goes to school, who goes shopping with parents, who attends a party with friends and who does sports. I am the same person when I am sad as when I am happy, I am able to recognize myself as possessing feelings of hatred or love toward someone. You could say that identity has to do with recognition in a temporal continuum: I am the same person despite the change. A subject who has achieved internal cohesion and a solid identity does not present major psychic breakdowns or splits. It is precisely this internal coherence that fails in borderline personality. The person is not able to see themselves in a cohesive way and shows dissociated, split psychic functioning. This feature of borderline personality disorder is also accompanied by a sense of unreality, a lack of genuine feeling, confusion and depersonalization. All these sensations are manifested in self-harm without suicidal intent, for example, in making cuts in the skin.

The diagnosis of borderline personality has increased substantially in recent years, from 2% of the population in 1995 to 3.5% today. The diagnosis is also being made at an increasingly younger age [20, 21]. The prevalence of borderline personality disorder is 11% among adolescents in outpatient psychiatric settings [22], while in inpatient psychiatric settings the rate among adults is generally higher, with studies showing prevalences of 35.6 and 32.8% [23, 24].

In relation to its conceptualization, this disorder has been theorized in different ways, on a spectrum ranging from a form of mood disturbance to psychosis. In 1953, R.P. Knight introduced the term "borderline," based on the idea—now abandoned—that some patients would be on the border between neurosis and psychosis. Its official use was established in the 1980s when it was included among the DSM-III axis II disorders, under the name of "borderline personality disorder." The most relevant diagnostic criteria of this pathology indicated in the DSM-V include a general pattern of instability and conflict in interpersonal relationships, identity problems (unstable self-image or sense of self) and chronic feelings of emptiness [25].

Research on BPD over time shows that the pattern of affective and behavioral instability, as well as the great difficulty in shaping identity, are elements that are always present when it comes to characterizing the essence of this personality type [21, 26–32].

However, the reflection of the relationship between the significant increment in the diagnosis of borderline conditions, the sociocultural transformations and the difficulties in the consolidation of identity, is still a pending task. As we have pointed out before, several authors have raised the urgency of rethinking the challenges and problems of our current time and their impact on personal identity, an aspect of our being that would be a necessary condition to find a place for ourselves in society.

The psychoanalyst Scalozub [33] tries to understand why this phenomenon occurs in our time by giving us a rather enlightening reading from psychoanalysis. According to her, it is crucial that nowadays the generational difference and asymmetry of the bond between parents and children is altered or erased. This fact often generates confusion in children compared to their parents, who have neglected their role as adult guides, an issue that can be observed, for example, in their eagerness to respond to the social demand for a desirable and youthful body image, which makes the marks of generational differences blurred.

The phenomenon would also lead to the experiences of previous generations being less appreciated and used by the offspring in the process of shaping their identity. Hence, their future appears uncertain, in the sense that only they would now have the task of becoming the main architects of their own identities. In a way, they are left alone when they do not yet have the maturity or experience to decide their future autonomously and without protective guidance.

4. Non-suicidal self-injury (NSSI)

In the last decade, the phenomenon of self-injury has become a relevant public and social health problem, whose clinical manifestation has been increasing and has affected the adolescent population to a greater extent [34, 35]. Including it in the DSM-V [25] as a specific nosological entity "requiring further investigation" has led to an increased interest in studying it. It consists of a direct and deliberate destruction of one's own body surface without lethal intent, such as cutting, burning, rubbing one's skin, hitting or biting oneself [36]. However, even if there is no suicidal intent, unintentional lethality is approximately 0.6% [37]. When an elevation in the frequency and severity of non-suicidal self-injury is observed, it becomes a predictor of suicide attempts [38].

NSSI should be approached from three levels: (1) descriptive; (2) comprehensive and (3) therapeutic. The first level includes information on symptoms and prevalences. At the comprehensive level, biological and psychological dimensions are incorporated, as well as the sociohistorical impact or influence, that is, "the epochal mark" or how society generates "footprints" at the psychic level during development.

Although NSSI is present in children, adolescents and adults, research shows a higher frequency in adolescence [39]. Likewise, an increase in its incidence has been observed in both the child-adolescent and adult population [40], a phenomenon that is increasingly being associated with the impact the uncontrolled use of social networks is having on the mental health of children and young people [41].

This phenomenon has become a public health problem with an increasing prevalence. In 2013, studies indicated that between 13 and 29% of adolescents had exhibited at least one NSSI behavior in their lives [42], a figure that rose in 2018 from 13 to 45% [43]. In clinical samples, the prevalence has also risen in recent years to 40–60% in adolescents and 20% in adults, with rates between 32 and 27% according to studies carried out in Spain.

Meta-analysis on the subject shows that the figure in this population increases from 50 to 72% [44]. It has also been observed that the behavior is self-limiting and disappears after a few years, although in 20% it persists after 5 years [45]. The age of onset is puberty, at the age between 10 and 15 [42, 46], and happens more in women than in men, with a ratio of 4:1 [47, 48].

The meta-analysis by Bresin and Schoenleber [49] indicates that women have a greater history of NSSI, and that the most evident difference is in the clinical population. Differences have also been observed in the method used for self-injury. Adolescent females use methods that involve bleeding (seeing blood), while adolescent males are more likely to hit or burn themselves. According to Doctors [50], for boys and men self-cutting would be a secondary phenomenon, more frequent in special circumstances (such as juvenile detention and prisons).

On a comprehensive level, NSSI is no accidental behavior, but an intentional one that becomes an addictive ritual that is mostly performed in solitude. It is paradoxical in nature, in the sense that it is simultaneously a greatly impulsive as well as a calculated act, triggered by experiences of deep helplessness when facing pain and that generates feelings of omnipotence, enabling one to go from suffering to relief [51]. In patients who cut themselves, at first glance it seems to be an impulsive act, but on closer inspection, we see a cut with very precise and ritualized calculation, from the instrument to be used to the physical space for the self-injurious behavior to take place. Also subject to calculation is the place on the body where the cut is generated, which is usually repeated (forearms, abdomen and inner thigh, areas that are not visible to others).

Feelings of helplessness are associated with a great psychological fragility that prevents the young person from managing their affections in a more satisfactory way, so they resort to a means that allows them to "sedate" these affections. This painful act would have greater control, as it is a self-generated physical suffering that can be governed [52]. This dynamic leads to the behavior generating omnipotence, since the effect that an anxiolytic could have, for example, is compensated for through self-harm. The paradox between suffering and relief is seen in the anguish suffered by the young person and the sensation of deep relief produced by the cut, trying to produce with this act a more pleasant emotional state and an escape from their suffering.

The cut, an aggressive and painful act, causes important psychic relief, even if temporary, which favors repetition. That is why NSSI is considered a repetitive way of escaping from significant emotional frustration, which constitutes a non-adaptive strategy for managing or regulating affects, in the absence of other psychological, affective or relational resources [53, 54].

Thus, NSSI can be understood as a resource to alleviate an unknown and unmanageable suffering, which cannot be identified or named, as it is not possible to put the overwhelming emotion into words. This resource of attacking the skin or the edge itself, as a way of bringing psychic pain to the terrain of a bodily ailment, more concrete and visible, would be maladaptive and risky.

Regarding the influence of epoch or culture, it is important to note that it is a complex phenomenon associated with a multiplicity of factors, necessary to consider in order to understand it properly. By reviewing and analyzing the codes of the time, to enrich the understanding, it is possible to ask why self-harm is so frequent today.

However, lately, self-harm is considered an early symptom of borderline personality disorder [55]. Epidemiological data show that an overwhelming "80% of BPD patients have had at least one episode of NSSI" ([56], p. 52).

As already mentioned, BPD is a condition fundamentally characterized by a fragility of the ego that is accompanied by great relational and affective instability. Today's society fails in its task of helping young people to work on their identity. Therefore, adolescents who are more fragile and have a more dysfunctional biography would have even more difficulty to successfully overcome the challenges of this era [19]. Cultural transformations and the consolidation of identity are tightly linked in a way described by philosophers and sociologists with great precision.

Côté [16] refers to an increment in subjective malaise associated with the particularities of late modernity, in the context of societies characterized by the overabundance of goods, high levels of consumption and an "accelerated" time or immediacy, whose increasing speed leads to poorer resting and reflection, which are necessary to understand oneself and the world. Young people who resort to self-harm and pain would be violently expressing a subjectivity where the body is marked because words are scarce or impotent in their symbolic function.

Today's youngsters frantically seek to "belong," to be part of some group that gives them identity, that helps them to know who they are, causing phenomena such as "urban tribes," extreme body modifications, all manifestations that would fulfill the function of leaving an indelible mark, something that does not disappear, which ultimately serves them to manage their identity [19].

In 1927 Heidegger warned of the dangers the "technical world" would bring and raised his fears about the "velociferous" nature of the future. This term condenses two concepts, velocitas and Lucifer, and alludes to the demonic character of the search for increasing speed that leads to the loss of rest and patience (necessary for thinking and reflection), causing intolerance to frustration and falling into presentness. The speed reaches such a point that everything must be done immediately. We know that intolerance to frustration and being trapped in the present without being able to transcend and achieve projects are common characteristics in addictive behavior, which could include NSSI [57, 58].

We cannot fail to mention the impact that social networks have had on the psyche of children and young people. Facebook, Instagram and TikTok, among the most popular, are digital platforms that have come to change the way we communicate and relate, present ourselves and make ourselves intelligible to others, and particularly impact the shaping of the child and adolescent psyche, in ways whose scope we have not yet managed to understand in depth [41].

In recent years, there has been an increment in research linking adolescent mental health and the use of social networks as well as interest in studying the presence of NSSI in these networks [59–61].

Literature shows that in many cases of NSSI, social media would reinforce or even perpetuate self-injurious behavior. A recent study on the type of Twitter user interactions found that:

> *"Twitter reinforces self-injurious behavior, mainly by gaining community recognition through likes. Interactions between self-harming individuals and health professionals on Twitter are minimal, if not non-existent. These social media posts seem to offer solutions to their distress as they exchange information with other peers, feel part of a group instead of isolated, get quick responses and believe they find an emotional outlet" ([35], pp. 238–239).*

Without wanting to present a biased and partial (catastrophic or celebratory) image of communication and information technologies, evidence shows that their indiscriminate and unmediated use carries a series of potential risks for the child and adolescent population (eating disorders, self-harm, effects of cyberbullying, etc.) [62, 63].

Along with the above, the importance of the role of parents and family is worth mentioning. Failing as an adult society or as parents, renouncing the complex task of caring for and exercising an authority that operates as a subjective support, necessary to maintain the social bond and shape the identity of the adolescent, is an act of abandonment that leaves young people in a situation of loneliness and psychic suffering, right at a time of the internal combat in which they are not able to take charge of their impulsive and aggressive forces. Baumann [64] delves into current orphanhood and grief, pointing out that "flying light produces joy, flying adrift is distressing" (pp. 68–69). In self-harm, therefore, an aggressive impulse could emerge, turned on oneself, on one's own skin, an extreme reaction in which one tries to discover the love that accompanies, according to Winnicott, destruction.

To treat borderline personality disorder and severe non-suicidal self-harm, recent studies recommend dialectical-behavioral therapy and mentalization-based therapy, because of their greater effectiveness [56], however, the effects of these therapies are small or medium [38].

In general, the therapeutic approach is recommended to be multimodal, starting with a rigorous clinical examination to investigate or rule out the presence of other pathologies, such as major depressive disorder. If the self-injurious behavior is related to depression, the treatment plan focuses on this disorder as well as the self-injurious behavior. Pharmacological interventions are based on neurobiological models of the opioid, dopaminergic and serotonergic systems to alleviate emotional distress [65]. Strict control of treatment is required, as these drugs can in certain cases produce unexpected or paradoxical reactions [66].

For the psychotherapeutic approach, the main objective would be to work on self-injurious behavior and depressive symptoms by working on the relationship with family history and the difficulty in identifying and expressing the patient's emotions. Achieving this would allow them to integrate their emotional pain and adapt to manage it. The family needs to be included in the process too, to restructure the family environment and relationships.

5. Adolescent drug abuse

The abusive use of drugs at this stage is tremendously harmful and can leave consequences in the young people's biography that are difficult to recover, such as unfulfilled life projects. It is precisely in adolescence when aspects of great importance for the future are defined when youngsters consciously and willingly assume the orientation that will give meaning to their lives. In this regard, Guidano [67] states that it is at this time of life when identity processes become increasingly complex and articulated to enable them to form a more comprehensive point of view about themselves and the world, from which they can begin to structure their life project. The fact that precisely at this stage young people take risks and consume drugs, thus putting their future at risk, is related to *biological, psychological* and *sociocultural* factors.

From a *biological* perspective, the most decisive thing is that the prefrontal cortex, a structure involved in judgment, planning, decision-making and self-control, is the last area to develop in the adolescent. This explains why young people take risks and are particularly vulnerable to drug abuse, and why consumption in this critical period can affect the propensity for future addictive behavior (Maturana in [68]).

At the same time, there are substances considered "sequence drugs" or "gateway drugs," because they produce neurobiological changes that will increase the response of the Central Nervous System (CNS) to other addictive substances, that is, the sequence in which the use of one substance precedes and increments the likelihood of the use of another illicit substance. The most studied are marijuana, tobacco and alcohol [69].

Regarding alcohol, according to studies by SENDA [70], in Chile 29.8% of youth consumed alcohol in the past month, women more than men (32.5 vs. 27.2%, respectively) and 64% of school students reported getting drunk at least once in the last month. In the pandemic, this figure dropped to 24% prevalence of consumption in the last month, which is attributed to greater parental control [71]. On the other hand, the prevalence of alcohol consumption in the last month in the university population is 68% (71% in men and 65% in women), while the level of drunkenness reaches 68.1%.

Especially adolescents are harmed by the abusive consumption of alcohol, since it begins at a very early age, right when their brain is in the process of maturing its neural networks, and causes brain damage at the level of the mitochondria—those responsible for producing the energy of all cells. This phenomenon has implications for memory development and learning. This damage, however, is not visible in the short term, as it remains silent for a long time and then manifests itself in adulthood [72].

As for abuse of other drugs, we are interested in analyzing marijuana consumption in greater depth, because of its high prevalence among Chilean adolescents, and because its increasing consumption in the global population is also alarming [70, 73]. This phenomenon has been evidenced throughout the region of the Americas and in Europe, with the United States being the country with the highest prevalence in adolescents, with 35.2% of students having consumed in the last year. This has led to a rise in the percentage of subjects addicted to this substance, which, in turn, has significantly increased the number of subjects who engage in psychosis due to consumption [74, 75]. This fact contributes the low perception of risk and the fact that the available marijuana is more potent than that existing in previous decades, since, through sophisticated biotechnology methods, cannabis plants can be genetically manipulated to obtain a higher concentration of tetrahydrocannabinol (THC) [76].

Common marijuana in the 1980s contained an average of 3% THC, while hashish (gummy resin from the flowers of female plants) can have up to 20% THC [77, 78]. This increment in THC content suggests that the consequences of marijuana use could be worse now than in the past. When the body receives external cannabinoids, which can also be synthetic (remedies made in laboratories) or phyto-cannabinoids (cannabinoids from the marijuana plant), our endocannabinoid system is tricked. Thus, the system becomes confused and reduces its own receptors, which leads to the subject needing more of the substance to achieve pleasure. Thus, the classic addiction circuit is triggered.

In Chile, a very active and lucrative market that has increased its profits in the last decade has contributed to these very high consumption figures and low-risk perception [70]. This reality places Chilean schoolchildren as the ones who consume the most tobacco, cocaine and marijuana in the Americas [79], and puts the future of our adolescents at risk, since the probability of becoming addicted if started before the age of 17 is high [80–84], in addition to the well-known damage it causes to the developing brain.

One of the most important studies on the effect of continued marijuana use on the brain, sponsored by the European community and conducted by several universities and research centers [85], concluded that marijuana in adolescents damages the brain even with low doses of consumption and interferes with the correct neuronal pruning that takes place at this stage of life. In turn, the study by Meier et al. [86] in which 1037 subjects who began using at the age of 14 were studied and evaluated at three different times, between the ages of 14 and 30, showed that those who smoked marijuana consistently during adolescence lost an average of 8 to 10 IQ points. That means, in terms of IQ, that the subject who was brilliant became normal and the normal one went down to borderline. This is the largest study ever conducted on the effect of continued marijuana use on the brain.

Recent scientific evidence [75, 87] shows the relationship between the rise in certain mental health disorders and the use of marijuana, specifically schizophrenia, mood disorders, panic attacks and suicide, largely due to the high concentrations of THC currently contained in the plant.

Respecting drug abuse in adolescence and its relationship with psychological factors, most noteworthy is not the individual or the circumstantial situations that could affect the increase in the probability of falling into consumption behavior, but those psychological phenomena common to the youth psyche that make them a population at risk. With formal thinking, which opens the possibility of abstract thought, another form of egocentrism arises in the adolescent, different from that of childhood and which marks one of the most constant characteristics of adolescence. The young person seeks to adapt their ego to the social environment and, at the same time, to adapt the environment to their ego, for which they think about the future activity that will allow them to transform this environment. Their egocentrism is reflected in the relative indifference they feel toward the point of view of the group they are trying to reform, attributing unlimited power to their thinking, a phenomenon that diminishes as they join social groups and in discussions with peers, since, through criticism, they discover the fragility of their own theories [88].

We could summarize the egocentrism of adolescent thinking through four phenomena: (1) criticism of authority figures, manifesting itself in a tendency to idealize and easily devalue people they held very high, feeling obliged to say so; (2) tendency to argue, motivated by a desire to practice their new ability to see the slightest nuances of a fact; (3) heightened self-awareness, as a phenomenon having to do with the "imaginary audience," which would be a kind of observer existing only in their mind and equally concerned with their behavior and thoughts. This leads to the assumption that anyone thinks the same way they do, e.g., they may react badly when discovering a strain on their clothes when going to a party or when asked to speak in class, because they think everyone is aware of their stain or of how they speak. This excessive "self-awareness" predisposes to distressing experiences during adolescence and that is why adults are advised not to ridicule or criticize them in public and (4) self-focus, or "personal myth," which refers to the conviction that they are special, that their experience is unique, and that they are not subject to the rules that govern others. This is a very important aspect of adolescent egocentrism, since it is responsible for many self-destructive conducts, to the extent that adolescents think they are magically protected from harm.

It is important to emphasize that the interplay of the different factors (biological, psychological and sociocultural) that intervene in whether or not a young person falls into risky behavior like drug abuse, will have an impact on their future personal project. In the specific case of marijuana, this abusive consumption would affect the experience of temporality, in the sense that the user is more focused on the immediate "presentized" here and now [57], without a more explicit connection between the past, the longing for the future and present praxis. Although the young person has goals, the abusive consumption of marijuana would affect their ability to anticipate the behavior to achieve such a project, leaving them unable to transcend the present, imprisoned in themselves, which is finally reflected in tasks not assumed, decisions not yet made regarding what to study, whether or not to prepare for this or that task, etc., which drastically affects the personal project [89].

Finally, regarding treatment, it is essential to be clear about when it is required, distinguishing whether abusive behavior or addiction is involved, for which we must place ourselves on a continuum, whose ultimate criterion is loss of control and risky use, of any substance, whether legal or illegal. According to the DSM-V, substance use disorders refer to a set of cognitive, physiological and behavioral symptoms indicating that an individual continues to use a substance despite the problems it causes. In this case, the person would spend good amounts of time obtaining the substance, using it or recovering from the effects. At the same time, tolerance would be developed, to the extent that the subject uses the drug more and increases their ability to eliminate the substance, or there is a desensitization of receptors which makes them need more substance to obtain the effect.

Young adolescents are a high-risk population, even though most get through the stage without developing an addiction. However, one must keep in mind that not just any young person falls into addiction, there are risk factors that contribute, like the environment (friends and parents), education, social vulnerability, the prevailing culture and of course, personality. Regarding this last variable, young people with a clear introversion (very shy or with social phobia), with low self-esteem or who seek a high level of sensation, would be at greater risk. Suffering from some degree of cognitive deficit, scattered attention, psychopathological alterations, depression, etc., also play a role [68].

Thus, many times what is behind a substance abuse behavior is the use of a dysfunctional strategy to cope with a stressful situation, so therapies should focus on finding more adaptive ways. The help of parents and/or relatives is important, as they are essential as a role model for the adolescent.

Psychological treatment is a fundamental aspect of the approach to substance abuse or addiction. This should focus not only on addiction but also on the reinforcing factors of the environment and on protective factors, like family relationships and activities carried out together (watching movies, cooking, etc.) or the stimulation of sports activities [90]. Literature shows that in the psychotherapeutic treatment of substance abuse or addiction, we find various intervention approaches, however, there is more empirical evidence that cognitive-behavioral therapies (individual or group) are more recommended for young people and adolescents and are the most used by professionals in clinical practice [91]. These approaches direct to the "development of strategies aimed at increasing personal control over oneself" (p. 24), with special attention to the analysis of ideas, beliefs, behavior and affections associated with substance use, as well as the reinforcement of coping skills in risk situations.

6. Eating disorders

Eating disorders (ED) can appear in childhood, but usually occur during adolescence. Their emergence is influenced by the prevailing lifestyle in the West and, when this behavior is prolonged over time, they become a medical condition.

According to the DSM-V and the Eleventh Edition of the International Statistical Classification of Diseases (ICD-11), the most common types of eating disorders are: (1) anorexia nervosa; (2) bulimia nervosa and (3) binge eating. Although all are complex mental health diseases that entail a high level of suffering, morbidity and mortality, severe disability, high comorbidity, therapeutic resistance and tendency to chronicity, the one with the most biomedical compromise is anorexia. In adolescents, the prevalence in females is 2.8% and in males 0.8%. In Chile, prevalence studies range from 3 [92] to 3.8% [93].

Anorexia nervosa consists of a significant loss of body mass due to a voluntary decision to lose weight by drastically restricting food intake [94]. It was first described in the nineteenth century by the Englishman Sir William Withey Gull, who published in the British Medical Journal the phenomenon observed in four female patients between 14 and 18 years of age who, without a demonstrable medical disease, suffer from anorexia, cachexia, bradycardia, amenorrhea, constipation and incomprehensible motor activity. Gull recognizes the psychic origin of this disease and renames it from "hysterical apepsia" to "anorexia nervosa" as he attributes it to psychic trauma.

Simultaneously France featured similar descriptions, with Charles Lasègue speaking in 1873 of a condition he called "hysterical anorexia," which occurred in young girls who refuse to eat but claim to feel well [95]. The interesting thing about this author is that he makes a sort of differential diagnosis, comparing the "hyper-activity" of these anorexic patients with the "passivity" of people who had suffered hunger in the Franco-Prussian War of 1871. Both Gull and Lassègue give complete descriptions of anorexic symptoms, and both consider hysteria as the cause of the disorder and call it hysterical anorexia. Freud, in his article "History of an infantile neurosis" (1918), interprets this illness as a "neurosis" that would occur in young people of pubertal age who would reject sexuality and link the picture to melancholy. Later, the condition disappeared from medical discussion and was thought to be caused by atrophy of the anterior lobe of the pituitary gland (Simmonds disease), and then re-emerged as an independent clinical entity in 1965, within the framework of an international congress held in Germany, in which psychiatrists, endocrinologists, anthropologists and sociologists gathered to address this pathology. In this meeting, a remarkable consensus was reached about the disease being related to the transformations of puberty, the conflict being bodily and not strictly of the alimentary function, and the etiopathogenesis and the clinical being different from neurotic processes [96]. Nowadays the view of the problem is more pragmatic and heterodox, considering that biological, psychological and social factors must influence the appearance of this disorder.

Anorexia has a severe impact on a biological level, with this being more severe in adolescence. The most significant damage is related to a compromise in growth and an impact on height, which is greater if the condition precedes the pubertal growth spurt. Anorexia nervosa is also associated with low BMD (bone mineral density) and deterioration of bone structure and strength, with a heightened risk of fractures, so the development of this disease in this period enlarges the risk of persistently compromised bone health. The degree of BMD impairment is strongly influenced by the longer duration of amenorrhea and the later age of menarche. Likewise, acute anorexia in adolescence can lead to a significant global decrease in gray and white matter in the brain, more pronounced in adolescents than in adults [97]. Finally, up to 80% of cases of anorexia show cardiovascular compromise, which can be mild and reversible or severe and life-threatening (they are responsible for a third of the deaths in this pathology) and become more significant as there is greater nutritional compromise [98].

Psychologically, there is consensus that this disorder is accompanied by a perfectionist and self-demanding personality profile, which seeks total control to achieve its goals, in this case, losing weight [1]. Contempt for the body would be accompanied by an excessive valuation of everything intellectual. They are always the best students, they reason admirably, they show extraordinary ability to lie, evade controls and achieve their goals of continuing to lose weight. As for the importance of the social factor, anorexia nervosa responds to the search for an ideal of beauty imposed by a fashion that promotes bodies of extreme thinness that would enable social and economic success to be achieved, an ambition that in the past, when this disorder occurred, was associated with the ascetic desire to possess non-corporeal characteristics, such as the emblematic case of Sor Juana Inés de la Cruz [95].

We can conclude that anorexia nervosa appeared with modernity (second half of the nineteenth century), grew slowly throughout the twentieth century to experience a sort of "boom" in the 1960s and continues to increase, albeit more slowly, until today. Although the literature shows that its prevalence has been extended to other age ranges [99], adolescence continues to be the vital period where this disorder appears most and forms an important public health problem that mainly affects young women. These young women seek, with an immovable will, to lose not only weight but also the feminine forms, as a way of rejecting bodily maturation and sexuality and, with it, the possibility of a satisfactory erotic life and motherhood.

Bulimia nervosa is a condition that consists of recurrent episodes of excessive intake of high-calorie foods, which ends up producing physical and psychological discomfort. As a compensatory behavior to this discomfort, people who suffer from this disorder self-induce purging behavior [100]. Until the early 1970s, the difference between anorexia nervosa and bulimia as two different diseases had not been established, and it was Doerr [101] who first described the condition under the name of "Hyperphagia and Vomiting Syndrome in Young Women," characterized by the overwhelming desire to eat large amounts of food. Regardless of its quality, the person would vomit. Later, in 1979, Gerald Russell published in the journal *Psychological Medicine* a paper on hyperorexia that, for some time, was considered the first description of bulimia nervosa as an independent entity and whose main symptom was the uncontrollable desire to ingest large amounts of food, followed by the induction to vomiting to avoid gaining weight, along with a morbid fear of obesity.

The age of onset of this disorder is usually around 16, as they usually hide the behavior earlier [102]. Hyperphagia and vomiting crises would initially occur in isolation and be episodic but finally become almost permanent behavior. Concomitantly, constipation, laxative abuse and increasingly intense and frequent dysthymic states were observed, with no significant weight gain or decrease. From a taxonomic point of view, this syndrome would belong, like anorexia, to the group of addictive behaviors, which also include obesity, alcoholism and drug addiction, which are largely culturally mediated [103].

Among the sociocultural factors, the particularities of our consumer society stand out, characterized by imperatives of extreme success, productivity and control, as well as by a "morbid culture of thinness" [104], which translates into ideals of female beauty (widely disseminated by the media), which would have a significant impact on adolescence, being this a critical stage of life characterized by greater psychological vulnerability [99]. This way, as to Turner [105], our consumer society would be permanently directing "contradictory social pressures on women (...) and an anxiety directed at the surface of the body in a system organized around narcissistic consumption" (p. 93).

For Doerr and Pellegrina [106], other characteristics of our current societies to help us understand the sociocultural framework in which these disorders appear, would be the predominance of technical-instrumental reason and the artificial, the virtual and the image or appearance, over reality. In these conditions, the body, which is experienced as a thing or an "enemy" that must be totally controlled, becomes a mere object manufactured "from instrumental reason, as something that can be modeled to give it any appearance that is exposed to the gaze" (p. 13). Linked to the above, "obscenity," typical of an information society, in which everything is hypertransparent, visible and incessantly exposed to the public gaze, would also be a key enabling us to get closer to the understanding, especially, of anorexia. Thus, the anorexic's body would be obscene, in the sense of being "staged":

> *Whether it is when they hide their body in large robes or when they show it disembodied, in the literal sense of the word, there is a human being in a scene, there is a predominance of appearance, an empire of image, to say, obscenity. Let us remember that "ob" in Latin means to be in front, in sight and "stage" is naturally derived from the scene ([107], p. 189).*

Likewise, for these authors, the hedonism of our time, resulting in a "loss of the religious sense" or transcendence of existence, would be paradigmatically exemplified in these disorders, shown to us as an existence fixed in the immediacy of an "enemy" or "prison" body that must be controlled, subdued or suppressed.

Finally, with regard to the therapeutic management of eating disorders, the earlier they are diagnosed and treated, the better the prognosis. Treatment should be carried out by interdisciplinary teams with experience in working with adolescents and specialization in eating disorders, to provide an effective intervention that includes nutritional and psychological management, the use of psychotropic drugs when indicated and addressing medical complications and psychiatric comorbidities [97]. The personality profiles of patients with anorexia or bulimia are very different from each other, as well as their biographies, so the therapies recommended must be adjusted to each case. Perhaps this is why the literature recommends different psychotherapeutic approaches, such as family therapy, cognitive-behavioral therapy and behavioral-dialectical therapy [108]. However, family therapy has the most scientific support for anorexia nervosa [109–111].

7. Discussion

In this chapter, we wanted to highlight that the understanding of the psychological characteristics of the most common disorders in adolescence can be enriched by considering the particularities of our current way of life and the sociocultural patterns of the behavior that it promotes.

In a world of contingencies, in which social and intergenerational bonds have been weakened and a presentist temporality has been installed, mobilized by the eagerness to consume objects that the image market offers as a promise of happiness and volatile identity—always changing and eternally unsatisfied—borderline disorders, self-harm, eating disorders and drug abuse can be seen as an expression of the malaise of subjectivity and the dynamics of contemporary culture.

In this general environment just described, it is not surprising that there is a rise in the diffusion of identity and the loss of a meaning or direction enabling life experiences to be articulated coherently.

Especially regarding the borderline personality, because of its high prevalence and different forms of presentation, the relationship between the pathology and our current society is made visible and characterized by the decline of the traditional institutions of socialization, whose mediation makes it possible for the new members of a society to be effectively incorporated into the culture (family, school and political or religious institutions).

The crisis of these institutions of socialization, with the subsequent lack of referents, would affect the process of consolidating the identity of the young person.

This could help to understand why young people in situations of greater psychological vulnerability carry out a search for identity or belonging through often dangerous and even openly self-destructive means, such as drug abuse or the various extreme interventions on the body, which they experience as a way of having something "forever" and that fulfill the function of a lasting brand that makes it possible to deny the expiry inherent to the passage of time, which is experienced in a more anguished way in an age in which acts lack a transcendent meaning.

There is consensus that the generalized increase of certain types of youth practices of body intervention can be understood as a way to achieve inclusion in a reference group and to have a magical experience of changing the self—resisting pain, feeling more powerful, improving self-esteem, etc. 2000 [33, 112–114].

In this context, the disorders reviewed here would be the extreme case of many young people's difficulty in attaining a successful consolidation of their identity, in the sense of achieving the experience of unity and continuity [115]. When the perception of the internal is experienced as fragile and somewhat chaotic, the elements of the external world (habits, fashions and belonging to homogeneous groups) acquire great importance, and there is a marked lack of preparation for adult social life. This gradually accentuates the structural insufficiency, leaving the subject at the mercy of despair, with an unintegrated adult identity with little possibility of joining a world of increasing complexity [116].

Author details

Anneliese Dörr[1]* and Paulina Chávez[2]

1 Medicine Faculty, Psychiatry and Mental Health Department, University of Chile, Chile

2 Faculty of Philosophy and Humanities, Department of Pedagogical Studies University of Chile, Chile

*Address all correspondence to: anneliesed@gmail.com

References

[1] Dörr O. Psiquiatría Antropológica, contribuciones a una psiquiatría de orientación fenomenológico-antropológica. Chile: Editorial Universitaria; 2017

[2] Torrey E. Schizophrenia and Civilization. New York, London: Jason Aronson Publishers; 1980

[3] Hoch A. Benign Stupors: A Study of a New Manic-Depressive Reaction Type. New York: The Macmillan Company; 1921

[4] Yap P. Phenomenology of affective disorders in Chinese and other cultures. In: De Reuck AV, Porter R, editors. Transcultural Psychiatry. Boston: Little Brown; 1965. pp. 84-114

[5] Retamal P, Fullerton C, Salinas P, Gillibrand R. Enfermedad Depresiva, Etiopatogenía, Clínica y Terapéutica. Chile: Ediciones Serie Roja Sonepsyn; 2021

[6] Maddaleno M, Munist M, Serrano C, Sílber T, Suárez E, Yunes J. La salud del adolescente y el joven. Washington, D.C.: Organización Panamericana de la Salud; 1995

[7] World Health Organization. World Health Report. 2021. Available from: https://www.who.int/es/news-room/fact-sheets/detail/adolescent-mental-health

[8] Manes F. Usar el cerebro, conocer nuestra mente para vivir mejor. Argentina: Paidós; 2015

[9] Manes F. El Cerebro del Futuro. ¿Cambiará la vida moderna nuestra esencia? Argentina: Paidós; 2018

[10] Zoja L. La muerte del prójimo. Buenos Aires: Fondo de Cultura Económica; 2015

[11] Bauman Z. Modernidad líquida. México: Fondo de Cultura Económica; 2003

[12] Novella EJ. Identidades inestables: el síndrome borderline y la condición postmoderna. Revista Latinoamericana de Psicopatología Fundamental. 2015;**18**(1):118-138. DOI: 10.1590/1415-4714.2015v18n1p118.9

[13] Han B-C. La sociedad del cansancio. España: Herder Editorial; 2017

[14] Han B-C. En el enjambre. Barcelona: Herder Editorial S.L; 2014

[15] Heidegger M. Serenidad. Barcelona: Serbal; 1994

[16] Côté J. Sociological perspectives on identity formation: The culture–identity link and identity capital. Journal of Adolescence. 1996;**19**(5):417-428. DOI: 10.1006/jado.1996.0040

[17] Lipovetsky G. La era del vacío. Barcelona: Anagrama; 1986

[18] Lasch C. The Culture of Narcissism. Nueva York: WW Norton; 1979

[19] Dörr A, Chávez P. Personalidad limítrofe: aportes de Martin Heidegger y James Côtè al problema de la identidad en nuestra época postmoderna. Actas Españolas de Psiquiatría. 2012;**40**(Supl. 2):29-34

[20] ARMAI-TP. Fundación Regional Murciana de Ayuda e Investigación del Trastorno Límite de Personalidad

ARMAI-TLP. 2016. Available from: www.fundacionarmaitlp.com

[21] Sharp C. Bridging the gap: The assessment and treatment of adolescent personality disorder in routine clinical care. Archives of Disease in Childhood. 2017;**102**(1):103-108. DOI: 10.1136/archdischild-2015-310072

[22] Chanen A, Jackson H, McGorry P, Allot K, Clarkson V, Yuen H. Two-year stability of personality disorder in older adolescent outpatients. Journal of Personality Disorders. 2004;**18**:526-541

[23] Ha C, Balderas JC, Zanarini MC, Oldham J, Sharp C. Psychiatric comorbidity in hospitalized adolescents with borderline personality disorder. The Journal of Clinical Psychiatry. 2014;**75**(5):457-464. DOI: 10.4088/JCP.13m08696

[24] Kaess M, von Ceumern-Lindenstjerna IA, Parzer P, Chanen A, Mundt C, Resch F, et al. Axis I and II comorbidity and psychosocial functioning in female adolescents with borderline personality disorder. Psychopathology. 2013;**46**:55-62. DOI: 10.1159/000338715

[25] American Psychiatric Association, editor. Diagnostic and Statistical Manual of Mental Disorders. 5th ed. Washington, DC: American Psychiatric Association; 2013

[26] Gunderson JG, Singer MT. Defining borderline patients: An overview. The American Journal of Psychiatry. 1975

[27] Bergeret J. Manual de Psicología Patológica. Barcelona: Masson; 1973

[28] Fairbairn W. An Object Relations Theory of the Personality. New York: Basic Books; 1952

[29] Kernberg O. Borderline personality organization. Journal of the American Psychoanalytic Association. 1967;**15**:641-685

[30] Knight R. Borderline states. Bulletin of the Menninger Clinic. 1953;**17**:1-12

[31] Rapaport D, Gill MM, Schafer R. Diagnostic Psychological Testing. Chicago: Year Book Publishers; 1946

[32] Koenigsberg H, Fan J, Ochsner KN, Liu X, Guise KG, Pizzarello S, et al. Neural correlates of the use of psychological distancing to regulate responses to negative social cues: A study of patients with borderline personality disorder. Biological Psychiatry. 2009;**66**(9):854-863. DOI: 10.1016/j.biopsych.2009.06.010

[33] Scalozub L. El protagonismo del cuerpo en la adolescencia. Rev de Psicoanálisis. 2007;**29**(2):377-391

[34] Baños J. Modelo explicativo de ansiedad generalizada y bullying como predictores de autolesiones no suicidas en adolescentes peruanos. MediSur. 2023;**21**(3):624-632

[35] Martínez E, Atauri D, Nicolás MA, Blanco M. Visualización e interpretación de las interacciones en los mensajes de autolesiones no suicidas en Twitter. Redes, Revista Hispana para el Análisis de Redes Sociales. 2023;**34**(2):238-253. DOI: 10.5565/rev/redes.996

[36] Zetterqvist M, Lundh LG, Dahlström Ö, Svedin CG. Prevalence and function of non-suicidal self-injury (NSSI) in a community sample of adolescents, using suggested DSM-5 criteria for a potential NSSI disorder. Journal of Abnormal Child Psychology. 2013;**41**(5):759-773. DOI: 10.1007/s10802-013-9712-5

[37] Halicka J, Kiejna A. Non-suicidal self-injury (NSSI) and suicidal: Criteria differentiation. Advances in Clinical and Experimental Medicine. 2018;**27**(2):257-261. DOI: 10.17219/acem/66353

[38] Kaess M, Koenig J, Bauer S, Moessner M, Fischer-Waldschmidt G, Mattern M, et al. Self-injury: Treatment, assessment, recovery (STAR): Online intervention for adolescent non-suicidal self-injury – Study protocol for a randomized controlled trial. Trials. 2019;**20**(1):425. DOI: 10.1186/s13063-019-3501-6

[39] Xiao Q, Song X, Huang L, Hou D, Huang X. Global prevalence and characteristics of non-suicidal self-injury between 2010 and 2021 among a non-clinical sample of adolescents: A meta-analysis. Frontiers in Psychiatry. 2022;**13**:912441. DOI: 10.3389/fpsyt.2022.912441

[40] Dörr Alamos A, Viani S. Self-injury in adolescents: Expression of subjective discontent in contemporary society. European Psychiatry. 2022;**65**(S1):S444-S445. DOI: 10.1192/j.eurpsy.2022.1129

[41] Abbasi J. Surgeon general sounds the alarm on social media use and youth mental health crisis. JAMA. 2023;**330**(1):11-12. DOI: 10.1001/jama.2023.10262

[42] Villarroel J, Jerez S, Montenegro A, Montes C, Igor M, Silva H. Conductas autolesivas no suicidas en la práctica clínica: Primera parte: conceptualización y diagnóstico. Revista chilena de neuro-psiquiatría. 2013;**51**(1):38-45. DOI: 10.4067/S0717-92272013000100006

[43] Vega D, Sintes A, Fernández M, Puntí J, Soler J, Santamaria P, et al. Revisión y actualización de la autolesión no suicida: ¿quién, cómo y por qué? Actas Españolas de Psiquiatría. 2018;**46**(4):146-155

[44] Lim K, Wong C, McIntyre R, Wang J, Zhang Z, Tran BX, et al. Global lifetime and 12-month prevalence of suicidal behavior, deliberate self-harm and non-suicidal self-injury in children and adolescents between 1989 and 2018: A meta-analysis. International Journal of Environmental Research and Public Health. 2019;**16**(22):4581. DOI: 10.3390/ijerph16224581

[45] Saíz MD, Alberdi I, Servá B, Baena R. Autolesión no suicida como entidad nosológica diferencial. In: Congreso Virtual Internacional de Psiquiatría, Psicología y Salud mental INTERPSIQUIS. XXIII Edición ed. 2022. Available from: http://psiqu.com/1-11854

[46] Cabrera De la Cruz N. Autolesiones no suicidas y variables sociodemográficas en adolescentes limeños. Avances en Psicología. 2021;**29**(1):59-77. DOI: 10.33539/avpsicol.2021.v29n1.2350

[47] Del Rosario M, Cancino M, Figueroa MR. Revisión sistemática de conductas autolesivas sin intención suicida en adolescentes. Revista Cubana de Salud Pública. 2018;**44**(4):200-216

[48] Frías A, Vázquez M, Del Real A, Sánchez C, Giné E. Conducta autolesiva en adolescentes: prevalencia, factores de riesgo y tratamiento. Cuadernos de Medicina psicosomática y psiquiatría de enlace. 2012;**103**:33-48

[49] Bresin K, Schoenleber M. Gender differences in the prevalence of nonsuicidal self-injury: A meta-analysis. Clinical Psychology Review. 2015;**38**:55-64

[50] Doctors S. Perspectivas del apego en el trabajo clínico con adolescentes y sus

figuras parentales. Clínica e Investigación relacional. 2013;7(2):296-307

[51] Mauer S, May N. Cortarse solo: Acerca de las autolesiones en la piel. Controversias en Psicoanálisis de Niños y Adolesecentes. 2015;**16**:1-6

[52] Di Agostino C, Fabi M, Sneider M. Autolesionismo. Quando la pelle è colpevolle. Roma: L'Asino d'oro edizioni; 2016

[53] Guadix MG, Almendros C, Mondragón LR, Pérez EM. Autolesiones online entre adolescentes españoles: Análisis de la prevalencia y de las motivaciones. Revista de Psicología Clínica Con Niños y Adolescentes. 2020;**7**(1):9-15. DOI: 10.21134/rpcna.2020.07.1.1)

[54] Sipos L, Alcindor P, Delgado A. Revisión bibliográfica de los efectos en el psiquismo de la conducta autolesiva como forma de manejar lo traumático en el acoso escolar. Revista de Psiquiatría Infanto-Juvenil. 2019;**36**(2):63. DOI: 10.31766/revpsij.v36n2

[55] Colle L, Hilviu D, Rossi R, Garbarini F, Fossataro C. Self-harming and sense of agency in patients with borderline personality disorder. Frontiers in Psychiatry. 2020;**11**:449. DOI: 10.3389/fpsyt.2020.00449

[56] Mollà L, Batlle S, Treen D, López J, Sanz N, Martín LM, et al. Autolesiones no suicidas en adolescentes: revisión de los tratamientos psicológicos. Revista de Psicopatología y Psicología Clínica. 2015;**20**(1):51-61. DOI: 10.5944/rppc.vol.1.num.1.2015.14408

[57] Dörr O. Adicción y temporalidad. Psicología Médica. 1980;**5**(3):381-397

[58] Spitzer M. Demencia Digital: el peligro de las nuevas tecnologías. Barcelona: Ediciones B; 2013

[59] Arendt F, Scherr S, Romer D. Effects of exposure to self-harm on social media: Evidence from a two-wave panel study among young adults. New Media & Society. 2019;**21**(11-12):2422-2442. DOI: 10.1177/1461444819850106

[60] Moss C, Wibberley C, Witham G. Assessing the impact of Instagram use and deliberate self-harm in adolescents: A scoping review. International Journal of Mental Health Nursing. 2022;**32**(1):14-29. DOI: 10.1111/inm.13055

[61] Picardo J, McKenzie SK, Collings S, Jenkin G. Suicide and self-harm content on Instagram: A systematic scoping review. PLoS One. 2020;**15**(9):e0238603. DOI: 10.1371/journal.pone.0238603

[62] Boyd, D. Digital self-harm and other acts of self-harassment. 2010. Available from: https://www.zephoria.org/thoughts/archives/2010/12/07/digital-self-harm-and-other-acts-of-self-harassment.htm

[63] Emma C. Unveiling self-harm behaviour: What can social media site twitter tell us about self-harm? A qualitative exploration. Journal of Clinical Nursing. 2017;**26**(11-12):1690-1704. DOI: 10.1111/jocn.13575

[64] Bauman Z. Amor líquido. Acerca de la fragilidad de los vínculos. España: Fondo de Cultura Económica; 2005

[65] Turner B, Austin S, Chapman A. Treating nonsuicidal self-injury: A systematic review of psychological and pharmacological interventions. Canadian Journal of Psychiatry. 2014;**59**(11):576-585. DOI: 10.1177/070674371405901103

[66] García M. Programa de intervención para el tratamiento de las autolesiones no suicidas en población adolescente. (Tesis fin de Máster en Psicología General Sanitaria Universidad). España:

Universidad Autónoma de Madrid; 2018. Available from: https://repositorio.uam.es/handle/10486/685289

[67] Guidano V. Complexity of the Self. A Developmental Approach to Psychopathology and Therapy. New York: The Guilford Press; 1987

[68] Almonte C, Montt E. Psicopatología Infantil y de la Adolescencia. Chile: Mediterráneo; 2019

[69] Fergusson D, Horwood L, Boden J. Cannabis use and other illicit drug use: Testing the cannabis gateway hypothesis. Addiction. 2006;**101**(4):556-569. DOI: 10.1111/j.1360-0443.2005.01322.x

[70] SENDA. Servicio Nacional para la Prevención y Rehabilitación del Consumo de Drogas y Alcohol. In: Décimo Tercer Estudio Nacional de Drogas en Población Escolar. 2019. Available from: https://www.senda.gob.cl/principales-resultados-del-decimo-tercer-estudio-nacional-de-drogas-en-poblacion-escolar-2019/

[71] SENDA. Servicio Nacional para la Prevención y Rehabilitación del Consumo de Drogas y Alcohol. In: Décimo Cuarto Estudio Nacional de Drogas en Población Escolar. 2021. Available from: https://www.senda.gob.cl/senda-da-a-conocer-resultados-del-14-estudio-de-drogas-en-poblacion-escolar/

[72] Tapia-Rojas C, Mira R, Torres A, Jara C. Alcohol consumption during adolescence: A link between mitochondrial damage and ethanol brain intoxication. Birth Defects Research. 2017;**109**(20):1623-1639. DOI: 10.1002/bdr2.1172

[73] United Nations Office on Drugs and Crime (UNODC). (2021). World Drug Report, 2021: Booklet 3: Drug market trends: Opioids, Cannabis. Available from: https://www.unodc.org/res/wdr2021/field/WDR21_Booklet_3.pdf

[74] Forti D et al. The contribution of cannabis use to variation in the incidence of psychotic disorder across Europe (EU-GEI): A multicentre case control study. The Lancet Psychiatry. 2019;**6**(5):427-436

[75] Hjorthøj C, Posselt CM, Nordentoft M. Development over time of the population-attributable risk fraction for Cannabis use disorder in schizophrenia in Denmark. JAMA Psychiatry. 2021;**78**(9):1013-1019. DOI: 10.1001/jamapsychiatry.2021.1471

[76] Ranganathan M, Skosnik P, D'Souza D. Marijuana and madness: Associations between cannabinoids and psychosis. Biological Psychiatry. 2016;**79**(7):511-513. DOI: 10.1016/j.biopsych.2016.02.007

[77] Loflin M, Earleywine M. A new method of cannabis ingestion:The dangers of dabs? Addictive Behaviors. 2014;**39**:1430-1433. DOI: 10.1016/j.addbeh.2014.05.013

[78] Volkow N, Baler R, Compton W, Weiss S. Adverse health effects of marijuana use. The New England Journal of Medicine. 2014;**370**(23):2219-2227. DOI: 10.1056/NEJMra1402309

[79] Organización de Estados Americanos. Informe sobre el Consumo de Drogas de las Américas. 2019. Available from: http://cicad.oas.org/Main/ssMain/HTML%20REPORT%20DRUG%202019/mobile/index.html

[80] Arias F, Szerman N, Vega P, Mesias B, Basuarte I, Morant C, et al. Abuso o dependencia al cannabis y otros trastornos psiquiátricos. Estudio Madrid sobre prevalencia de patología

dual. Actas Españolas de Psiquiatría. 2013;**41**(2):122-129

[81] Large M, Sharma S, Compton MT, Slade T, Nielssen O. Cannabisuse and earlier onset of psychosis: A systematic meta-analysis. Archives of General Psychiatry. 2011;**68**:555-561. DOI: 10.1001/archgenpsychiatry.2011.5

[82] Pattij T, Wiskerke J, Schoffelmeer AN. Cannabinoid modulation of executive functions. European Journal of Pharmacology. 2008;**585**(2-3):458-463. DOI: 10.1016/j.ejphar.2008.02.099

[83] Pope H, Gruber A, Hudson J, Cohane G, Huestis M, Yurgelun-Todd D. Early-onset cannabis use and cognitive deficits: What is the nature of the association? Drug and Alcohol Dependence. 2003;**69**(3):303-310. DOI: 10.1016/S0376-8716(02)00334-4

[84] Zalesky A, Solowij N, Yücel M, Lubman D, Takagi M, Harding I, et al. Effect of long-term cannabis use on axonal fibre connectivity. BRAIN, Journal of Neurology. 2012;**135**:2245-2255. DOI: 10.1093/brain/aws136

[85] Orr C, Spechler P, Cao Z, et al. Grey matter volume differences associated with extremely low levels of Cannabis use in adolescence. The Journal of Neuroscience. 2019;**39**(10):1817-1827. DOI: 10.1523/JNEUROSCI.3375-17.2018

[86] Meier MH, Caspi A, Ambler A, Harrington H, Houts R, Keefe RS, et al. Persistent cannabis users show neuropsychological decline from childhood to midlife. Proceedings of the National Academy of Sciences of the United States of America. 2012;**109**(40):2657-2664. DOI: 10.1073/pnas.1206820109

[87] Gobbi G, Atkin T, Zytynski T, Wang S, Askari S, Boruff J, et al. Association of Cannabis use in adolescence and risk of depression, anxiety, and suicidality in young adulthood: A systematic review and Meta-analysis. JAMA Psychiatry. 2019;**76**(4):426-434. DOI: 10.1001/jamapsychiatry.2018.4500

[88] Dörr A, Gorostegui ME, Bascuñán ML. Psicología General y Evolutiva. Buenos Aires: Editorial Mediterráneo; 2008

[89] Dörr A, Espinoza A, Acevedo J. Vivencia de la temporalidad en adolescentes consumidores habituales de marihuana. Rev. Actas Españolas de Psiquiatría. 2014;**42**(2):49-56

[90] Libuy N, Ibáñez C, Araneda AM, Donoso P, Contreras L, Guajardo V, et al. Community-based prevention of substance use in adolescents: Outcomes before and during the COVID-19 pandemic in Santiago, Chile. Prevention Science: The Official Journal of the Society for Prevention Research. 2023:1-11. DOI: 10.1007/s11121-023-01539-9

[91] Sánchez-Hervás E, Tomas V. Intervención psicológica en conductas adictivas. Trastornos Adictivos. 2001;**3**(1):21-27. DOI: 10.1016/S1575-0973(01)70004-9

[92] Vicente B, Saldivia S, De la Barra F, Melipillán R, Valdivia M, Kohn R. Salud mental infanto-juvenil en Chile y brechas de atención sanitarias. Revista médica de Chile. 2012;**140**:447-457. DOI: 10.4067/S0034-98872012000400005

[93] Granillo MT, Grogan-Kaylor A, Delva J, Castillo M. Eating disorders among a community-based sample of Chilean female adolescents. Journal of Research on Adolescence. 2011;**21**(4):762-768. DOI: 10.1111/j.1532-7795.2010.00733.x

[94] Gil E, Sanz J, Pujol J. Gestión de Poder y constitución de Subjetividad en la Práctica Psicológica: un Análisis de las Definiciones Clínicas de Anorexia. Madrid: Biblioteca Nueva; 2000

[95] Fernández AM. Historia de la anorexia nerviosa. MoleQla. 2015;**20**:15-17

[96] Turon V. Aproximación histórica y evolución conceptual de los trastornos de la conducta alimentaria. In: Moreno P, editor. (Presidencia)XI Congreso virtual de Psiquiatria, Psicología y Salud Mental. España: INTERPSIQUIS; 2010

[97] Gaete V, López C. Trastornos de la conducta alimentaria en adolescentes. Una mirada integral. Revista chilena de pediatría. 2020;**91**(5):784-793

[98] Spaulding-Barclay MA, Stern J, Mehler PS. Cardiac changes in anorexia nervosa. Cardiology in the Young. 2016;**26**(4):623-628. DOI: 10.1017/S104795111500267X

[99] Rivarola MF, Penna F. Los factores socioculturales y su relación con los trastornos alimentarios e imagen corporal. Revista Intercontinental de Psicología y Educación. 2006;**8**(2):61-72

[100] Losada A, Lioy B. Etiología y prevención de bulimia nerviosa y anorexia nerviosa. Psicología para América latina. 2018;**30**:26-43

[101] Doerr O. Síndrome de hiperfagia y vómito en la mujer joven. Revista chilena de neuro-psiquiatría. 1972;**11**(2):27-41

[102] Golden NH, Schneider M, Wood C, Daniels S, Abrams S, Corkins M, et al. Preventing obesity and eating disorders in adolescents. Pediatrics. 2016;**138**(3)

[103] Doerr O. About a particular type of oral perversion in the female: Hyperphagia folowed by vomiting. International Journal of Eating Disorders. 1994;**16**(2):117-132

[104] Vandereycken W. The sociocultural roots of the fight against fatness: Implications for eating disorders and obesity. Eating Disorders. 1993;**1**(1):7-16. DOI: 10.1080/10640269308248262

[105] Turner B. The Body and Society: Explorations in Social Theory. Oxford: Basil Blackwell; 1984

[106] Doerr O, Pelegrina H. Phenomenology of corporeality (and spatiality) of anorexia nervosa with a reference to the problem of its temporality. In: Stanghellini G, Tewes C, editors. Time and Body. UK: Cambridge University Press; 2020. pp. 263-281

[107] Dörr O. La anorexia nerviosa y la post modernidade. Psicopatologia Fenomenológica Contemporânea. 2016;**5**(2):185-194. DOI: 10.37067/rpfc.v5i2.996

[108] Loucas C, Fairburn C, Whittington C, Pennant M, Stockton S, Kendall T. E-therapy in the treatment and prevention of eating disorders: A systematic review and meta-analysis. Behaviour Research and Therapy. 2014;**63**:122-131. DOI: 10.1016/j.brat.2014.09.011

[109] Lock J. Treatment of adolescent eating disorders: Progress and challenges. Minerva Psichiatrica. 2010;**51**(3):207-216

[110] Lock J. An update on evidence-based psychosocial treatments for eating disorders in children and adolescents. Journal of Clinical Child and Adolescent Psychology. 2015;**44**(5):707-721. DOI: 10.1080/15374416.2014.971458

[111] Resmark G, Herpertz S, Herpertz-Dahlmann B, Zeeck A.

Treatment of anorexia nervosa-new evidence-based guidelines. Journal of Clinical Medicine. 2019;**8**(2):153. DOI: 10.3390/jcm8020153

[112] Groschwitz R, Plener P, Kaess M, Schumacher T, Stoehr R, Boege I. The situation of former adolescent self-injurers as young adults: A follow-up study. BMC Psychiatry. 2015:15-160. DOI: 10.1186/s12888-015-0555-1

[113] Pelento ML. Los tatuajes como marcas: Ruptura de los lazos sociales y su incidencia en la construcción de la subjetividad individual y social. Revista de Psicoanálisis. 1999;**56**(2):283-297

[114] Reisfeld S. Tatuajes: una mirada psicoanalítica. Buenos Aires: Amorrortu; 2005

[115] Bateman AW, Fonagy P, editors. Handbook of Mentalizing in Mental Health Practice. Washington, DC: American Psychiatric Publishing, Inc; 2012

[116] Bernardo EG. Control de emociones e impulsos en las personalidades borderline. Aperturas psicoanalíticas. 2000;**6**

Chapter 4

Disorders Associated with Stress

Yasodha Rohanachandra

Abstract

Major changes to the concept of disorders specifically associated with stress have been made since the introduction of the latest revision of the International Classification of Diseases (ICD-11). With the ICD-11, a separate entity titled complex post-traumatic stress disorder (PTSD) was introduced to the classification systems for the first time, to include those who have suffered repeated, sustained and multiple forms of trauma, which is commonly associated with childhood abuse. The ICD-11 also includes an entity called prolonged grief disorder, to differentiate the boundaries between normal and atypical grief. Since the release of the ICD-11, there has been much discussion about the validity, utility, reliability and cross-cultural comparison of these disorders, as well as the comparability of these diagnoses with the DSM-V categories. This chapter aims to summarize the latest evidence on the disorders associated with stress, with special relevance to children and adolescents.

Keywords: post-traumatic stress disorder, complex post-traumatic stress disorder, prolonged grief disorder, disorders associated with stress, stress related disorders

1. Introduction

The hallmark of the disorders associated with stress, is that these disorders occur as a direct consequence of exposure to stress or trauma. Hence, this category of disorders differs from others, in that the diagnosis not only requires the presence of certain symptomatology but also requires the causative factor, namely the presence of an identifiable trauma that led to the development of these symptoms.

The Diagnostic and Statistical Manual, 5th edition (DSM-V) includes PTSD, acute stress disorder, adjustment disorder and other specified Trauma-and-Stressor-related disorders as Trauma-and-Stress-Related disorders [1]. Similar to DSM-V, the International Classification of Diseases, 10th edition (ICD-10) also includes these three disorders as reactions to severe stress [2]. However, in contrast to the ICD-10, reactive attachment disorder and disinhibited social engagement disorder are also included as Trauma-and-Stress-Related disorders in the DSM-V, whereas these are included as behavioral and emotional disorders with onset usually occurring in childhood and adolescence, in the ICD-10.

With the introduction of the International Classification of Diseases, 11th Edition (ICD-11) in 2018, there have been major changes to the concept of disorders specifically associated with stress [3]. With the ICD-11, a separate entity titled Complex PTSD was introduced to the classification systems for the first time, to include those who have suffered repeated, sustained and multiple forms of trauma. The ICD-11

DSM-V **Trauma-and-stress-related disorder**	ICD-10 **Reaction to severe stress, and adjustment disorders**	ICD-11 **Disorders specifically associated with stress**
313.89 Reactive attachment disorder *313.89* Disinhibited social engagement disorder *309.81* Post-traumatic stress disorder (PTSD) *308.3* Acute Stress Disorder *309* Adjustment disorder *309.89* Other specified trauma-and-stress-related disorder	*F43.1* Post-traumatic stress disorder *F43.2* Adjustment disorders *F43.8* Other reactions to severe stress *F43.9* Reaction to severe stress, unspecified	*6B40* Post-traumatic stress disorder (PTSD) *6B41* Complex post-traumatic stress disorder (CPTSD) *6B42* Prolonged grief disorder *6B43* Adjustment disorder *6B44* Reactive attachment disorder *6B45* Disinhibited social engagement disorder *6B4Y* Other specified disorders specifically associated with stress *6B4Z* Disorders specifically associated with stress, unspecified

Table 1.
Classification of disorders associated with stress across classification systems.

also includes an entity called prolonged grief disorder to differentiate the boundaries between normal and atypical grief. The diagnosis of adjustment disorders had also been reformulated in the ICD-11 [3]. Furthermore, ICD-11 also included reactive attachment disorder and disinhibited social engagement disorder as disorders associated with stress, in keeping with the DSM-V (**Table 1**).

This chapter aims to summarize the latest evidence on the disorders associated with stress, with special relevance to children and adolescents.

2. Diagnostic classification

2.1 Post-traumatic stress disorder (PTSD)

PTSD was first introduced to the classification systems in 1980, in the Diagnostic and Statistical Manual, 3rd edition (DSM-III) [4]. Since its conception, it has undergone several revisions in 1987 in the DSM-III-R, in 2000 in the DSM-IV, and finally in 2013 for the DSM-V.

According to the DSM-V criteria, diagnosis of PTSD is complex and requires the presence of one or more symptoms in criterion A-C, two or more symptoms in criterion D-E and symptoms to be present for more than 1 month, with clinically significant distress or functional impairment [1] (**Table 2**).

Evidence has shown that in preschool children, diagnostic criteria for PTSD need to be developmentally sensitive and focused on behavior changes, to line with the limited cognitive and verbal expressive skills in younger children [5]. Taking this into consideration, the DSM-V has separate diagnostic criteria for the diagnosis of PTSD in children younger than 6 years [1]. The diagnostic criteria for preschoolers in the DSM-V acknowledge that the intrusive memories of the trauma need not be distressing to children younger than 6 years. In addition, instead of needing symptoms of both avoidance and negative alterations in cognition and mood, the DSM-V only requires the presence of either symptoms of avoidance or negative altercations of cognition and mood in younger children. Furthermore, the inability to remember

1. Exposure to actual or threatened death, serious injury, or sexual violence in one (or more) of the following ways:
    1. Directly experiencing the traumatic event(s).
    2. Witnessing, in person, the event(s) as it occurred to others.
    3. Learning that the traumatic event(s) occurred to a close family member or close friend. In cases of actual or threatened death of a family member or friend, the event(s) must have been violent or accidental.
    4. Experiencing repeated or extreme exposure to aversive details of the traumatic event(s) (e.g., first responders collecting human remains; police officers repeatedly exposed to details of child abuse). *Note*: Criterion A4 does not apply to exposure through electronic media, television, movies, or pictures, unless this exposure is work related.
2. Presence of one (or more) of the following intrusion symptoms associated with the traumatic event(s), beginning after the traumatic event(s) occurred:
    1. Recurrent, involuntary and intrusive distressing memories of the traumatic event(s). *Note*: In children older than 6 years, repetitive play may occur in which themes or aspects of the traumatic event(s) are expressed.
    2. Recurrent distressing dreams in which the content and/or effect of the dream are related to the traumatic event(s). *Note*: In children, there may be frightening dreams without recognizable content.
    3. Dissociative reactions (e.g., flashbacks) in which the individual feels or acts as if the traumatic event(s) were recurring. (Such reactions may occur on a continuum, with the most extreme expression being a complete loss of awareness of present surroundings.) *Note*: In children, trauma-specific reenactment may occur in play.
    4. Intense or prolonged psychological distress at exposure to internal or external cues that symbolize or resemble an aspect of the traumatic event(s).
    5. Marked physiological reactions to internal or external cues that symbolize or resemble an aspect of the traumatic event(s).
3. Persistent avoidance of stimuli associated with the traumatic event(s), beginning after the traumatic event(s) occurred, as evidenced by one or both of the following:
    1. Avoidance of or efforts to avoid distressing memories, thoughts or feelings about or closely associated with the traumatic event(s).
    2. Avoidance of or efforts to avoid external reminders (people, places, conversations, activities, objects, situations) that arouse distressing memories, thoughts or feelings about or closely associated with the traumatic event(s).
4. Negative alterations in cognitions and mood associated with the traumatic event(s), beginning or worsening after the traumatic event(s) occurred, as evidenced by two (or more) of the following:
    1. Inability to remember an important aspect of the traumatic event(s) (typically due to dissociative amnesia, and not to other factors such as head injury, alcohol or drugs).
    2. Persistent and exaggerated negative beliefs or expectations about oneself, others, or the world (e.g., "I am bad," "No one can be trusted," "The world is completely dangerous," "My whole nervous system is permanently ruined").
    3. Persistent, distorted cognitions about the cause or consequences of the traumatic event(s) that lead the individual to blame himself/herself or others.
    4. Persistent negative emotional state (e.g., fear, horror, anger, guilt or shame).
    5. Markedly diminished interest or participation in significant activities.
    6. Feelings of detachment or estrangement from others.
    7. Persistent inability to experience positive emotions (e.g., inability to experience happiness, satisfaction or loving feelings).
5. Marked alterations in arousal and reactivity associated with the traumatic event(s), beginning or worsening after the traumatic event(s) occurred, as evidenced by two (or more) of the following:
    1. Irritable behaviour and angry outbursts (with little or no provocation), typically expressed as verbal or physical aggression toward people or objects.
    2. Reckless or self-destructive behaviour.
    3. Hypervigilance.
    4. Exaggerated startle response.
    5. Problems with concentration.
    6. Sleep disturbance (e.g., difficulty falling or staying asleep or restless sleep).
6. Duration of the disturbance (Criteria B, C, D and E) is more than 1 month.
7. The disturbance causes clinically significant distress or impairment in social, occupational or other important areas of functioning.
8. The disturbance is not attributable to the physiological effects of a substance (e.g., medication and alcohol) or another medical condition.

Table 2.
DSM-V. Criteria for PTSD.

important aspects of the event and persistent and negative beliefs about self, others or the world have been removed as a diagnostic criterion for those younger than 6 years, as preschool children may not be developmentally capable of experiencing such symptoms. The wording of some symptoms has also been changed, to make detection of symptoms easier. For example, feelings of detachment or estrangement have been worded as social withdrawal in the criteria for preschool children.

In the ICD-11, the diagnosis of PTSD requires symptoms from three clusters of (A) re-experiencing the traumatic event or events in the form of vivid intrusive memories, flashbacks, or nightmares; (B) avoidance of thoughts, memories, activities, situations, or people reminding of the event or events; and (C) persistent perceptions of heightened current threat, indicated by hypervigilance or an enhanced startle reaction [3]. ICD-11 also requires that the symptoms need to be present for at least several weeks and cause significant functional impairment. The criterion that the onset should be within 6 months of exposure to the event, which was included in ICD-10, has been removed from the ICD-11 [3]. Unlike the DSM [5], the ICD does not provide a list of specific symptoms and does not specify the number of symptoms in each category that is needed for a diagnosis. Instead, the ICD provides a broad overview of the disorder and the essential requirements for a diagnosis.

2.2 Complex PTSD (C-PTSD)

The term complex PTSD was first proposed by Herman, in 1992. Herman argued that the diagnosis of PTSD mostly relates to survivors of relatively circumscribed traumatic events and fails to capture the effects of prolonged, repeated trauma, where the victim is in a state of captivity and is unable to flee [6]. The diagnosis of "Enduring personality change after a catastrophic experience" in ICD-10 [3] and "Disorders of Extreme Stress Not Otherwise Specified" (DESNOS), which was included in the Appendix to DSM-IV [7], have both attempted to capture the effects of repeated exposure to trauma. However, for years, there have been concerns about the validity of complex PTSD as a separate diagnostic entity, as its symptomatology often overlaps with other psychiatric disorders such as PTSD as well as with certain personality disorders.

The ICD-11 has included complex PTSD into the classification systems for the first time. The ICD-11 suggests that complex PTSD is likely to develop following exposure to an event or series of events of an extremely threatening or horrific nature, which are prolonged or repetitive in nature and where escape if either difficult or impossible [3]. Such events may include repeated sexual or physical abuse in childhood, prolonged domestic violence, torture, slavery and genocide campaigns. The ICD-11 diagnostic criteria do not specify the type of trauma needed for the diagnosis to be made [3].

The diagnosis of complex PTSD in ICD-11 requires all diagnostic requirements for PTSD, i.e., re-experience, hypervigilance and avoidance to have been present at some point following the exposure to the trauma. In addition, symptoms from three other categories are required for a diagnosis. These include (A) severe and pervasive problems in affect regulation; (B) persistent beliefs about oneself as diminished, defeated or worthless, accompanied by deep and pervasive feelings of shame, guilt or failure related to the traumatic event; and (C) persistent difficulties in sustaining relationships and in feeling close to others [3]. These symptoms are collectively referred to as "disturbance of self-organization". The diagnoses of PTSD and complex PTSD are mutually exclusive. That is, if a person is diagnosed with complex PTSD, he cannot receive a diagnosis of PTSD at the same time.

Unlike the ICD-11, the DSM-V had tried to include the effects of prolonged and repetitive trauma within the diagnosis of the PTSD itself, by expanding the diagnostic criteria of PTSD, to include the symptom clusters of negative alternations in mood and cognitions, and by including a dissociative subtype to capture some aspects of disturbance of affect and self-perception. This has allowed a large number of symptom profiles to be categorized into a single category of PTSD, decreasing the utility of the disorder in treatment planning.

ICD-11 does not have separate criteria for the diagnosis of complex PTSD in children and adolescents. However, clinicians should keep in mind that the expression of symptoms may vary according to the developmental age. For example, in children, affect dysregulation may manifest as temper tantrums and dissociation may present as inattention or daydreaming.

2.3 Prolong grief disorder

The experience of persistent and disabling grief has been described and classified in the literature under several names, such as abnormal grief, pathological grief and complicated grief disorder. DSM-5 included persistent complex bereavement disorder

a. The death, at least 12 months ago, of a person who was close to the bereaved (for children and adolescents, at least 6 months ago).

b. Since the death, there has been a grief response characterized by one or both of the following, to a clinically significant degree, nearly every day or more often for at least the last month:
   1. Intense yearning/longing for the deceased person
   2. Preoccupation with thoughts or memories of the deceased person (in children and adolescents, preoccupation may focus on the circumstances of the death)

c. As a result of the death, at least three of the following eight symptoms have been experienced to a clinically significant degree since the death, including nearly every day or more often for at least the last month:
   1. Identity disruption (e.g., feeling as though part of oneself has died)
   2. Marked sense of disbelief about the death
   3. Avoidance of reminders that the person is dead (in children and adolescents, may be characterized by efforts to avoid reminders)
   4. Intense emotional pain (e.g., anger, bitterness, sorrow) related to the death
   5. Difficulty with reintegration into life after the death (e.g., problems engaging with friends, pursuing interests, planning for the future)
   6. Emotional numbness (i.e., absence or marked reduction in the intensity of emotion, feeling stunned) as a result of the death
   7. Feeling that life is meaningless as a result of the death
   8. Intense loneliness (i.e., feeling alone or detached from others) as a result of the death

d. The disturbance causes clinically significant distress or impairment in social, occupational or other important areas of functioning.

e. The duration and severity of the bereavement reaction clearly exceeds expected social, cultural or religious norms for the individual's culture and context.

f. The symptoms are not better explained by major depressive disorder, post-traumatic stress disorder, or another mental disorder, or attributable to the physiological effects of a substance (e.g., medication and alcohol) or another medical condition

Table 3.
DSM-5. TR criteria for prolonged grief disorder.

as a "condition for further study" [1]. The ICD-11 and the Diagnostic and Statistical Manual of Mental Disorders 5, Text Revision (DSM-5 TR) [8] have introduced the diagnostic category of "prolonged grief disorder" (PGD) into the diagnostic systems for the first time (**Table 3**).

For a diagnosis of PGD, the ICD-11 requires the presence of (A) persistence pervasive grief response (e.g., longing for the diseased, persistent preoccupations with the diseased) and (B) intense emotional pain (e.g., sadness, guilt, anger, denial, blame, difficulty accepting the death, feeling one has lost a part of one's self, an inability to experience positive mood, emotional numbness, difficulty in engaging with social or other activities) (C). These symptoms need to have been present for a minimum of 6 months and should have resulted in functional impairment.

The DSM-5 TR criteria differs from the ICD-11 criteria in that the DSM-5 TR requires the symptoms to have been present for more than 12 months, in contrast to the cut-off of 6 months in the ICD-11. Both classification systems include symptoms of yearning or preoccupation with thoughts or memories of the deceased. In addition to the yearning and preoccupation, the DSM criteria requires at least three further symptoms that need to be present in order to make a diagnosis [3, 8]. There is evidence that since ICD-11 has fewer criteria for the diagnosis of PGD, the prevalence rates of PGD maybe higher when using the ICD classification compared to the DSM classification.

Certain modifications may be needed when applying these criteria to children and adolescents. It is suggested that identity disruption in children and adolescents may manifest as feeling different from others (e.g., feeling weird or different from peers due to being motherless), rather than as feeling as though a part of oneself has died, as in adults [9]. It has also been hypothesized that the criteria of needing to have a marked sense of disbelief about death may not be relevant to children, as young children do not understand the permanency of death. Furthermore, difficulty in reintegration into life may manifest in children as a failure to acquire developmental milestones. In addition, young children may express intense yearning through their wishes to physically reunite with their loved one through fantasies of dying. This may not indicate suicidal thinking, but rather, as a way of expressing the pain of separation, through their concrete thinking [9].

There have been several criticisms against including PGD as a separate diagnosis in the classification systems. There have been concerns about whether this would result in the medicalization of normal grief and the inappropriate use of pharmacotherapies [10]. The validity of the diagnosis across cultures has also been questioned, given the variation in the expression of grief among different cultures. It has also been suggested that labelling grief as a psychiatric disorder, could lead to stigmatization of the affected individuals. However, others have argued that since the symptoms listed in PGD can be reliably identified, shown to be distinct from other psychiatric disorders such as depression, PTSD and anxiety, and respond to grief-specific rather than other (e.g., depression-focused) interventions, PGD warrants a separate diagnosis [10]. There is also emerging evidence that PGD symptoms have distinct neurobiological correlates, which further supports a separate diagnosis.

3. Epidemiology

3.1 PTSD versus complex PTSD

There is limited evidence comparing the prevalence of PTSD and CPTSD among children and young people in the general population. The first such study was done in Lithuania, and it revealed the prevalence of CPTSD (11.6%) [11] to be higher than the prevalence of PTSD (10.4%). Similar patterns were seen in studies from Northern Ireland (CPTSD 3.4%; PTSD 1.5%) [12] and Japan (CPTSD 4.1%; PTSD 2.3%) [13]. These findings suggest that CPTSD may be more prevalent among children and young people than PTSD [12]. These findings also oppose the previous beliefs that PTSD is commoner in community samples than CPTSD.

Studies have assessed the difference between the two disorders in terms of risk factors. While some studies indicate that cumulative trauma is a predictor of PTSD, some found that cumulative trauma did not discriminate between PTSD and CPTSD [11, 14]. However, interpersonal trauma was found to be associated with CPTSD [11, 14, 15]. Certain socio-demographic factors such as unemployment, minority status, lower education, living alone and being unmarried have been reported to carry a higher risk of CPTSD [16, 17]. Furthermore, social factors such as financial difficulties, family conflicts, mental illness in the family and lack of social support were found to be particularly associated with CPTSD in adolescents [11]. In addition, loneliness was also reported to have a greater association with CPTSD than PTSD. Having special educational needs has been identified as a unique risk factor for CPTSD in adolescents exposed to trauma [12]. This may be due to the vulnerability of children with low intellectual functioning to trauma exposure or their reduced capacity to adapt to traumatic events. Bullying was also shown to be associated more with CPTSD than PTSD [11].

3.2 Prolonged grief disorder

A recent meta-analysis found the prevalence of PGD in adults to range between 9.8% following natural disasters, to 49% following unnatural loss [18, 19]. Data on the prevalence of PGD in children and adolescents is limited, but the available data suggests that it ranges between 7 and 10% [20].

Evidence on risk factors associated with a higher risk of prolonged grief mostly comes from studies done on adult populations. These suggest that maladaptive thoughts (e.g., self-blame), avoidance, lack of social support and pre-existing mental health problems, especially mood disorders, carry a higher risk of developing PGD [21–23]. Socio-demographic factors such as female gender, older age, and lower socio-economic status are also shown to be associated with prolonged grief [24]. With regard to the nature of the death, bereavement by sudden losses such as suicide, homicide or accidents is thought to predispose to PGD [25]. Exposure to childhood adversity has also been identified as a risk factor for PGD [26]. The limited studies carried out in children and adolescents suggest that, similar to adult populations, the female gender is a risk factor for the development of PGD in children [27, 28]. In contrast to adults, children who were bereaved due to a prolonged illness of a loved one were at a higher risk of developing PGD compared to those who were bereaved by sudden natural death [29]. This suggests that children and adults differ in their experience of the circumstances surrounding death. It has been suggested that prolonged illness gives rise to longer exposure to traumatic memories, contributing to a higher risk of PGD in children. In addition, due to the common belief that sudden deaths are more traumatic than deaths following prolonged illness, children bereaved through prolonged illness may receive less social support compared to those bereaved through sudden death. Furthermore, not receiving accurate information and their limited capacity to understand the circumstances around the death may make children believe that they could have prevented the death. This in turn can make children and adolescents more vulnerable to develop PGD [29]. Other factors that have been found to be associated with a higher risk of PGD in children and adolescents include exposure to interpersonal conflicts, personal history of depression, family history of anxiety disorders and peritraumatic stress [27–29].

4. Differential diagnosis

4.1 PTSD and CPTSD

There have been concerns about the discriminant validity of CPTSD from borderline personality disorder (BPD), as both disorders share the symptoms clusters of disturbances of self-organization. However, the manifestation of these clusters differs between the two disorders. In BPD, there is an unstable sense of self, whereas in CPTSD, there is a persistent negative sense of self. The relational difficulties in BPD are characterized by volatile pattern of interactions, where the person rapidly changes from idealizing to devaluing a person, in contrast to CPTSD, where the person generally avoids relationships. In BPD, the affect dysregulation is often triggered by the fear of abandonment or rejection, whereas in CPTSD, it is a manifestation of difficulty in maintaining emotional equilibrium [30]. Furthermore, the diagnosis of CPTSD requires the presence of trauma and associated re-experiencing, avoidance and heightened threat perception, which is not a diagnostic criterion of BPD. Moreover, self-harming behaviors, which are a part of diagnostic criteria for BPD, is not a requirement for the diagnosis of CPTSD [30]. Several studies have supported the discriminant validity of the CPTSD and BPD diagnoses. Evidence suggests that the relationship between CPTSD and BPD is the same as in any other two psychiatric diagnoses [31]. That is, the two disorders share conceptual similarity, there is some correlation between the constructs at a dimensional level, they share similar risk factors, and there is a high comorbidity between the two disorders.

4.2 Prolonged grief disorder

There are several overlapping features between PGD and depression. Both disorders share sadness, social isolation/withdrawal, guilt and sleep disturbances. However, the low mood in PGD is more often reported to occur as waves of sadness, in contrast to the generalized low mood in depression. Guilt experienced in PGD is often related to the circumstances surrounding the death (e.g., what could have been done to prevent the death), in contrast to more generalized guilt in depression [25, 32]. Although both conditions may have social isolation, in depression, this is often due to poor motivation, whereas in PGD it is most likely an attempt to avoid reminders of the deceased (e.g., avoidance of previously shared activities or friends). While suicidal thoughts can occur in both disorders, in depression, it is usually in the context of hopelessness and worthlessness, whereas in PGD, it is mostly due to wishes of joining the deceased.

PGD and PTSD can also share several features such as intrusive thoughts or images of the death, avoidance related to the death, emotional numbness and sleep disturbances. However, in PTSD, the predominant emotion is fear, whereas in PGD, yearning and sadness are the prominent emotions [25, 33]. Although both disorders show avoidance, in PTSD, it serves to reduce exposure to potential threat, whereas in PGD, it is to avoid painful memories and reminders of the permanency of the loss. In addition, symptoms of hypervigilance are thought to be associated more with PTSD than with PGD [25, 33].

5. Comorbidities

5.1 PTSD versus CPTSD

Studies examining the psychiatric comorbidities among children with PTSD and CPTSD are sparse. Studies from adult populations show PTSD and CPTSD to be highly comorbid with depression, generalized anxiety disorder (GAD), dissociative disorder, somatic symptom disorder, suicidality, substance use, quasi-psychotic symptoms and chronic illness [31, 34, 35]. It has been found that depression GAD, and substance use show greater comorbidity with CPTSD than with PTSD [36]. BPD has also been shown to be comorbid with CPTSD. Studies show that the presence of BPD as a comorbidity of CPTSD is higher than CPTSD occurring as a comorbidity of BPD. In keeping with the findings from adults, the available studies on adolescents suggests that CPTSD is associated with higher levels of depression, anxiety, self-harm, suicidal ideation, somatization disorder and eating disorder compared to PTSD, especially in boys [36]. In addition, children and adolescents with CPTSD are known to have greater neurocognitive deficits, namely deficits in spatiotemporal visual attention and working memory, than those with PTSD [37]. This suggests that CPTSD is associated with a higher risk of psychiatric burden and may require a longer course of treatment compared to PTSD.

5.2 Prolonged grief disorder

Previous literature shows PGD to be highly comorbid with other psychiatric disorders, with up to 75% having comorbid mental health problems [38]. Studies have shown depression and PTSD to have the highest rates of comorbidity [25]. This may be due to the shared risk factors (e.g., female gender, exposure to traumatic events) or shared symptoms (e.g., intrusive thoughts, feelings of hopelessness, suicidal thoughts) between these disorders [39, 40]. PGD is also highly comorbid with anxiety disorders, with generalized anxiety disorder being the most common comorbid anxiety disorder [38]. Up to 80% of those with PGD are also known to suffer from long-term poor sleep [33]. Other sleep disorders such as poorer sleep quality, difficulties in falling asleep, shorter duration of sleep and night-time awakenings, are also shown to be associated with PGD [33]. PGD is also known to be comorbid with suicidal ideation and behaviors, increased substance use, general health impairments and a higher risk of all-cause mortality [25].

6. Screening

6.1 PTSD and complex PTSD

Several instruments are available to screen for the presence of PTSD in children and adolescents. However, assessment of CTPSD in children and adolescents is a challenge, as most tools assess the impact of a single trauma as opposed to exposure to multiple traumatic events, and that the number of tools available to assess complex developmental trauma is limited.

The Children's Revised Impact of Event Scale (CRIES), The Child PTSD Symptom Scale (CPSS) and The UCLA PTSD Reaction Index for DSM-IV, revision 1 (UCLA CPTSD-RI) are three of the scales that are considered reliable and valid tools to screen for PTSD in children and adolescents [41–43]. All three scales have self-report versions. The UCLA CPTSD-RI also has a parent report version and the CPSS has an interviewer administered version as well. The CRIES and CPSS are validated for children and adolescents between 8 and 18 years. The CRIES has two versions with 8 items and 13 items and both are considered to be equally reliable for screening of PTSD.

A recent meta-analysis reported that the International Trauma Questionnaire (ITQ) is the instrument that has been most widely investigated to measure CPTSD [44]. The ITQ has shown validity and reliability across several populations (i.e., general population, veterans, psychiatric outpatients, refugees and children in foster care) in different counties [44]. The ITQ also has the ability to distinguish between PTSD and CPTSD. The ITQ is a self-report measure, consisting of 18 items, which have been developed to be consistent with the organizing principles of the ICD-11 [45]. The ITQ also has a separate version for children and adolescents (ITQ-CA), to be used in children and adolescents between 7 and 17 years. The ITQ is freely available and has been translated into several languages. However, as all self-report measures, the ITQ is affected by response bias [44].

The International Trauma Interview (ITI), Symptoms of Trauma Scale (SOTS) or Complex PTSD Item Set additional to the Clinician-Administered PTSD Scale (COPISAC) have been recommended for the assessment of PTSD and CPTSD in adults, where self-report measures are deemed unsuitable [44]. The ITI is a semi-structured interview consisting of two parts, which assess PTSD symptoms and symptoms of disturbances in self-organization (DSO), respectively. The ITI has been investigated in two studies, and is thought to have promising results in its validity in diagnosing CPTSD [44]. However, it is recommended that further studies in other populations including children and adolescents are needed in order to establish its validity [41]. SOTS is a 12 item semi-structured interview, which is a screening tool which can also be used to measure improvement. Two studies have assessed its validity in screening for PTSD [46]. There is only preliminary evidence for its reliability and validity and further replication studies are recommended prior to it being used in clinical settings [44]. COPISAC was devised by adding an additional set of items to the already existing instrument, the Clinician-Administered PTSD Scale (CAPS) [47]. While the ITQ and ITI align with ICD-11, COPISAC was designed to align with both DSM-5 and ICD-11. However, at present, there is only limited evidence for the use of this instrument in screening for CPTSD and further validation studies are required [41]. To date, there are no instruments to assess the presence of CPTSD in children and adolescents.

6.2 Prolonged grief disorder

A meta-analysis of the instruments used to assess PGD provided evidence for 11 instruments to demonstrate good reliability and validity in measuring symptom severity, or for screening or diagnosis of PGD in adults.

This review recommends the 5-item Brief Grief Questionnaire (BGQ) as the shortest reliable tool for screening for PGD. Other screening tools demonstrated to have good psychometric properties were the Inventory of Complicated Grief (ICG), Indicator of Bereavement Adaption-Cruse Scotland (IBACS) and Traumatic Grief Inventory Self-Report Version (TGI-SR) [48, 49]. In addition to screening for PGD, the ICG and TGI-SR can also be used to assess symptom severity [50]. The Persistent Complex Bereavement Inventory (PCBI) and Indicator of Bereavement Adaption-Cruse Scotland (IBACS) (part II) have been reported as other reliable self-report tools to assess the symptom severity of PGD [50]. The ICG, TGI-SR, PCBI and IBACS are all short, with less than 20 items, which makes it user-friendly and easy to administer. The Two-Track Bereavement Questionnaire for Complicated Grief (TTBQ-CG31) and Inventory of Complicated Grief (ICG-R) have also been identified as a reliable tool to measure symptoms severity, but takes a longer time to administer, given that they consist of 30 or more items. There are no instruments at present which cover all ICD-11 criteria for PGD [50]. However, the TGI-SR can be used to diagnose PGD in accordance with the DSM criteria. All the evidence about screening tools for PGD is from studies carried out on adult populations, and to date, there are no studies on screening instruments that can be used to detect PGD in children and adolescents.

7. Prognosis

7.1 PTSD versus complex PTSD

Literature on the prognosis of children and adolescents with a diagnosis of PTSD is sparce. Evidence from adult populations shows that compared to PTSD, those with CPTSD are more likely to have long-term functional impairment and higher symptom burden. Those with CPTSD are reported to have higher levels of work-related impairment, and the working capacity of those with CPTSD changed little with treatment [51]. Patents with CPTSD were twice as likely to have received suspended working capacity than those with PTSD.

There is abundant evidence which shows PTSD to be associated with poorer physical health (i.e., greater musculoskeletal pain, cardio-respiratory problems, gastrointestinal problems), more physical health complaints and poorer health-related quality of life [52]. The use of medical services is also known to be higher in those with PTSD compared to those without. Overall, there is evidence that PTSD is a risk factor for higher rates of all-cause mortality and behavioral-cause mortality [53].

7.2 Prolonged grief disorder

There is ample evidence on the long-term effects of bereavement. Bereavement is shown to be associated with an increased use of health care services, increased health care costs, sudden death and death from all causes [54]. However, the research examining the long-term impact of prolonged grief disorder, especially in children and adolescents, is limited. Available evidence suggests that prolonged grief disorder is associated with poorer quality of life in bereaved individuals [55].

8. Treatment

8.1 PTSD and CPTSD

8.1.1 Psychological interventions

8.1.1.1 Trauma-focused CBT

Trauma-focused CBT (TF-CBT) has the most evidence for effectiveness in children with trauma-related symptoms. More than 25 randomized controlled trials demonstrate TF-CBT to be superior to wait-list, treatment as usual and active treatment [56]. Some trials have found the improvements to be more pronounced when the therapy was carried out in group settings and when the treatment was completed. Several studies have also found TF-CBT to have medium-to-high effect sizes on emotion dysregulation, interpersonal problems, and negative self-concept [57]. However, the improvements in emotional dysregulation were shown to be more rapid in those with acute trauma compared to chronic trauma [58]. There is also evidence that TF-CBT improves dissociation and internalizing and externalizing symptoms in children [59]. TF-CBT has also been shown to improve prosocial behaviors [49]. Therefore, TF-CBT is recommended as the first-line treatment for trauma-related symptoms in international guidelines. However, some studies have found that 16–40% of children continue to meet the diagnostic criteria of PTSD, even after completing TF-CBT [60].

There is some evidence that TF-CBT is effective in the treatment of CPTSD as well as PTSD. The evidence comparing its efficacy for PTSD and CPTSD is controversial, with some studies showing no difference in the response rate for PTSD and CPTSD, while some have found the response rate to be higher for CPTSD [57, 61]. The available evidence suggests that the recommended duration of therapy is not sufficient to treat those with CPTSD and that a longer duration of treatment is needed [62]. It is thought that the difficulty in engaging clients with CPTSD and the longer time needed to build a good therapeutic relationship may contribute to the need for a longer duration of therapy. Therefore, these studies have highlighted the need to develop guidelines specifically for CPTSD.

So far, no socio-demographic factors have been identified as determinants of treatment outcomes in TF-CBT [62], but comorbid depression was found to predict poor treatment response [63, 64]. Although adverse effects to TF-CBT is not common, there are reports of a minority of patients experiencing worsening of PTSD symptoms, depression or functional impairment [62].

8.1.1.2 Exposure therapy

Exposure therapy (ET) may take the form of prolonged exposure (PE) or narrative exposure therapy (NET). A modified version of NET is available for children, referred to as kid narrative exposure therapy (KIDNET). A recent meta-analysis showed ET to be effective in trauma-related symptoms and depressive symptoms in children and adolescents, especially those 14 years or older [65]. ET was shown to be more effective for children and adolescents with exposure to a single trauma, compared to those with multiple traumas. With regard to the type of ET, PE was shown to be superior to NET and KIDNET. However, ET did not perform well in terms of acceptability, and the quality of life at the end of treatment was not reported to be significantly improved [65].

8.1.1.3 Eye Movement Desensitization and Reprocessing therapy (EMDR)

Several meta-analyses have shown the effectiveness of EMDR in reducing trauma-related symptoms in children and adolescents. EMDR is shown to be effective in not only improving trauma symptoms but also anxiety symptoms, depressive symptoms and behavioral problems [66]. One meta-analysis has shown EMDR to be more effective than CBT, but this finding has not been replicated [67]. EMDR has been shown to be effective in both single and multiple traumas and in various types of traumas including child abuse and disasters.

8.1.1.4 Phase-based treatment

The Expert Consensus Treatment Guidelines for CPTSD in Adults [68] have recommended a phase-based approach to the treatment of CPSTD. This includes an initial phase of skills training in affect regulation, followed by a second phase of exposure-based treatment. There is evidence that this phase-based approach to treatment is superior to treatments that do not involve either one of these phases of treatment [63]. However, given the scarcity of data on the child and adolescent populations, further evidence is needed to assess the effectiveness of phase-based treatment in this population.

8.1.2 Pharmacological interventions

There is limited evidence for pharmacotherapy for PTSD and CPTSD in children and adolescents. Studies have compared the effectiveness of TF-CBT plus sertraline to TF-CBT plus placebo; and the effectiveness of sertraline to placebo for PTSD have found no significant difference in the outcome between these groups [69, 70]. There is some evidence from open-labeled uncontrolled case series and case reports of the effectiveness of atypical antipsychotics (risperidone, quetiapine), mood stabilizers (carbamazepine) and anti-adrenergic agents (guanfacine, clonidine, propranolol) [71]. Effectiveness of D-cycloserine in enhancing exposure therapy has also been assessed but reported to have no difference from placebo [72]. More recent studies have examined the effectiveness of prazosin and found that prazosin was helpful in improving sleep, intrusive thoughts, negative cognitions, mood and hyperarousal [73].

8.1.3 Treatment guidelines

A review of 14 guidelines for the management of PTSD found that around one-third of the guidelines recommend psychological therapy over pharmacological therapy, as the first line in the management of PTSD [74]. CBT was recommended as the first-line psychological treatment in all guidelines, and SSRIs were recommended as the first-line pharmacotherapy. Most guidelines have failed to include targeted treatment for the nightmares associated with PTSD, and Prazosin has been discussed in some [74]. However, clinicians are advised to keep in mind that guidelines are not appropriate for all patients, and clinical judgment should be prioritized when tailoring treatment to individual patients.

8.2 Prolonged grief disorder

The evidence base for effective psychological interventions for PGD is limited and is mostly based on adult populations. In children and adolescents, a group therapy programme called the Family Bereavement Programme (FBP), which addresses parenting skills and the child's coping skills, is shown to be effective in reducing immediate as well as long-term outcomes in children bereaved through parental loss [75]. There is also evidence of a group therapy programme in reducing grief, depression and anxiety symptoms in children and adolescents bereaved as a consequence of war [76]. However, both of these studies do not examine the effectiveness of these interventions in the treatment of PGD diagnosed in accordance with the ICD-11 criteria.

Two recent studies have assessed the effectiveness of a new CBT termed "Grief-Help". Grief-Help consists of nine sessions of manualized individual CBT treatment, which is combined with five sessions of parental counseling. An open trial with ten participants has shown this treatment to be effective in reducing self-rated symptoms of PDG, depression and PTSD [77]. The efficacy of this intervention is also supported by a randomized controlled trial (RCT), which compared "grief-help" with supportive counseling. This study found "Grief-help" to be superior to supportive psychotherapy in reducing PGD symptoms, depression and internalizing problems [78]. Given the limited evidence, more research needs to focus on designing interventions for PGD in children and adolescents.

9. Conclusions

The concept of disorders associated with stress has been evolving over the years. However, the evidence on this topic in children and adolescents is limited, and most evidence comes from adult populations. Further studies should be carried out in the child and adolescent population, especially with regard to effective treatment.

Author details

Yasodha Rohanachandra[1,2]

1 Child and Youth Mental Health Services, Latrobe Regional Health, Australia

2 Faculty of Medicine Nursing and Health Sciences, School of Rural Health, Monash University, Australia

*Address all correspondence to: yasodha_mk@yahoo.com; Yasodha.Rohanachandra@lrh.com.au

References

[1] American Psychiatric Association. Diagnostic and Statistical Manual of Mental Disorders: DSM-5. Washington, DC: American Psychiatric Association; 2013

[2] World Health Organization. International Classification of Diseases, Tenth Revision (ICD-10) Classifications of Mental and Behavioural Disorder: Clinical Descriptions and Diagnostic Guidelines. Geneva: World Health Organization; 1992

[3] World Health Organization. International Classification of Diseases, Eleventh Revision (ICD-11), Classifications of Mental and Behavioural Disorder: Clinical Descriptions and Diagnostic Guidelines. Geneva: World Health Organization; 2018

[4] American Psychiatric Association. Diagnostic and Statistical Manual of Mental Disorders. Washington, DC: American Psychiatric Association; 1985

[5] Va.gov: Veterans Affairs [Internet]. 2013. Available from: https://www.ptsd.va.gov/professional/treat/specific/ptsd_child_under6.asp

[6] Herman JL. Complex PTSD: A syndrome in survivors of prolonged and repeated trauma. Journal of Traumatic Stress. 1992;**5**(3):377-391. DOI: 10.1002/jts.2490050305

[7] American Psychiatric Association. Diagnostic and Statistical Manual of Mental Disorders: DSM-IV. Washington, DC: American Psychiatric Association; 1994

[8] Diagnostic and Statistical Manual of Mental Disorders: DSM-5-TR. Washington, DC: American Psychiatric Association Publishing; 2022

[9] Alvis L, Zhang N, Sandler IN, Kaplow JB. Developmental manifestations of grief in children and adolescents: Caregivers as key grief facilitators. Journal of Child & Adolescent Trauma. 2023;**16**(2):447-457

[10] Eisma MC. Prolonged grief disorder in ICD-11 and DSM-5-TR: Challenges and controversies. The Australian and New Zealand Journal of Psychiatry. 2023;**57**(7):944-951

[11] Daniunaite I, Cloitre M, Karatzias T, Shevlin M, Thoresen S, Zelviene P, et al. PTSD and Complex PTSD in adolescence: Discriminating factors in a population-based cross-sectional study. European Journal of Psychotraumatology. 2021;**12**(1). DOI: 10.1080/20008198.2021.1890937:1890937

[12] Redican E, Hyland P, Cloitre M, McBride O, Karatzias T, Murphy J, et al. Prevalence and predictors of ICD-11 posttraumatic stress disorder and complex PTSD in young people. Acta Psychiatrica Scandinavica. 2022;**146**(2):110-125

[13] Kazlauskas E, Jovarauskaite L, Abe K, Brewin CR, Cloitre M, Daniunaite I, et al. Trauma exposure and factors associated with ICD-11 PTSD and complex PTSD in adolescence: A cross-cultural study in Japan and Lithuania. Epidemiology and Psychiatric Sciences. 2022;**31**:e49

[14] Haselgruber A, Sölva K, Lueger-Schuster B. Symptom structure of ICD-11 complex posttraumatic stress disorder (CPTSD) in trauma-exposed foster children: Examining the International Trauma Questionnaire – Child and adolescent version (ITQ-CA). European Journal of Psychotraumatology. 2020;**11**(1). DOI: 10.1080/20008198.2020.1818974

[15] Kazlauskas E, Zelviene P, Daniunaite I, Hyland P, Kvedaraite M, Shevlin M, et al. The structure of ICD-11 PTSD and complex PTSD in adolescents exposed to potentially traumatic experiences. Journal of Affective Disorders. 2020;**265**:169-174. DOI: 10.1016/j.jad.2020.01.061

[16] Hyland P, Murphy J, Shevlin M, Vallières F, McElroy E, Elklit A, et al. Variation in post-traumatic response: The role of trauma type in predicting ICD-11 PTSD and CPTSD symptoms. Social Psychiatry and Psychiatric Epidemiology. 2017;**52**(6):727-736. DOI: 10.1007/s00127-017-1350-8

[17] Perkonigg A, Höfler M, Cloitre M, Wittchen HU, Trautmann S, Maercker A. Evidence for two different ICD-11 posttraumatic stress disorders in a community sample of adolescents and young adults. European Archives of Psychiatry and Clinical Neuroscience. 2016;**266**:317-328

[18] Djelantik AM, Smid GE, Mroz A, Kleber RJ, Boelen PA. The prevalence of prolonged grief disorder in bereaved individuals following unnatural losses: Systematic review and meta regression analysis. Journal of Affective Disorders. 2020;**265**:146-156

[19] Lundorff M, Holmgren H, Zachariae R, Farver-Vestergaard I, O'Connor M. Prevalence of prolonged grief disorder in adult bereavement: A systematic review and meta-analysis. Journal of Affective Disorders. 2017;**212**:138-149

[20] Harrison L, Harrington R. Adolescents' bereavement experiences. Prevalence, association with depressive symptoms, and use of services. Journal of Adolescence. 2001;**24**(2):159-169

[21] Eisma MC, Stroebe MS, Schut HA, Stroebe W, Boelen PA, van den Bout J. Avoidance processes mediate the relationship between rumination and symptoms of complicated grief and depression following loss. Journal of Abnormal Psychology. 2013;**122**(4):961

[22] Simon NM, Pollack MH, Fischmann D, Perlman CA, Muriel AC, Moore CW, et al. Complicated grief and its correlates in patients with bipolar disorder. Journal of Clinical Psychiatry. 2005;**66**(9):1105-1110

[23] Sung SC, Dryman MT, Marks E, Shear MK, Ghesquiere A, Fava M, et al. Complicated grief among individuals with major depression: Prevalence, comorbidity, and associated features. Journal of Affective Disorders. 2011;**134**(1-3):453-458

[24] Kersting A, Brähler E, Glaesmer H, Wagner B. Prevalence of complicated grief in a representative population-based sample. Journal of Affective Disorders. 2011;**131**(1-3):339-343

[25] Szuhany KL, Malgaroli M, Miron CD, Simon NM. Prolonged grief disorder: Course, diagnosis, assessment, and treatment. Focus. 2021;**19**(2):161-172

[26] Vanderwerker LC, Jacobs SC, Parkes CM, Prigerson HG. An exploration of associations between separation anxiety in childhood and complicated grief in later life. The Journal of Nervous and Mental Disease. 2006;**194**(2):121-123

[27] Kaplow JB, Howell KH, Layne CM. Do circumstances of the death matter? Identifying socioenvironmental risks for grief-related psychopathology in bereaved youth. Journal of Traumatic Stress. 2014;**27**(1):42-49

[28] Melhem NM, Day N, Shear MK, Day R, Reynolds CF, Brent D. Predictors of complicated grief among adolescents exposed to a peer's suicide. Journal of Loss and Trauma. 2004;**9**(1):21-34

[29] Revet A, Suc A, Auriol F, Djelantik AM, Raynaud JP, Bui E. Peritraumatic distress predicts prolonged grief disorder symptom severity after the death of a parent in children and adolescents. European Journal of Psychotraumatology. 2021;**12**(1): 1936916

[30] Cloitre M, Garvert DW, Weiss B, Carlson EB, Bryant RA. Distinguishing PTSD, complex PTSD, and borderline personality disorder: A latent class analysis. European Journal of Psychotraumatology. 2014;**5**(1):25097

[31] Hyland P, Shevlin M, Fyvie C, Karatzias T. Posttraumatic stress disorder and complex posttraumatic stress disorder in DSM-5 and ICD-11: Clinical and behavioral correlates. Journal of Traumatic Stress. 2018;**31**(2):174-180

[32] Malgaroli M, Maccallum F, Bonanno GA. Symptoms of persistent complex bereavement disorder, depression, and PTSD in a conjugally bereaved sample: A network analysis. Psychological Medicine. 2018;**48**(14):2439-2448

[33] Lancel M, Stroebe M, Eisma MC. Sleep disturbances in bereavement: A systematic review. Sleep Medicine Reviews. 2020;**53**:101331

[34] Maercker A, Cloitre M, Bachem R, Schlumpf YR, Khoury B, Hitchcock C, et al. Complex post-traumatic stress disorder. The Lancet. 2022;**400**(10345):60-72

[35] Karatzias T, Hyland P, Bradley A, Cloitre M, Roberts NP, Bisson JI, et al. Risk factors and comorbidity of ICD-11 PTSD and complex PTSD: Findings from a trauma-exposed population based sample of adults in the United Kingdom. Depression and Anxiety. 2019;**36**(9):887-894

[36] Lipschitz DS, Winegar RK, Hartnick E, Foote B, Southwick SM. Posttraumatic stress disorder in hospitalized adolescents: Psychiatric comorbidity and clinical correlates. Journal of the American Academy of Child & Adolescent Psychiatry. 1999;**38**(4):385-392

[37] Shin YJ, Kim SM, Hong JS, Han DH. Correlations between cognitive functions and clinical symptoms in adolescents with complex post-traumatic stress disorder. Frontiers in Public Health. 2021;**9**:586389

[38] Simon NM, Shear KM, Thompson EH, Zalta AK, Perlman C, Reynolds CF, et al. The prevalence and correlates of psychiatric comorbidity in individuals with complicated grief. Comprehensive Psychiatry. 2007;**48**(5):395-399

[39] Cole MG, Dendukuri N. Risk factors for depression among elderly community subjects: A systematic review and meta-analysis. American Journal of Psychiatry. 2003;**160**(6):1147-1156

[40] Xue C, Ge Y, Tang B, Liu Y, Kang P, Wang M, et al. A meta-analysis of risk factors for combat-related PTSD among military personnel and veterans. PLoS One. 2015;**10**(3):e0120270

[41] Perrin S, Meiser-Stedman R, Smith P. The Children's revised impact of event scale (CRIES): Validity as a screening instrument for PTSD. Behavioural and Cognitive Psychotherapy. 2005;**33**(4):487-498

[42] Foa EB, Johnson KM, Feeny NC, Treadwell KR. The child PTSD symptom scale: A preliminary examination of its psychometric properties. Journal of Clinical Child Psychology. 2001;**30**(3):376-384

[43] Li Y, Zhou Y, Chen X, Fan F, Musa G, Hoven C. Post-traumatic stress disorder in children and adolescents: Some

recent research findings. Psychosomatic Medicine. 2020;**13**

[44] Seiler N, Davoodi K, Keem M, Das S. Assessment tools for complex post-traumatic stress disorder: A systematic review. International Journal of Psychiatry in Clinical Practice. 2023;**13**:1-9

[45] Cloitre M, Shevlin M, Brewin CR, Bisson JI, Roberts NP, Maercker A, et al. The international trauma questionnaire: Development of a self-report measure of ICD-11 PTSD and complex PTSD. Acta Psychiatrica Scandinavica. 2018;**138**(6):536-546

[46] Ford JD, Mendelsohn M, Opler LA, Opler MG, Kallivayalil D, Levitan J, et al. The symptoms of trauma scale (SOTS): An initial psychometric study. Journal of Psychiatric Practice. 2015;**21**(6):474

[47] Lechner-Meichsner F, Steil R. A clinician rating to diagnose CPTSD according to ICD-11 and to evaluate CPTSD symptom severity: Complex PTSD item set additional to the CAPS (COPISAC). European Journal of Psychotraumatology. 2021;**12**(1):1891726

[48] Shear KM, Jackson CT, Essock SM, Donahue SA, Felton CJ. Screening for complicated grief among project liberty service recipients 18 months after September 11, 2001. Psychiatric Services. 2006;**57**(9):1291-1297

[49] O'Callaghan P, McMullen J, Shannon C, Rafferty H, Black A. A randomized controlled trial of trauma-focused cognitive behavioral therapy for sexually exploited, war-affected Congolese girls. Journal of the American Academy of Child & Adolescent Psychiatry. 2013;**52**(4):359-369

[50] Treml J, Kaiser J, Plexnies A, Kersting A. Assessing prolonged grief disorder: A systematic review of assessment instruments. Journal of Affective Disorders. 2020;**274**:420-434

[51] Brenner L, Köllner V, Bachem R. Symptom burden and work-related impairment among patients with PTSD and complex PTSD. European Journal of Psychotraumatology. 2019;**10**(1):1694766

[52] Pacella ML, Hruska B, Delahanty DL. The physical health consequences of PTSD and PTSD symptoms: A meta-analytic review. Journal of Anxiety Disorders. 2013;**27**(1):33-46

[53] Flood AM, Boyle SH, Calhoun PS, Dennis MF, Barefoot JC, Moore SD, et al. Prospective study of externalizing and internalizing subtypes of posttraumatic stress disorder and their relationship to mortality among Vietnam veterans. Comprehensive Psychiatry. 2010;**51**(3):236-242

[54] Hendrickson KC. Morbidity, mortality, and parental grief: A review of the literature on the relationship between the death of a child and the subsequent health of parents. Palliative & Supportive Care. 2009;**7**(1):109-119

[55] Maccallum F, Bryant RA. A network approach to understanding quality of life impairments in prolonged grief disorder. Journal of Traumatic Stress. 2020;**33**(1):106-115

[56] Thielemann JF, Kasparik B, König J, Unterhitzenberger J, Rosner R. A systematic review and meta-analysis of trauma-focused cognitive behavioral therapy for children and adolescents. Child Abuse & Neglect. 2022;**134**:105899

[57] Sachser C, Keller F, Goldbeck L. Complex PTSD as proposed for ICD-11: Validation of a new disorder in children and adolescents and their response to trauma-focused cognitive behavioral therapy. Journal of Child Psychology and Psychiatry. 2017;**58**(2):160-168

[58] Sharma-Patel K, Brown EJ. Emotion regulation and self blame as mediators and moderators of trauma-specific treatment. Psychology of Violence. 2016;**6**(3):400

[59] Hébert M, Amédée LM. Latent class analysis of post-traumatic stress symptoms and complex PTSD in child victims of sexual abuse and their response to trauma-focused cognitive Behavioural therapy. European Journal of Psychotraumatology. 2020;**11**(1):1807171

[60] Stallard P. Psychological interventions for post-traumatic reactions in children and young people: A review of randomised controlled trials. Clinical Psychology Review. 2006;**26**(7):895-911

[61] Ross SL, Sharma-Patel K, Brown EJ, Huntt JS, Chaplin WF. Complex trauma and trauma-focused cognitive-behavioral therapy: How do trauma chronicity and PTSD presentation affect treatment outcome? Child Abuse & Neglect. 2021;**111**:104734

[62] Melegkovits E, Blumberg J, Dixon E, Ehntholt K, Gillard J, Kayal H, et al. The effectiveness of trauma-focused psychotherapy for complex post-traumatic stress disorder: A retrospective study. European Psychiatry. 2023;**66**(1):e4

[63] Cloitre M, Garvert DW, Weiss BJ. Depression as a moderator of STAIR narrative therapy for women with post-traumatic stress disorder related to childhood abuse. European Journal of Psychotraumatology. 2017;**8**(1):1377028

[64] Ehlers A, Grey N, Wild J, Stott R, Liness S, Deale A, et al. Implementation of cognitive therapy for PTSD in routine clinical care: Effectiveness and moderators of outcome in a consecutive sample. Behaviour Research and Therapy. 2013;**51**(11):742-752

[65] Huang T, Li H, Tan S, Xie S, Cheng Q, Xiang Y, et al. The efficacy and acceptability of exposure therapy for the treatment of post-traumatic stress disorder in children and adolescents: A systematic review and meta-analysis. BMC Psychiatry. 2022;**22**(1):1-2

[66] Moreno-Alcazar A, Treen D, Valiente-Gomez A, Sio-Eroles A, Perez V, Amann BL, et al. Efficacy of eye movement desensitization and reprocessing in children and adolescent with post-traumatic stress disorder: A meta-analysis of randomized controlled trials. Frontiers in Psychology. 2017;**8**:1750

[67] Rodenburg R, Benjamin A, de Roos C, Meijer AM, Stams GJ. Efficacy of EMDR in children: A meta-analysis. Clinical Psychology Review. 2009;**29**(7):599-606

[68] Cloitre M, Courtois CA, Charuvastra A, Carapezza R, Stolbach BC, Green BL. Treatment of complex PTSD: Results of the ISTSS expert clinician survey on best practices. Journal of Traumatic Stress. 2011;**24**(6):615-627. DOI: 10.1002/jts.20697

[69] Cohen JA, Mannarino AP, Perel JM, Staron V. A pilot randomized controlled trial of combined trauma-focused CBT and sertraline for childhood PTSD symptoms. Journal of the American Academy of Child & Adolescent Psychiatry. 2007;**46**(7):811-819

[70] Robb AS, Cueva JE, Sporn J, Yang R, Vanderburg DG. Sertraline treatment of children and adolescents with posttraumatic stress disorder: A double-blind, placebo-controlled trial. Journal of Child and Adolescent Psychopharmacology. 2010;**20**(6):463-471

[71] Smith P, Dalgleish T, Meiser-Stedman R. Practitioner review: Posttraumatic stress disorder and its treatment in children and adolescents. Journal of Child Psychology and Psychiatry. 2019;**60**(5):500-515

[72] Schnurr PP, Friedman MJ, Engel CC, Foa EB, Shea MT, Chow BK, et al. Cognitive behavioral therapy for posttraumatic stress disorder in women: A randomized controlled trial. Journal of the American Medical Association. 2007;**297**(8):820-830

[73] Keeshin BR, Ding Q, Presson AP, Berkowitz SJ, Strawn JR. Use of prazosin for pediatric PTSD-associated nightmares and sleep disturbances: A retrospective chart review. Neurology and Therapy. 2017;**6**:247-257

[74] Martin A, Naunton M, Kosari S, Peterson G, Thomas J, Christenson JK. Treatment guidelines for PTSD: A systematic review. Journal of Clinical Medicine. 2021;**10**(18):4175

[75] Sandler IN, Ayers TS, Wolchik SA, Tein JY, Kwok OM, Haine RA, et al. The family bereavement program: Efficacy evaluation of a theory-based prevention program for parentally bereaved children and adolescents. Journal of Consulting and Clinical Psychology. 2003;**71**(3):587

[76] Layne CM, Saltzman WR, Poppleton L, Burlingame GM, Pašalić A, Duraković E, et al. Effectiveness of a school-based group psychotherapy program for war-exposed adolescents: A randomized controlled trial. Journal of the American Academy of Child & Adolescent Psychiatry. 2008;**47**(9):1048-1062

[77] Spuij M, Dekovic M, Boelen PA. An open trial of 'grief-help': A cognitive–behavioural treatment for prolonged grief in children and adolescents. Clinical Psychology & Psychotherapy. 2015;**22**(2):185-192

[78] Boelen PA, Lenferink LI, Spuij M. CBT for prolonged grief in children and adolescents: A randomized clinical trial. American Journal of Psychiatry. 2021;**178**(4):294-304

Chapter 5

The Impact of Social Media on Adolescent Mental Health

Milton Anguyo, Joel Masete, Magdalen Akia and Henry Drasiku

Abstract

This chapter delves into the profound impact of social media on the mental well-being of twenty first-century adolescents. It intricately explores the extensive engagement of young individuals with various social media platforms and critically analyses its potential implications for their psychological health. The discussion encompasses a spectrum of dimensions, including the alarming prevalence of cyberbullying, the detrimental influence of distorted body image perceptions, the pervasive fear of missing out (FOMO), and the concerning addictive tendencies associated with social media usage. Furthermore, the chapter sheds light on the optimistic side of social media, elucidating its capacity to foster online support communities and spearhead campaigns promoting mental health awareness. Ultimately, this exploration culminates in a strategic roadmap designed to cultivate a balanced and constructive relationship with social media. The outlined strategies aim to empower adolescents with the tools necessary to harness the benefits of these platforms while proactively mitigating the potential adverse consequences discussed earlier. By adopting these strategies, individuals, caregivers, educators, and policymakers collectively strive to cultivate a digital environment that safeguards and enhances the mental well-being of our future generations.

Keywords: social media, adolescent mental health, cyberbullying, mental health awareness, online support

1. Introduction

Adolescence often referred to as the pivotal bridge between childhood and adulthood, stands as a remarkably transformative developmental phase. This period is characterized by multifaceted changes, encompassing the emergence of self-identity, the cultivation of intricate social interactions, and the profound expansion of emotional horizons. It serves as a dynamic canvas upon which individuals experiment with their self-concept, establish connections with peers, and embark on the journey of self-discovery.

In recent times, the emergence of social media platforms has indelibly altered the landscape within which adolescents navigate these critical transitions. Social media, with its expansive virtual realms, has ushered in unprecedented ways of communication and interaction, dramatically altering the dynamics of relationships and self-presentation. The digital age has witnessed an exponential surge in the use of platforms that enable instant sharing, engagement, and networking, providing adolescents with a potent toolkit to express themselves, connect with peers, and explore the intricacies of the world around them.

Within this context, this chapter embarks on an exploration of the intricate interplay between social media use and the mental well-being of adolescents. As these platforms become integral components of adolescents' lives, they wield the power to shape self-perceptions, amplify social connections, and leave an indelible imprint on emotional experiences. Our examination delves into both the positive and negative dimensions of this interconnection, aiming to present a comprehensive view that encapsulates the nuances of this relationship.

From the vantage point of understanding the multifaceted impacts, we delve into the ways in which social media's influence extends to various facets of adolescent mental health. We unravel how these platforms have the potential to engender positive effects like fostering mental health awareness and nurturing supportive virtual communities. Simultaneously, we confront the darker aspects, ranging from the pernicious repercussions of cyberbullying to the haunting specter of FOMO, all of which can cast long shadows over the fragile mental landscapes of adolescents.

Through an exploration of these dichotomies, we aspire to equip readers with a holistic understanding of the intricate interplay between social media and adolescent mental health. This inquiry calls us to re-evaluate our perspectives, prompting us to proactively harness the transformative potential of these digital realms while also devising strategies to safeguard the emotional and psychological well-being of the young minds that traverse them. In navigating this complex terrain, we aim to empower stakeholders—ranging from adolescents themselves to educators, parents, and policymakers—to embark on a collective journey toward nurturing a digital landscape that fosters resilience, empowerment, and holistic mental health.

2. The influence of social media on adolescent mental health

Social media platforms have become integral to the lives of adolescents, shaping their self-perception, interpersonal relationships, and psychological well-being.

2.1 Cyberbullying and its impact

The rise of cyberbullying in the digital age has emerged as a significant and distressing concern for the mental health of adolescents. This section delves into the various forms of cyberbullying, its prevalence, and the profound emotional toll it takes on young individuals.

Cyberbullying encompasses a range of aggressive behaviors that are conducted through electronic communication platforms such as social media, text messages, and online forums. These behaviors include hurtful comments, derogatory messages, sharing private information without consent, and even threats of harm. With the anonymity provided by the online world, aggressors are often emboldened to engage in harmful actions that they might not consider in face-to-face interactions. According to a study conducted by Hinduja and Patchin [1], approximately 34% of adolescents have reported being victims of cyberbullying [1]. Oliveira et al. [2] examined the correlation between screen time activities and bullying among Brazilian adolescents

DOI: http://dx.doi.org/10.5772/intechopen.1003060

and found out that higher social media use is associated with a greater likelihood of bullying victimization, particularly among males.

The emotional consequences of cyberbullying are profound and far-reaching. Victims of cyberbullying often experience heightened levels of stress, anxiety, and depression. They are subjected to a continuous barrage of hurtful messages and attacks, making it difficult for them to escape the torment even in the confines of their own homes. The emotional distress can spill over into their physical well-being, leading to disrupted sleep patterns, loss of appetite, and even psychosomatic symptoms. Importantly, bystanders who witness cyberbullying are also impacted emotionally, experiencing feelings of guilt, helplessness, and discomfort as they witness the suffering of their peers [1].

Addressing the menace of cyberbullying requires a multifaceted approach. Schools, parents, and policymakers must collaborate to implement stringent anti-bullying measures, educate adolescents about responsible online behavior, and create safe reporting mechanisms for victims. Additionally, fostering empathy and digital citizenship among adolescents can help cultivate a culture of respect and kindness in the digital sphere. By acknowledging and addressing the detrimental impact of cyberbullying on adolescent mental health, society can take a decisive step toward nurturing a supportive and safe digital environment.

2.2 Body image concerns and social media

The advent of social media platforms has ushered in an era of unprecedented visual exposure, which has in turn significantly influenced body image perceptions among adolescents. This subsection delves into the intricate connection between pervasive social media imagery and the alarming rise of body image dissatisfaction among young individuals.

Social media platforms are flooded with images that project idealized and often unrealistic body standards. Adolescents are bombarded with pictures of perfectly sculpted bodies, flawless skin, and curated appearances that propagate a narrow definition of beauty. This relentless exposure cultivates an environment where young individuals internalize these unrealistic standards, leading to heightened body dissatisfaction and a skewed self-perception. A study by Cao et al. [3] highlights the role of unrealistic beauty ideals portrayed on social media platforms and their negative impact on adolescents' self-perception and psychological well-being. Another study by Fardouly et al. [4] underscores this phenomenon, indicating that exposure to images of thin and idealized bodies on social media is associated with increased body dissatisfaction and an elevated likelihood of engaging in unhealthy weight control behaviors.

The impact of these skewed body image perceptions on mental health is substantial. Adolescents who internalize these unrealistic beauty ideals are at a higher risk of developing body dimorphic tendencies, low self-esteem, and symptoms of depression and anxiety. The constant comparison to the "perfect" bodies portrayed on social media fosters negative self-comparisons and fuels feelings of inadequacy. Moreover, the pressure to conform to these standards can lead to extreme behaviors such as crash dieting, excessive exercise, and even the development of eating disorders.

Counteracting the detrimental effects of social media on body image requires a concerted effort from various stakeholders. Promoting media literacy among adolescents can empower them to critically analyze and deconstruct the images they encounter. Encouraging body positivity and self-acceptance can help adolescents develop a healthier relationship with their bodies and reject unrealistic beauty ideals. Moreover, fostering open conversations about body image within families, schools, and communities can contribute to dismantling harmful stereotypes and promoting a culture of self-love and acceptance.

2.3 Fear of missing out (FOMO)

The pervasive nature of social media platforms has given rise to a unique phenomenon known as the Fear of Missing Out (FOMO), which contributes significantly to feelings of inadequacy and anxiety among adolescents. This section delves into the intricacies of FOMO, its implications for mental health, and strategies to mitigate its impact.

FOMO is driven by the incessant updates and posts on social media platforms that showcase peers' activities, experiences, and social interactions. Adolescents experience a gnawing fear of being excluded from the events and moments that others seem to be enjoying. The constant stream of images depicting social gatherings, outings, and adventures can make adolescents feel left out and disconnected. A study done in China investigated the relationship between cyber victimization, non-suicidal self-injury, depression, and school connectedness among Chinese adolescents. The Finding was that cyber victimization was positively associated with non-suicidal self-injury, mediated by depression, and this link is stronger for adolescents with low school connectedness. [5]. Another study by Przybylski et al. [6] highlights the correlation between FOMO and lower life satisfaction, as well as mood disturbances among adolescents [6].

The implications of FOMO on adolescent mental health are far-reaching. The fear of being excluded can evoke feelings of loneliness, inadequacy, and sadness. Adolescents may perceive their own lives as mundane in comparison to the seemingly exciting experiences showcased on social media. This perception can undermine their self-esteem and lead to a heightened sense of social isolation. Moreover, the constant comparison to the curated lives of peers can contribute to a distorted self-perception and a constant sense of dissatisfaction.

To mitigate the impact of FOMO, adolescents and those who support them can adopt strategies that foster healthy digital habits. Encouraging adolescents to set limits on their social media use, practice mindfulness, and engage in offline activities that bring joy can help reduce the grip of FOMO. Additionally, educators and parents can promote open discussions about the curated nature of social media and the importance of valuing real-life experiences over virtual ones. By cultivating self-awareness and resilience, adolescents can navigate the digital landscape with a healthier perspective, minimizing the detrimental effects of FOMO on their mental well-being.

2.4 Addiction and mental health

The rise of social media addiction has sparked concerns about its impact on adolescent mental health. This section explores the signs, causes, and consequences of excessive social media use on psychological well-being, shedding light on the potential risks and avenues for intervention.

The allure of social media lies in the instantaneous gratification it offers through notifications, likes, and comments. This constant feedback triggers dopamine responses in the brain, creating a reward loop that fosters addictive behaviors. Adolescents find themselves increasingly drawn to their devices, seeking validation and affirmation through the digital realm. A study by Kuss and Griffiths [7] suggests that addictive social media use is linked to higher levels of anxiety, depression, and feelings of loneliness among adolescents [7] meanwhile [8] carried a study on this similar topic and found out that evidence supports social contagion in gun violence, bullying, cyberbullying, violent offending, and suicide. They therefore argued that social learning, identification with significant others, and the normalization of specific norms play a role.

The consequences of social media addiction on mental health are concerning. Excessive social media use can lead to a neglect of real-world relationships, hinder academic performance, and exacerbate feelings of social isolation. The constant need for validation in the form of likes and comments can create a sense of emptiness and dissatisfaction when these expectations are not met. Moreover, the addictive cycle can disrupt sleep patterns, impact concentration, and contribute to heightened stress levels.

Addressing social media addiction requires a comprehensive approach that involves education, awareness, and moderation. Adolescents, along with their families and educators, can benefit from understanding the signs of addiction and the importance of setting healthy boundaries. Encouraging digital detoxes, where individuals disconnect from screens periodically, can help break the addictive cycle. Promoting face-to-face interactions, engaging in hobbies, and fostering a balanced lifestyle can redirect adolescents' focus away from the virtual world and toward nurturing their mental and emotional well-being.

2.5 Positive aspects: mental health awareness and online support

Contrary to its negative reputation, social media platforms can play a constructive role in addressing adolescent mental health challenges. This section highlights the positive potential of social media by examining the impact of online support communities and mental health awareness campaigns.

Online support communities provide a virtual refuge for adolescents grappling with mental health issues. These digital spaces offer a sense of belonging, where individuals can share their experiences, fears, and triumphs without fear of judgment. The study by Tu et al. [9] examined the positive aspects of social media in promoting mental health awareness and providing online support communities also Vannucci and Ohannessian [10] demonstrated that online peer support can significantly reduce symptoms of depression in adolescents, providing them with a valuable avenue for seeking advice and validation. Moreover, the anonymity offered by these communities can create a safe space for adolescents who may feel hesitant to open up in traditional face-to-face settings. Cao et al. [3] also explored the impact of childhood trauma on adolescent cyberbullying, mediated by emotional intelligence and online social anxiety. Concludes that childhood trauma is positively associated with cyberbullying, and emotional intelligence and online social anxiety play mediating roles.

Social media also serves as a powerful platform for mental health awareness campaigns. Advocacy groups, organizations, and individuals leverage the reach of social media to challenge stigma and spread knowledge about mental health. By sharing personal stories, testimonials, and informational content, social media fosters open conversations that normalize discussions about mental health. Adolescents can access resources, information about available support, and learn coping strategies from experts and peers alike. This proactive approach can contribute to early intervention and destigmatization of mental health challenges.

To harness the positive potential of social media for mental health, adolescents and those who support them must actively engage in fostering a supportive digital community. Educators can incorporate digital citizenship education into curricula, guiding students on ethical and responsible online behavior. Parents can stay informed about the platforms their children use and promote open conversations about online experiences. Mental health professionals can leverage social media to share evidence-based strategies for coping and seeking help. By recognizing social media's potential as a force for good, society can create a virtual ecosystem that nurtures adolescent mental health and encourages mutual support.

In conclusion, social media's influence on adolescent mental health is a complex and multifaceted issue. From the detrimental impact of cyberbullying and body image concerns to the challenges posed by FOMO and addiction, adolescents face a range of pressures and risks in the digital realm. However, the positive potential of social media should not be underestimated. Online support communities and mental health awareness campaigns showcase the platform's capacity to foster understanding, empathy, and empowerment. By cultivating responsible online behaviors, promoting media literacy, and embracing the power of digital connectivity for positive change, society can pave the way for a healthier digital landscape that supports the mental well-being of adolescents in the 21st century.

3. Strategies for healthy social media use

To navigate the intricate landscape of social media, adolescents need guidance and strategies for healthy usage.

3.1 Digital literacy and media literacy education

Empowering adolescents with digital literacy skills is crucial in enabling them to navigate the complex landscape of social media responsibly. Digital literacy equips adolescents with the ability to critically evaluate online content, discern credible information from misinformation, and understand the implications of their online actions. Media literacy education provides them with the tools to recognize biased narratives, identify fake news, and engage with social media content in a discerning manner.

Incorporating digital and media literacy education into school curricula can equip adolescents with the skills they need to engage critically with the content they encounter. This education helps them understand the motives behind viral trends, recognize the potential for manipulation, and make informed decisions about what to engage with and share. Research by Livingstone and Sefton-Green [11] emphasizes the importance of media literacy education in promoting responsible and ethical online behavior among adolescents [11].

3.2 Setting healthy boundaries

Encouraging adolescents to establish healthy boundaries with social media is essential to prevent excessive usage and its associated negative effects. Adolescents can benefit from setting time limits for their social media interactions, designating device-free zones and times (such as during meals or before bedtime), and scheduling regular digital detoxes. By setting these boundaries, adolescents can strike a healthier balance between their online and offline lives. Cao et al. [3] in their study carried out from four schools in Shandong province, China emphasized the need to establish healthy boundaries for screen time and suggested strategies such as limiting device use and digital detoxes [3].

Research by Primack et al. [12] suggests that setting limits on social media use is associated with improved psychological well-being and reduced symptoms of depression and anxiety among adolescents. Educators and parents can play a pivotal role in modeling and encouraging these healthy digital habits, helping adolescents develop healthier relationships with their devices and social media platforms.

3.3 Promoting positive online communities

Creating and nurturing positive online communities focused on mental health discussions can provide adolescents with a supportive and safe space to share their experiences and seek advice. Educators, parents, and policymakers can collaborate to establish and oversee these communities, ensuring that they are moderated and free from harmful content.

Online platforms that promote mental health awareness and provide evidence-based resources can play a crucial role in supporting adolescents' well-being. These platforms can provide accurate information, coping strategies, and resources for seeking help. Research by Moreno et al. [13] suggests that online interventions can effectively promote mental health literacy and awareness among adolescents, a similar idea was also echoed by Tu et al. [9].

By fostering a culture of empathy, mutual support, and open dialog within these communities, adolescents can find comfort in knowing that they are not alone in their struggles. Furthermore, these communities can contribute to reducing the stigma associated with mental health challenges and promoting a culture of acceptance and understanding.

4. Conclusions

This chapter has delved into the intricate relationship between social media and adolescent mental health, revealing both positive and negative impacts. While social media offers unprecedented connectivity, it also poses risks like cyberbullying, body image concerns, FOMO, and addiction. Yet, it is important to note that social media is not solely detrimental; it can foster online support communities and mental health awareness.

To navigate this landscape, digital literacy is crucial for discerning reliable information from misinformation. Encouraging healthy boundaries, both in screen time and emotional investment, promotes balance. Positive online communities can provide safe spaces for mental health discussions.

In essence, social media's influence on adolescents is multifaceted. By understanding its dynamics and utilizing strategies for responsible use, we can promote both healthy digital engagement and mental well-being. Through collective efforts, adolescents can thrive in the digital age with resilience and positive mental health outcomes.

Acknowledgements

We extend our heartfelt gratitude to all those who contributed to the development of this chapter on the impact of social media on adolescent mental health. Our appreciation goes to our families, including our wives and children, for their unwavering support and understanding throughout this endeavor. Your patience and encouragement have been invaluable.

We would also like to express our sincere thanks to the faculty and staff of Gulu University and Kampala International University for providing us with a conducive environment for research and learning.

Our heartfelt thanks go to the reviewers who provided insightful feedback and suggestions, which greatly enhanced the quality of this chapter

Conflict of interest

The authors declare no conflict of interest.

Notes/thanks/other declarations

We want to express our deep gratitude to the individuals who shared their stories and experiences related to social media and adolescent mental health. Your willingness to open up and discuss these important topics contributed immensely to the authenticity and relevance of this chapter.

Additionally, we extend our appreciation to our colleagues and friends who engaged in thoughtful discussions and provided valuable insights that enriched our perspective on this subject.

Lastly, our sincere thanks to the editorial team and publisher for their guidance and support throughout the publication process. Your dedication to the dissemination of knowledge is greatly appreciated.

This chapter would not have been possible without the collective effort of all those mentioned above. Thank you for being an integral part of this journey.

Appendix A: resources for healthy social media use

This appendix provides a curated list of online resources, websites, and tools that offer guidance and support for adolescents and their caregivers on navigating social media in a healthy and responsible manner. The resources cover a range of topics, including digital literacy, mental health awareness, and strategies for setting healthy boundaries with social media.

1. *Digital Literacy Resources*

   - [Digital Literacy Institute] (https://www.digitalliteracyinstitute.org/): Offers free online courses and tutorials on developing digital literacy skills, including evaluating online information and media critically.

   - [FactCheck.org] (https://www.factcheck.org/): A non-profit organization that provides resources for fact-checking and verifying online information.

2. *Mental Health Awareness Platforms*

- [NAMI: National Alliance on Mental Illness] (https://www.nami.org/): A leading organization dedicated to raising awareness about mental health, providing resources for adolescents and caregivers.

- [Psych Central Forums] (https://forums.psychcentral.com/): An online community where individuals can discuss mental health challenges, seek advice, and share personal experiences.

3. *Guides for Setting Healthy Boundaries*

- [Screen Time Guidelines from the American Academy of Pediatrics] (https://www.healthychildren.org/English/media/Pages/default.aspx): Offers guidelines and recommendations for managing screen time for children and adolescents.

- [Center for Humane Technology] (https://www.humanetech.com/): Provides tools and resources for fostering healthier relationships with technology, including tips for digital detoxes.

Appendix B: case studies

This appendix presents in-depth case studies that delve into real-life scenarios illustrating the concepts discussed in the chapter. Each case study offers a nuanced exploration of the relationship between social media and adolescent mental health, providing readers with practical examples and insights to enhance their understanding.

Case study 1: Addressing cyberbullying

Background:

Emily, a 16-year-old high school student, found herself increasingly targeted by hurtful comments and malicious rumors on social media platforms. Struggling with the emotional toll of cyberbullying, Emily's self-esteem began to plummet, affecting her overall mental well-being.

Analysis:

This case study delves into the various forms of cyberbullying Emily experienced, such as derogatory comments, exclusion from online groups, and the spreading of false information. The emotional impact on Emily's mental health is examined, including feelings of anxiety, depression, and isolation. We explore how Emily's support network, including friends, family, and school counselors, played a vital role in providing emotional support and strategies for coping with the negative effects of cyberbullying.

Strategies:

The case study highlights the importance of open communication between adolescents and their support systems. We discuss how Emily's school implemented anti-bullying policies and educated students about responsible online behavior. Additionally, we explore the role of digital literacy in recognizing and addressing cyberbullying, as well as providing resources for seeking help and reporting online harassment.

This case study provides a real-life scenario of cyberbullying and offering strategies for support and coping, it was supported by a study done by [14].

Case study 2: Overcoming fear of missing out (FOMO)

Background:

Alex, a 17-year-old aspiring artist, frequently found himself comparing his life to the curated and seemingly perfect lives of his peers on social media. This led to feelings of inadequacy and anxiety as he constantly feared missing out on experiences others appeared to be enjoying.

Analysis:

In this case study, we delve into Alex's struggle with the fear of missing out (FOMO) and how it impacted his mental well-being. We explore the psychology behind FOMO, discussing the role of social comparison and the illusion of idealized lives on social media. The emotional toll of constant comparison and anxiety is examined, along with its potential to contribute to stress and self-esteem issues.

Strategies:

The case study focuses on strategies Alex and his support network employed to mitigate the effects of FOMO. We discuss the importance of setting healthy boundaries for social media use, including designated "offline" times and practicing mindfulness techniques. Furthermore, we explore how fostering a strong sense of identity, self-worth, and appreciation for offline experiences helped Alex build resilience against the negative impact of FOMO. These strategies were similar to the ones provided in the study by [15] and they found out that controlling for emotional symptoms and other victimization led to a reduction in the effect.

Author details

Milton Anguyo[1*], Joel Masete[1], Magdalen Akia[2] and Henry Drasiku[3]

1 Gulu University, Uganda

2 Yumbe Hospital, Uganda

3 Kampala International University, Uganda

*Address all correspondence to: miltonanguyoosk@gmail.com

References

[1] Hinduja S, Patchin JW. Cyberbullying: A review of the legal issues facing educators. Preventing School Failure: Alternative Education for Children and Youth. 2018;**55**(2):71-78

[2] Oliveira BN, Dos Santos PC, da Costa BGG, Malheiros LEA, Lopes MVV, Silva KS. Screen time correlates of bullying perpetration and victimization in Brazilian adolescents. Journal of Child and Adolescent Trauma. 2023;**16**(3): 607-613. DOI: 10.1007/s40653-023-00515-3-00515-3

[3] Cao G, Wei X, Liu J, Li X. The association between childhood trauma and adolescent cyberbullying: Chain mediating roles of emotional intelligence and online social anxiety. Frontiers in Psychiatry. 2023;**14**:1184382. DOI: 10.3389/fpsyt.2023.1184382

[4] Fardouly J, Diedrichs PC, Vartanian LR, Halliwell E. Social comparisons on social media: The impact of Facebook on young women's body image concerns and mood. Body Image. 2015;**13**:38-45

[5] Liu S, Wu W, Zou H, Chen Y, Xu L, Zhang W, et al. Cybervictimization and non-suicidal self-injury among Chinese adolescents: The effect of depression and school connectedness. Frontiers in Public Health. 2023;**11**:1091959. DOI: 10.3389/fpubh.2023.1091959

[6] Przybylski AK, Murayama K, DeHaan CR, Gladwell V. Motivational, emotional, and behavioral correlates of fear of missing out. Computers in Human Behavior. 2013;**29**(4):1841-1848

[7] Kuss DJ, Griffiths MD. Online social networking and addiction—A review of the psychological literature. International Journal of Environmental Research and Public Health. 2017;**8**(9): 3528-3552

[8] Martínez V, Jiménez-Molina Á, Gerber MM. Social contagion, violence, and suicide among adolescents. Current Opinion in Psychiatry. 2023;**36**(3): 237-242. DOI: 10.1097/YCO.0000000000000858

[9] Tu W, Jiang H, Liu Q. Peer victimization and adolescent Mobile social addiction: Mediation of social anxiety and gender differences. International Journal of Environmental Research and Public Health. 2022;**19**(17): 10978. DOI: 10.3390/ijerph191710978

[10] Vannucci A, Ohannessian CM. Social media use subgroups differentially predict psychosocial well-being during early adolescence. Journal of Youth and Adolescence. 2019;**49**(8):1758-1773

[11] Livingstone S, Sefton-Green J. The Class: Living and Learning in the Digital Age. New York: New York University Press; 2016

[12] Primack BA, Shensa A, Sidani JE, Whaite EO, Lin LY, Rosen D, et al. Social media use and perceived social isolation among young adults in the U.S. Emerging Trends in the Social and Behavioral Sciences. 2017;**3**(1):46-57. DOI: 10.1002/9781118900772.etrds0381

[13] Moreno MA, Jelenchick LA, Egan KG, Cox E, Young H, Gannon KE, et al. Feeling bad on Facebook: Depression disclosures by college students on a social networking site. Depression and Anxiety. 2016;**33**(4): 323-331. DOI: 10.1002/da.22466

[14] Catone G, Signoriello S, Pisano S, Siciliano M, Russo K, Marotta R, et al.

Epidemiological pattern of bullying using a multi-assessment approach: Results from the Bullying and Youth Mental Health Naples Study (BYMHNS). Child Abuse & Neglect. 2019;**89**:18-28. DOI: 10.1016/j.chiabu.2018.12.018

[15] Catone G, Marotta R, Pisano S, Lennox B, Carotenuto M, Gritti A, et al. Psychotic-like experiences in help-seeking adolescents: Dimensional exploration and association with different forms of bullying victimization – A developmental social psychiatry perspective. International Journal of Social Psychiatry. 2017;**63**(8):752-762. DOI: 10.1177/0020764017733765

Chapter 6

Addressing Homophobic, Biphobic and Transphobic Bullying in Educational Contexts

Jonathan Glazzard

Abstract

This chapter addresses homophobic, biphobic and transphobic (HBT) bullying in schools, colleges and universities. It provides a useful definition of this kind of bullying and provides guidance to schools, colleges and universities to support them in recognising and addressing it. Educational institutions play a critical role in protecting all children from bullying. Bullying, which is based on protected characteristics such as perceived or actual sexual orientation or gender identity, is a form of discrimination which contravenes the Equality Act (2010) in the United Kingdom (UK) and therefore schools, colleges and universities have a legal duty to eradicate it. Schools in the UK are required by law to have an anti-bullying policy. This should provide clear guidance to staff on how to recognise homophobic, biphobic and transphobic bullying and how to address it. Protecting children from harm is the responsibility of all members of staff. It is therefore critical that staff undertake professional learning and development to help them identify the signs of HBT bullying and to empower them to address it.

Keywords: LGBTQ+, bullying, homophobia, biphobia, transphobia

1. Introduction

Although schools need to have robust policies and practices in relation to HBT bullying, it is important to remember that this constitutes one strand of the whole institutional approach to Lesbian, Gay, Bisexual, Trans/transgender, Queer, Questioning and other non-normative identities (LGBTQ+) inclusion. Addressing bullying is essential but focusing solely on this aspect when it happens can be reactive. Adopting a proactive approach to LGBTQ+ inclusion through shaping the development of positive attitudes towards sexuality and gender identity should reduce the number of bullying incidents that take place. There is a need to educate perpetrators of bullying about why prejudice is wrong rather than punishing them.

IntechOpen

2. What is homophobic, biphobic and transphobic bullying?

Homophobia is a hatred, fear and irrational dislike of individuals who have non-normative gender identities and sexualities. Homophobic, biphobic or transphobic bullying is bullying that a victim feels has been directed at them because of their actual or perceived sexual orientation or gender identity. It can take a variety of forms. These include physical and verbal abuse, inappropriate use of language and casual banter, being excluded from participation, online bullying and a range of forms of micro-aggressions. These include verbal and non-verbal exchanges such as laughing, smirking and eye contact between perpetrators or moving away from someone. This results in the victim feeling that these responses are related to their actual or perceived sexuality or gender identity. Homophobic, biphobic and transphobic bullying is motivated by prejudice based on a person's actual or perceived sexuality or gender identity.

3. Micro-aggressions

Micro-aggressions were originally discussed in the context of race but have since been extended to other minoritised identities. Micro-aggressions are subtle forms of discrimination and arguably are a form of bullying. In the context of LGBTQ+ young people, micro-aggressions might take a range of forms, including moving away from someone because of their gender or sexual orientation, socially excluding someone or making casual remarks in the presence of an LGBTQ+ individual which perpetrators pass off as banter or simply a joke. Making a casual comment or expressing casual humour about someone, in their presence because they are (or perceived to be) LGBTQ+, is an example of a micro-aggression. The problem with micro-aggressions is that they are difficult to 'call-out' because perpetrators will often not admit that their behaviour is homophobic, biphobic or transphobic. It is therefore critical that all students and staff understand what constitutes a micro-aggression and educators need appropriate training to enable them to challenge micro-aggressions when they occur in educational spaces.

4. Minority stress and bullying

Meyer's [1] model of minority stress provides a useful conceptual framework to further our understanding of bullying. The model assumes that all individuals are exposed to general stressors. However, Meyer argues that individuals with minoritised identities (for example, LGBTQ+ individuals) are exposed to two additional stressors. Meyer categorises these into distal stressors and proximal stressors.

Distal stressors originate externally to the individual, but they impact them. Bullying is an example of a distal stressor. It originates from other people (perpetrators), but it is targeted at an individual (the victim). It can have an adverse impact, including negative mental health outcomes for those individuals who are victims of bullying. Proximal stressors, in contrast, are internal stressors. The stressors originate within the individual because minoritised individuals and groups *anticipate* that they will be victim of bullying and other forms of discrimination. In the case of LGBTQ+ populations, the anticipation that something negative (for example, bullying) will occur can result in a range of adverse behaviours, including concealment, internalised homophobia, biphobia, or transphobia. Therefore, LGBTQ+ individuals might negotiate their personal identities by masking them or concealing them to reduce their exposure to bullying. In addition, LGBTQ+ individuals might witness prejudice-based bullying and start to self-stigmatise. When this occurs, they may start to dislike themselves and they may internalise the negative messages about their non-normative identities. The impacts of anticipating being bullied can lead to a range of adverse effects, including negative mental health outcomes. LGBTQ+ individuals may limit their social opportunities, avoid going into public and avoid accessing unsupervised spaces because of the fear that they will be exposed to bullying and other forms of discrimination. This anticipation that a negative incident might occur does not mean that it will occur. It creates internal psychological distress within potential victims who are always 'on guard' and who are constantly self-monitoring their identities so that they do not stand out.

The problem with Meyer's model is that it places the emphasis on victims of bullying to solve the problems. The model assumes that negative experiences, such as bullying, can be mitigated by minoritised individuals forming groups or collectives to gain solidarity, support and positive affirmation of identity. Although this may be a helpful response, it does not place a duty on educational institutions to address the bullying systemically. Educational institutions need robust policies which focus on educating young people about all forms of bullying, why bullying is wrong, and how to recognise and respond when bullying is witnessed. The policies should also outline how victims will be supported and the interventions in place to support perpetrators.

5. Young people's experiences of bullying

Research has demonstrated the prevalence of HTB bullying in primary schools. The Stonewall *Teacher's Report* identified that:

- 45% of primary school teachers have reported that their pupils have experienced homophobic bullying.
- 70% of primary school teachers have reported that they have heard the use of homophobic language in their school.
- More than 80% of primary school teachers have had no training on how to tackle homophobic bullying.
- Primary school teachers often link HBT bullying to gender stereotypes [2].

Data on the extent of HBT bullying in secondary schools presents a concerning picture. In 2017, Stonewall published a report into the experiences of LGBTQ+ young people in school. The key findings were alarming:

- Nearly half of LGBTQ+ students (45%)—including 64% of transgender students—are bullied in school for being LGBTQ+.
- Most LGBTQ+ students (86%) are regularly exposed to negative language.
- Nearly one in ten transgender students (9%) experience death threats at school.

- Approximately seven in ten LGBTQ+ students (68%) report that teachers fail to challenge or rarely challenge homophobic, biphobic and transphobic language when they hear it.

- Two in five LGBTQ+ students (40%) are never taught LGBTQ+-related content at school.

- Around three in four LGBTQ+ students (77%) do not experience a curriculum which addresses trans or transgender content.

- More than half of LGBTQ+ students (53%) say that there is no adult at school that they can talk to [3].

Research by the charity *Just Like Us* [4] in 2021 found that:

- Young people are twice as likely to experience bullying (43% compared to 21% of their non-LGBT+ peers) and this is not always reported to a teacher.

- Half (51%) of LGBT+ young people reported that they had experienced anxiety.

- Bisexual and pansexual young people are more likely to have experienced cyberbullying.

- Bisexual young people are more likely to have experienced sexual harassment, including unwanted sexual touching.

In Further and Higher Education, a report [5] found that in Scotland, not all staff were trained to address discriminatory language and banter and trans students perceived that they had more negative experiences of further and higher education than LGB students, including experiencing bullying and harassment. There are implications for leaders of institutions. Leaders should ensure that college and university staff are trained in identifying banter and other forms of bullying and know how to respond to it. There should be a clear policy which outlines how incidents should be addressed and documented. Adequate provision of well-being services should be prioritised so that victims of bullying can gain the support that they need.

6. Sense of belonging

Students are unlikely to experience a sense of belonging if they are experiencing bullying. Deci and Ryan [6], through their self-determination theory, illustrate the vital role that 'connectedness' plays in facilitating human flourishing. Bullying can adversely impact on students' capacities to connect to other people and to the institution.

7. Bullying and self-esteem

Mruk's [7] two-dimensional model of self-esteem demonstrates that self-esteem is the product of self-worth and self-competence. Self-worth relates to the view that a person forms of themselves. This view is informed by the perspectives of others, including peers, parents and teachers. Self-competence relates to the ability to accomplish tasks. Where self-worth and self-competence are high, overall self-esteem is also high. When individuals are low in both dimensions, overall self-esteem is low. However, if individuals are high in a single dimension and low in the other, this can result in defensive self-esteem. Individuals who experience bullying may experience adverse effects on their self-worth. If they start to develop a poor sense of self, this can impact on their engagement with their studies and lead to students withdrawing from courses or not engaging with course content. In turn, this can also adversely impact their self-competence.

8. Interventions

Research demonstrates that a variety of interventions show promise [8]. These include the following:

Inclusive curricula: Integrating LGBTQ+-related content in the curriculum is a universal intervention which seeks to educate all students about the importance of diversity and respect for all. In addition, including this content in the curriculum fosters a culture on inclusion by making all identities visible, thus promoting a sense of belonging and connectedness.

Film/drama interventions: Involving students in making films, documentaries or drama productions to highlight the experiences of LGBTQ+ people can be a powerful way of developing students' understanding about banter, the impact of bullying on LGBTQ+ people and appropriate ways of responding to bullying.

Mentoring: Providing LGBTQ+ people with access to a mentor can be a powerful way of providing support. Older students (who may be LGBTQ+ themselves, or allies) can be matched with younger LGBTQ+ students. This can provide opportunities for peer-to-peer talk and advice.

Staff training: Training all staff to recognise HBT bullying is vital. Staff should be trained in how to intervene/respond to bullying and how to have conversations with victims and perpetrators. In addition, staff should be appropriately trained in how to structure a conversation with a student if a student discloses their identity to them.

Social and emotional learning: Lessons which explicitly educate students in school about empathy, and relationships and increase their awareness about the impact that their own emotions can have on others may be useful in fostering a culture of inclusion [8].

9. Legislation

In the UK, the Equality Act (2010) places a legal duty on all educational institutions to prevent direct and indirect discrimination against individuals with a protected characteristic. Sexual orientation and gender reassignment are protected characteristics. Gender reassignment is not solely a medical process which takes place when an individual changes their gender. It can also be a social process. When an individual starts to live as a different gender, for example, by changing their name, dress or pronouns, they are starting the process of gender reassignment. Therefore, although students in school cannot receive medical intervention, they can still be classed as having a protected characteristic. Bullying is a form of direct discrimination and if educational institutions do not address bullying, this is a breach of the Equality Act.

The Equality Act also includes the Public Sector Equality Duty, which places a responsibility on educational institutions to foster good relations between groups of people, including those with and without protected characteristics. Educational institutions cannot promote good relations if they (a) do not tackle bullying and (b) do not make visible minoritised identities through the curriculum and the educational environment.

10. Key points

This chapter has emphasised:

- How schools, colleges and universities can support staff in recognising and addressing HBT bullying.
- The legal duties placed on educational institutions in relation to the Equality Act (2010) and anti-bullying policies.
- The importance of staff undertaking professional learning and development within the context of HBT bullying.

11. Conclusions

This chapter has addressed homophobic, biphobic and transphobic (HBT) bullying in schools, colleges and universities. It has also provided guidance to schools to support them in recognising and addressing it. The legal duties placed on educational institutions in the UK by the Equality Act (2010) have been outlined and explained in relation to sexual orientation and gender reassignment. The legal requirement of schools, colleges and universities to have an anti-bullying policy has also been highlighted and guidance has been given on what this policy should include. Additionally, this chapter has emphasised the importance of staff undertaking professional learning and development in relation to identifying the signs of and addressing HBT bullying.

Acknowledgements

The author declares no conflict of interest.

DOI: http://dx.doi.org/10.5772/intechopen.1005376

Author details

Jonathan Glazzard
University of Hull, Hull, UK

*Address all correspondence to: j.glazzard@hull.ac.uk

References

[1] Meyer IH. Prejudice, social stress, and mental health in lesbian, gay, and bisexual populations: Conceptual issues and research evidence. Psychological Bulletin. 2003;**129**:674-697

[2] Stonewall. The Teachers' Report. 2015. Available from: https://www.stonewall.org.uk/resources/teachers-report-2014-0?gad_source=1&gclid=EAIaIQobChMInMP1waS6hQMVIJZQBh3dMgW-EAAYASAAEgKxLvD_BwE

[3] Stonewall. School Report: The experiences of lesbian, gay, bi and trans young people in Britain's schools in 2017. 2017. Available from: https://www.stonewall.org.uk/system/files/the_school_report_2017.pdf

[4] Just Like Us, Growing up LGBT+: The impact of school, home and coronavirus on LGBT+ young people. 2021. Available from: https://www.justlikeus.org/wp-content/uploads/2021/11/Just-Like-Us-2021-report-Growing-Up-LGBT.pdf

[5] Stonewall. Experiences of LGBT People in Post 16 Education. (nd). Available from: https://www.eis.org.uk/Content/images/equality/LGBT/Post%2016%20-%20Stonewall%20Scotland,%20web.pdf

[6] Deci EL, Ryan RM. Intrinsic Motivation and Self-Determination in Human Behavior. Berlin: Springer Science & Business Media; 1985. DOI: 10.1007/978-1-4899-2271-7

[7] Mruk C. Self-Esteem Research, Theory and Practice. London: Free Association Books; 1999

[8] Amadori A, Intra FS, Taverna L, et al. Systematic review of intervention and prevention programs to tackle homophobic bullying at school: A socio-emotional learning skills perspective. International Journal of Bullying Prevention. 2023. DOI: 10.1007/s42380-023-00198-2

Chapter 7

The Intersection of Gender and Mental Well-Being among Adolescents in Pakistan: Challenges, Strategies, and Future Recommendations

Ambreen Tharani, Zahra Tharani, Sharifa Lalani, Razia Bano Momin and Shireen Shehzad Bhamani

Abstract

This chapter delves into the nexus of mental well-being, gender dynamics, and contextual intricacies in Pakistan. Acknowledging mental health's foundational role in human development, particularly during the post-COVID-19 landscape, immense need of comprehensive mental health action plans, with a focus on late adolescents and young adults is highlighted. The narrative unfolds the complex web of adolescent mental health challenges, woven by individual attributes, behaviors, and socioeconomic conditions. Adolescence emerges as a pivotal phase for identity exploration, marked by activities challenging established gender norms. Gender, viewed as a sociocultural construct and a dynamic continuum, is explored in its role in shaping behaviors and expectations. The chapter underscores the early imprinting of gender roles through familial, peer, and cultural channels. With a commitment to understanding these dynamics deeply, the chapter aims to offer nuanced insights. The overarching objective is to inform future research, influence policies, and guide interventions fostering mental well-being in Pakistan's diverse and globalized society.

Keywords: adolescent, gender roles, mental health, challenges, strategies, Pakistan

1. Introduction

The fortification of mental well-being is a key pillar in the panorama of human development, shaping our minds and how we interact with the world, our skills in managing interpersonal relationships, and our resilience in facing adversities. The significance of this facet of human experience cannot be overstated, as the repercussions of inadequate mental health reverberate throughout society.

In recent years, post-COVID-19 mental health has received a lot of limelight in public health policy. In 2013, a resolution was passed by the World Health

Organization (WHO) that called for a comprehensive mental health action plan for the next years to be followed in each country [1]. The population that was targeted to receive more attention was late adolescents and young adults. It is considered that half of all mental health issues may exhibit in adulthood, but the seeds are usually sown by age 14 [2]. Worldwide, approximately 14% of individuals, aged 10–19, have an experience with a mental disorder, contributing to 13% of the overall disease burden in this age bracket. Primary contributors to illness and disability in adolescents are depression, anxiety, and behavioral disorders. Furthermore, suicide stands as the fourth most prevalent cause of mortality among those aged 15–29 [3]. It is an enigma to see that mental health concerns are the most common ones and yet are the most taboo topic to be discussed [4, 5].

Adolescent mental health challenges arise from the intricate and dynamic interplay of individual attributes and behaviors, such as genetic elements, emotional and social intelligence, and so on. More factors such as social and economic conditions, including social support, financial dependency and paucity, and educational opportunities, further drag toward the compromised mental health pitfall. The larger sociocultural environment, influenced by factors such as national-level social and economic policies, further impacts mental well-being [5]. The interactions could be turbulent or self-motivated resulting in either safeguarding or posing risks to mental health.

Adolescence is a period of curiosity, experimentation, and learning about their identity. In this age period, boys and girls indulge in activities, which might not conform with socially constructed gender behaviors. Gender is a sociocultural construct that presets characteristics that are considered suitable and acceptable by society to be exhibited by men and women, such as norms, demeanor, and forethought [6, 7]. Gender is considered as a continuum; it is a self-concept that everyone develops during their personal development, and therefore, it is subject to change [8]. Gender roles are ingrained from an early age through socialization and education received by boys and girls. This cultural upbringing and learning occurs within the family setting, among friends and peers and are also influenced by cultural representations in the arts, media, and religion [9–11]. A study on school-going adolescents aged 15–18 years in Pakistan reported that 53.2% of the 400 students suffered from depression and anxiety [12].

This chapter seeks to navigate the multifaceted terrain of gender, mental health, and the unique contextual realities of Pakistan with a deep commitment to understanding these intricate links. By offering this comprehensive exploration, we aspire to provide a deeper and more nuanced understanding of the complexities inherent to this intersection. We aim to shed light on these complexities and offer insights that can inform future research, shape policies, and guide interventions aimed at promoting mental well-being in a diverse and globalized society.

2. Cultural aspect and mental health

In Pakistan, the relationship between gender and the mental health of adolescents is a complicated and multidimensional topic [13]. This section will examine the cultural aspects contributing to adolescents' mental health in the Pakistani context, covering the "what," "how," "when," and "why" of these realities. This analysis will lay the groundwork for comprehending the opportunities and difficulties in tackling this important problem in the Pakistani context. The prevalent gender preferences and role expectations are a crucial cultural aspect that has a major impact on the mental wellness of adolescents in Pakistan [14]. Pakistan's cultural customs and conventions frequently impose strict gender roles with distinct expectations for men and women. These demands place a great deal of strain on teenagers, who may experience disorientation and identity crises as they explore their own identities and go through sexual transitions. For example, in Pakistan, conventional gender roles typically require men to earn the family's living, while women should concentrate on taking care of the home. Young boys and girls who might not fit into these roles are under tremendous strain due to this inflexible gender split, which can cause stress and mental health problems. Furthermore, adolescents, particularly girls, are subjected to harsh expectations due to the strongly rooted concept of "honor" in Pakistani society. If they feel that their acts would bring dishonor to their families, they may experience great emotional pain. Depression and anxiety may arise from this.

The secrecy and stigma that surround conversations regarding gender-related concerns and mental health in Pakistani families and communities is another important factor [15]. Many adolescents find it challenging to open up about their mental health concerns due to the prevailing social stigma. This silence, combined with the absence of mental health and role transition education in the curriculum, exacerbates the problem. Adolescents are left to seek informal and often inappropriate resources for information, which can lead to the spread of incorrect and harmful beliefs about mental health and gender roles. For example, discussing openly mental health issues and challenges in adopting the gender-specific role expected by society, is considered taboo in many Pakistani families. Adolescents who experience depression or anxiety may fear seeking help and prefer to suffer in silence. Moreover, the topic of sexual education is often completely avoided, leading adolescents to rely on unreliable sources, like peers or the internet, for information. This can result in misconceptions and anxiety about sexual health.

In addition, adolescents in Pakistan often turn to the internet for information about mental health and gender-related topics. Unfortunately, they can encounter misleading and harmful content, which may worsen their mental health. Peer pressure is also a significant concern. Adolescents may receive advice and information from friends who may not be well-informed, leading to harmful decisions or behaviors. These pressures and misleading information can negatively impact their mental well-being.

These examples illustrate the real-world implications of gender and cultural dynamics, emphasizing the pressing need for sensitive and context-specific strategies to address the challenges of gender and mental well-being among adolescents in Pakistan [13–15]. By acknowledging these challenges and understanding the local context, researchers and mental health practitioners can develop more effective interventions and support systems tailored to the unique cultural landscape of Pakistan. This approach holds the potential to significantly contribute to the enhancement of mental health outcomes for young individuals in the country.

3. Socioeconomic aspect and mental health

Following the discussion on the cultural aspects and their relationship to mental health, exploring the relationship between socioeconomic variables and adolescence mental health is critical, because it leads to a greater understanding of the complicated difficulties that young adults experience. As individuals negotiate cultural standards and socioeconomic status, the development and maintenance of social interactions are crucial in forming their identity and frequently result in internal and external conflicts. Peers from higher socioeconomic status may have an influence on their friends and this could lead to copying and risk-taking behaviors such as substance abuse and thrill-seeking.

Additionally, there is a common assumption that lower socioeconomic status (SES) correlates with increased mental health problems in adolescence. In countries like Pakistan, where adolescence is typically at school or college, financial dependence on family can contribute to feelings of helplessness and depression affecting self-esteem. A supportive family environment, however, can mitigate mental health challenges, irrespective of socioeconomic status. A longitudinal study included 426 adolescents revealed that self-efficacy exhibited a modest protective effect against mental health problems in those belonging to low-income homes, while social support showed a similar effect for adolescents from higher-income families [16]. Additionally, a positive family environment emerged as a factor associated with lower mental health problems in adolescence, irrespective of socioeconomic status.

Moreover, in Pakistani culture, adolescence are considered as minors and they are not being involved in decision-making, if they try to speak and express their viewpoint, then they are being shunned. A qualitative study was done in 19 adolescents aged 11–17 years, highlighting their strong desire for decision-making, self-expression, decision-making autonomy, emphasizing the importance of achieving dreams for good mental health [17]. Conversely, in low-income eastern cultures, male teenagers may take on a paternal role, especially in situations when there is a lack of financial support for the family. This position and obligation frequently result in early school dropout, low-paying employment, and the abandonment of personal goals, all of which exacerbate mental health issues.

The above examples convey complex interplay between socioeconomic factors and adolescent mental health is essential for devising targeted interventions.

4. Recommendations and way forward

Gender and mental health realities in Pakistan call for thoughtful interventions that need to be interweaved at various levels such as individual, society, and government. It is crucial to prioritize mental well-being and use gender-sensitive approaches to tackle challenges faced by adolescents in Pakistan and nurture them as resilient individuals.

4.1 Addressing as a fundamental fabric of society

The societal pressures and gender-specific roles imposed on adolescents can lead to disparities and psychological stress [18]. Addressing those might require a complete societal shift, however, a few steps can serve as a whistle-blower and sensitize Pakistani society to thoughtfully invest in the mental health of future generations. Indeed, in Pakistan, there is a need to establish an inclusive society that is adolescents-centered and actively supports and promotes gender equality. As a first step, we need to instill equality and mutual respect in the next generation to embrace connectedness and positive values. Additionally, it requires settling their bewilderment regarding the understanding of gender norms, roles, and relationships. It is also critical to implement public awareness campaigns which challenge gender stereotypes and encourage gender sensitivity. By challenging negative attitudes and advocating fair treatment for everyone, regardless of gender, such activities can help to promote a more inclusive society and empowerment.

DOI: http://dx.doi.org/10.5772/intechopen.1003953

4.2 Promoting a gender-inclusive environment

Family environment and early years of education make an important contribution to how gender-inclusive society is shaped. The family has a significant role in normalizing the alteration of gender roles prescribed by society [19]. A helping hand from a male member of the family in home tasks, for example, and an economic contribution from a female member of the family should be acceptable. Also, it is equally important to create a gender-inclusive educational environment that teaches the significance of being flexible in relationships. The positive role demonstration with such examples will have a profound effect on creating an optimistic approach and unconditional acceptance of the sex individual is born. Educators play a critical role, particularly those who teach at primary schools. Their persistent guidance and mentorship will assist individuals in how social and personal relationships should be managed respectfully. This will promote the mental well-being of adolescents and allow them to enjoy freedom as an individual and reciprocate the same for others, without connecting roles imposed by society that are a possible obstacle to enjoying the freedom of living respectfully. However, one needs to be vigilant about how much freedom is internalized and practiced without breaching the ethical and moral values that are ingrained as a part of Eastern (Pakistani) culture. Equal opportunity to be part of entrepreneurship programs for financial independence can be a positive approach.

4.3 Positive use of media

The increased usage of digital media can play an important part in supporting a positive attitude shift by providing diverse and positive depictions of men and women while confronting stereotypes. By generating appropriate debate and relaying examples of empowerment, the media may influence public opinion and increase understanding of how gender equality can enhance teenage mental health in Pakistan. Additionally, films, drama series, and other social media platforms can depict inclusive debates and good effects of gender equality. Highlighting this important agenda through the media will reach the entire society.

4.4 Building resilience

Building a gender-inclusive society in Pakistan that has a promising effect on the mental health of adolescents will be a long journey. However, building resilience in children can enhance adolescent mental health and empower them to avoid gender biases and promote equality [18]. Moreover, it empowers individuals to handle and overcome stressors related to gender, as well as helps them navigate through these situations. We should also be mindful of an increasing trend of internal migration among adolescents in Pakistan to attain higher education or for climate reasons [20]. Therefore, self-care, communication, and life skills building are a few examples that need to be integral components in such training to strengthen adolescents' emotional well-being and help them cope with uncertainties in daily living. Creating accessible safe spaces for adolescents where they can openly discuss gender-related issues can be helpful.

4.5 Research and policy implications

Pakistan is moving forward in terms of integrating various policy-level measures to create gender quality in Pakistan. This includes the development of the National

Gender Policy Framework [21] and creating better representation of women in the national assembly and leadership at the federal level. However, integration at ground level is yet to be considered with the fact that gender discrimination is deeply rooted in our society, like in decision-making dynamics, shared inheritance, and power structures within households and communities [18]. Youth in the country can be whistle-blowers to bring a slow and progressive transition that is grounded within societies and serves as a "bottom-up" approach. Future research needs to consider this important agenda to understand how these measures and policies have influenced the mental health of adolescents. Those insights will be instrumental in informing future research and interventions to promote resilience and mental well-being among adolescents.

5. Conclusions

In conclusion, the intricate meshwork of culture, socioeconomic factors, gender dynamics, adolescence, and their intersectionality provides a comprehensive lens through which we understand the complex landscape of mental health. As adolescents navigate the subtle balance between societal expectations and personal aspirations, cultural influences, economic circumstances, and gender norms interweave into the fabric of their mental well-being. Recognizing the interconnectedness of these elements is crucial for developing thorough strategies that foster mental health resilience in adolescents. Embracing diversity and acknowledging the unique challenges faced by individuals at the intersection of these factors is essential for promoting a more inclusive and detailed understanding of mental health in the context of adolescence. This comprehensive approach not only aids in cultivating a supportive environment but also lays the foundation for informed interventions that consider the diverse needs of this pivotal stage in human development.

Conflict of interest

The authors declare no conflict of interest.

Author details

Ambreen Tharani*, Zahra Tharani, Sharifa Lalani, Razia Bano Momin and Shireen Shehzad Bhamani
School of Nursing and Midwifery, Aga Khan University School of Nursing and Midwifery, Karachi, Pakistan

*Address all correspondence to: ambreen.tharani@aku.edu

References

[1] Saxena S, Funk M, Chisholm D. World health assembly adopts comprehensive mental health action plan 2013-2020. The Lancet. 2013;**381**:1970-1971. DOI: 10.1016/S0140-6736(13)61139-3

[2] Hewlett E, Moran V. Making Mental Health Count: The Social and Economic Costs of Neglecting Mental Health Care. Paris: OECD Publishing; 2014. DOI: 10.1787/9789264208445-en

[3] World Health Organization (WHO). Mental Health of Adolescents. 2021. Available from: https://www.who.int/news-room/fact-sheets/detail/adolescent-mental-health [Accessed: November 15, 2023]

[4] Williams B, Pow J. Gender differences and mental health: An exploratory study of knowledge and attitudes to mental health among Scottish teenagers. Child and Adolescent Mental Health. 2007;**12**(1):8-12. DOI: 10.1111/j.1475-3588.2006.00413.x

[5] Van Droogenbroeck F, Spruyt B, Keppens G. Gender differences in mental health problems among adolescents and the role of social support: Results from the Belgian health interview surveys 2008 and 2013. BMC Psychiatry. 2018;**18**(1):1-9. DOI: 10.1186/s12888-018-1591-4

[6] Jewkes R, Flood M, Lang J. From work with men and boys to changes of social norms and reduction of inequities in gender relations: A conceptual shift in prevention of violence against women and girls. The Lancet. 2015;**385**:1580-1589. DOI: 10.1016/S0140-6736(14)61683-4

[7] Rafiq N, Tharani Z, Jetha Z, Saeed Ali T. Intimate partner violence through the lens of gender, finance, and ethics. In: Martin CR, Preedy VR, editors. Handbook of Anger, Aggression, and Violence. Cham: Springer; 2023. DOI: 10.1007/978-3-030-98711-4_188-1

[8] Thande NK, Wang M, Curlin K, Dalvie N, Mazure CM. The influence of sex and gender on health: How much is being taught in medical school curricula? Journal of Women's Health. 2019;**28**(12):1748-1754. DOI: 10.1089/jwh.2018.7229

[9] Amin A, Chandra-Mouli V. Empowering adolescent girls: Developing egalitarian gender norms and relations to end violence. Reproductive Health. 2014;**11**(1):1-3

[10] García-Díaz V, Lana-Pérez A, Fernández-Feito A, Bringas-Molleda C, Rodríguez-Franco L, Rodríguez-Díaz FJ. Sexist attitudes and recognition of abuse in young couples. Atencion Primaria. 2017;**50**(7):398-405

[11] Kelly J, Payton E. A content analysis of local media framing of intimate partner violence. Violence Gender. 2019;**6**(1):47-52

[12] Ibbad S, Baig LA, Ahmer Z, Shahid F. Prevalence of anxiety and depression in high school students of Karachi, Pakistan. Pakistan Journal of Medical Sciences. 2022;**38**(4Part-II):916

[13] Ali S, Riaz MN, Riaz MT, Aslam MF. Gender and mental health in the Pakistani context: An overview. Journal of Mental Health and Social Inclusion. 2017;**21**:112-127

[14] Khan S, Ahmed S. The impact of gender norms on adolescent mental health in the Pakistani context:

A qualitative study. International Journal of Adolescence and Youth. 2018;**23**:422-436

[15] Siddiqui N, Ali AS. Breaking the silence: Addressing mental health taboo in Pakistani society. Journal of Cultural Diversity. 2020;**27**:34-42

[16] Maurer J, Meyrose AK, Kaman A, et al. Socioeconomic status, protective factors, and mental health problems in transition from adolescence to emerging adulthood: Results of the longitudinal BELLA study. Child Psychiatry & Human Development. 2023:1-12. DOI: 10.1007/s10578-023-01582-1

[17] Lukoševičiūtė-Barauskienė J, Žemaitaitytė M, Šūmakarienė V, Šmigelskas K. Adolescent perception of mental health: It's not only about oneself, It's about others too. Children (Basel). 2023;**10**:1109. DOI: 10.3390/children10071109

[18] World Health Organization (WHO), the United Nations Children's Fund (UNICEF). Helping Adolescents Thrive Toolkit. 2021. Available from: https://iris.who.int/bitstream/handle/10665/341327/9789240025554-eng.pdf [Accessed: October 28, 2023]

[19] World Health Organization (WHO). Promoting Adolescent well-being. Available from: https://www.who.int/activities/promoting-adolescent-well-being [Accessed: November 2, 2023]

[20] UN Women. UN Women Pakistan. Available from: https://asiapacific.unwomen.org/en/countries/pakistan#:~:text=Despite%20these%20challenges%2C%20Pakistan%20has,Ordinance%20(2020)%20and%20the%20Domestic [Accessed: October 28, 2023]

[21] Government of Pakistan (GoP). National Gender Policy Framework [Report]. 2022. Available from: https://www.pc.gov.pk/uploads/report/NGPF.pdf [Accessed: November 1, 2023]

Section 2

Therapeutic Strategies

Chapter 8

Alternatives to Foster Care

Patricia Crittenden, Steve Farnfield, Susan Spieker, Andrea Landini, Monica Oxford, Katrina Robson, Siw Karlsen, Helen Johnson, Vicki Ellis and Zoe Ash

Abstract

It is unequivocally clear that separating children from parents through foster care is harmful. We offer several safe alternatives to foster care, including new assessment tools focusing on family strengths and parents' readiness to learn and six interventions tailored to local needs. These alternatives keep children with their parents while under child protection supervision. All cost substantially less than foster care. The alternatives had several characteristics in common. Child needs, especially safety, were met. Parents worked with professionals in structuring new services, resulting in co-created bespoke services with a wide buy-in in each community. Using the new tools, the alternatives were assessed for strengths and parental readiness before intervening so that success was promoted. The best services combined individual learning and group activities, especially activities that involved exercise, outdoor green-time, and social engagement. They also offered 24/7 availability and affiliated with a university to provide better program design and evidence of outcomes. We discuss the impediments to accepting alternatives to foster care, and call for policy makers, judges, supervisors, and managers, as well as case workers, to reduce the use of foster care by using safe alternatives that strengthen families.

Keywords: separation, fostering families, supportable families, foster care, protecting children, protecting families

1. Introduction

There have always been children whose parents could not care adequately for them. In this chapter we offer a rationale for keeping children at home with parents whose parenting skills are less than their children need them to be, together with examples of how to do this safely.

The chapter is structured in five parts. Part 1 reviews the history of removing children from their parents to establish that foster care was the well-intended solution to both dangerous child care and institutionalization. Part 2 describes early initiatives to prevent separations and foster care. Part 3 offers assessment tools that could help professionals to identify family strengths and, thus, avoid using foster care. The heart of this chapter is Part 4 in which we describe six alternatives to foster care; the strength of these examples is that they were developed and implemented by clinicians

 IntechOpen

under real life conditions. Part 5 closes with a set of recommendations for alternatives to foster care intended for child protection workers, managers, and supervisors, educational and clinical professionals, and attorneys and judges. For an overview, some readers might want to begin with Part 5. We also address possible reasons why the use of foster care continues to increase in spite of the greater efficacy and reduced cost of home-based alternatives. Because separation and foster care cause iatrogenic harm that hurts both families and professionals, we close by urging everyone to use their professional capacity to support alternatives to foster care.

2. A brief history of separating children from their parents

Child removal to protect children from harmful parental care can be traced back to nineteenth century child rescue societies [1]. These professional societies had quasi legal authority to remove children from dangerous homes and place them into foster or residential care.

Bowlby's attachment theory had a massive influence on the move from institutional to foster care. Nevertheless, Bowlby was very concerned about the harm done to children by separating them from their parents [2]. His theory became increasingly popular, but its practical application has been patchy [3]. Since the mid-twentieth century, child care practice in the US, Canada, Australia, and the UK has prioritized the use of foster care over residential care. The pace of change, however, was uneven; for example, the number of fostered children in the US overtook those in residential care in 1950, but this did not happen in England until the 1970s.

Now it is clear that removing children from their attachment figures causes harm because it involves separating attached children from the person they trust [4, 5]. It is also painful to parents (both biological and foster) and the professionals who must physically carry out the separations. In fact, we think it is so counter to professionals' motivations for working in child protection that it might contribute to burnout, high rates of turnover in staff and foster carers, [6] and even to moral injury [7].

Foster care is intended to protect children from mistreatment by their parents. Since publication of *The Battered Child Syndrome* [8], millions of families in the United States have been investigated for child abuse and neglect, and nearly half a million children are in foster care [9]. Neglect is by far the most common form of maltreatment [10], and is highly linked to poverty, mental illness, substance abuse [11, 12], and intergenerational neglect [13]. Although the use of foster care in the US has dropped, it still disproportionally impacts minority children [14]. In the UK, use of foster care has doubled from 1994 to 2023 as child protection agencies have become more risk averse following the highly publicized deaths of children left in parental care [15]. In effect, UK policy has been made by way of multiple single case events rather than by systemic appraisal. Canada does not report national statistics for children in care. However, provinces with high percentages of First Nations people also have high rates of removing children from parental care [16], suggesting that minority status might affect placement decisions.

Two generations after Helfer and Kempe's work on the physical abuse of children, as many as a quarter of parents who were "protected" by being raised in foster care are having their own children placed in foster or adoptive care [17]. In other words, being in foster care as a child might contribute to multi-generational harm. The outcomes for fostered children in the UK can be so poor that they have been described as a silent crisis [18].

Crittenden and Spieker's review of a century of research documents evidence of harm to children from being separated from their parents [4, 5]. In 242 studies, separating children from their parents was evidenced to be unequivocally harmful, with not one study reporting positive effects. Strikingly, harm from separation is not one of the factors that legislation mandates be considered by courts before separating children from their parents or by child protection personnel in carrying out such separations [19]. This is important because placement in foster care causes a cascade of additional possible separations: changes of school, loss of siblings and friends, repeated brief separations during parental visitation, and, in every case that does not result in adoption by the foster parents, separation from the foster parents. Many foster children are placed multiple times as placements break down. With each separation and change of placement, children become more distressed and less likely to remain permanently in the next placement [20]. One study of fostered toddlers reported that by 18 months they averaged 2.7 caregiver separations since birth [21]. It is important to note that, although separation always causes harm, that harm must be balanced against the risk of permanent injury or death if the child is left at home.

When children are transported to family visitations by aides who are strangers to them, there is risk that children will come to accept strangers as safe and approved participants in their lives. Such acceptance is like the 'indiscriminate attachment' of institutionalized young children [22] which bodes poorly for children's attachment to caregivers and, later, adult partners. Another risk lies in the way separations are performed, often abruptly without adequate time for transition and emotional preparation for both children and adults. We conclude that, despite the intention to protect children, the child protection bureaucracy and policy often harms children.

The number of children entering foster care still outstrips the number of foster carers and professionals available to help them, even though administrative budgets are increasing faster than placements [23]. This suggests that the child welfare bureaucracy has become ineffective, self-sustaining, and vulnerable to market exploitation. The introduction of marketization, increased outsourcing, and the split between purchasers of services and providers of services, has become a concern for many [11, 24]. This has also brought increased regulation in the form of targets and performance measures in social work, instrumentalizing practice with families and reducing the amount of face-to-face time that social workers spend with them [25–27]. For example, despite clear evidence of the harm of institutionalization, in England there was a 9% increase in the number of children's homes between 2022 and 2023 [28]. The provision of residential care in the UK is dominated by a small number of private firms that have been criticized for promoting their services too strongly and making excessive profits [29].

Legislation supporting foster care has created a huge bureaucracy of child protection professionals, police, expert witnesses, attorneys, and judges that cost immense sums of money [30]. Unfortunately, this bureaucracy is caught in a self-defeating loop whereby failures in the system are met with increased bureaucracy. For example, each time there is a death that might have been prevented, the regulations guiding professionals' decision-making are tightened and more children are placed in care – to protect both the children and the professionals. Alternatives to foster and residential care are urgently needed.

The alternatives to foster care that we offer include: (1) assessing needs and planning services around parent's readiness to learn, or their *zone of proximal development* (ZPD) [31] rather than *children's needs* that might exceed parents' current caregiving abilities; (2) ways to keep children safe while their parents are learning more appropriate ways to care for them, and (3) alternatives to foster care when parents cannot change at all or in a timely way. We note, however, underlying racial bias and structural and institutional inequality in the application of child welfare policy results in racial more foster placement of minority children. This topic needs separate attention and is not covered in this chapter (see [14] for discussion). In this chapter we do, however, address economic issues to demonstrate that transferring funds from foster care and child welfare to alternatives to foster care might both lower costs and increase the efficacy of intervention. As one social worker recalled about proceedings with a mother of three young children:

> *The court case went on for over 2 years. One day I did a quick calculation of the cost of these proceedings and concluded that we could have paid for a nanny to go into the family home until the children had reached 18 with the money spent on trying to keep these children from their mother (Joanne James, personal email communication, Nov. 7, 2023).*

3. Initiatives to prevent separations and foster placement

Early efforts to prevent foster care have added to our understanding of how to keep children safe in unsafe homes.

3.1 Improving parent competency and parent-child relationships

In the early 1970's one of us (Crittenden) ran parent groups for mothers under child protection supervision [1]. The groups were primarily educational, using home visits and weekly group viewing of their own mother-child videos, taken just prior to the meeting. Later this would be called a 'hybrid model' using 'video-feedback'; at the time it was a logical way to combine the social advantages and observational learning of a group with the power of individualized attention. In each home visit, the mother was commended for something she did in the group meeting (even just showing up), reinforced for something she did during this home visit, and given a suggestion of something she could try based on the video or what was happening right then in the home. The group discussions were regulated to be in each mother's ZPD. Mothers served as positive examples for each other, and reflective processing occurred without children being present.

The group teaching included learning to communicate more effectively with professionals – as a way of gaining agency with them. An unexpected outcome was that the mothers made friends in the group and began to help each other outside of group meetings, for example with child care, and to meet each in town and at medical appointments. A social network was formed. Unlike formal parent education, the topics for discussion were selected ad hoc based on mothers' immediate concerns and problems. Because the groups were on-going with members joining and leaving at different times, as mothers gained skills, they became leaders to their peers. There was also a strong element of what Robson later formalized as co-production (see below) in which the mothers strongly influenced the topics and structure of the home visits and group meetings. The limited data indicated that the *parental* intervention was successful for *children's* development [32]. But when passed to another group leader, it was difficult to write directions for what was spontaneously generated, and the groups were soon discontinued. Understanding the role of leadership might be important [33].

A series of pre-post evaluations of teaching techniques using the mother-infant videos [34] demonstrated that positive reinforcement did not change parental behavior and self-rating scales led to improvement on the rated behavior. Role playing in which mothers first pretended to be a child and then the mother led to dramatic improvements in mother's dyadic synchrony; today we might call this 'embodied empathy'. Strikingly, instructional material attuned to mothers' reading skill and need for images made no difference in maternal behavior at all and demonstrations or modeling of desired behavior *reduced* mothers' dyadic synchrony with their children. Later research using these videos revealed that maltreated children often used false positive affect and compulsive compliance [35]. It should be noted that this service was not university-based, did not have research funding, and none of the professionals were trained to do research. But knowing what was effective – and what was not – was important and so research was done and reported. Moreover, every mother was invited to participate in future research that she was told would be unlikely to help her but might help other families. Almost every mother signed consent to be contacted for this research, showing willingness to give of themselves to help others.

3.2 Court procedures to divert children from foster care

Keeping children in their extended families is generally better than placing them in stranger care in terms of fewer psychological and behavioral problems, less placement disruption and higher reunification rates with birth parents [36]. Several court-based procedures have been developed to promote 'kin care.' Family Group Conferences originated in New Zealand as a means of reducing the high number of Maori children in care. Following traditional Maori decision-making, family group conferences decide who in the family can best look after a child. This idea is now used in many countries, with fewer children whose families had kin conferences going into care than other children [37]. UK courts use Special Guardianship Orders to give relatives legal custody of a child without adoption. In a decade, the number of such orders has overtaken the number of adoptions [38], with lower disruption rates and lower costs than foster care [39]. Nevertheless, there is concern that this reduces permanency. American Family Drug Treatment Courts promote permanence during care proceedings by having parents with addiction attend a court service using a non-adversarial approach from a multi-disciplinary team specializing in addiction. The same judge deals with their case throughout and conducts regular reviews without attorneys. The 5-year effect is generally positive [40] with four times as many children reunited with their parents as matched comparison children and half as many placed in foster care [41].

Northern Ireland attempts to obtain more accurate, non-adversarial evidences by jointly instructing expert witnesses; all parties to the proceedings generate the list of questions for expert witnesses, including a final question "Is there anything else you think the court needs to know regarding the placement of the children?" Witnesses are paid by equal contributions from all parties, thus ensuring that witnesses have no monetary loyalty of any person or outcome. When Family Functional Formulations (see 4.2 below) are offered, the assessor is almost never called to deliver testimony in court. The courts have been generous with funds for thorough assessment but coming so late in the process of supporting families, preventive work that could have been done earlier is often no longer possible at the time of court proceedings. Such thorough assessment is highly recommended but would be better placed near intake when preventive work can best be accomplished.

3.3 Readiness for change

Finally, rather than using parenting assessments to determine whether children should be removed to foster care, a pioneer project in the UK used assessment to identify parents' readiness for specific services, leading to more attuned service delivery, improvement in outcomes, and reduced costs [41]. Using Sure Start funding, this assessment-for-intervention protocol led to services based on parents' skills, needs, and readiness to learn. This idea developed into brief Screening Functional Formulations and diagnostic Family Functional Formulations. Although the data indicated positive outcomes, this UK program was discontinued when the entire Sure Start initiative was defunded.

3.4 Normative approaches seeking change through mandated programs

In 2010 the Italian government, in collaboration with the University of Padova and with several local administration and social services, launched the Program of Intervention for the Prevention of Institutionalization (P.I.P.P.I) [42]. The goals were to update interventions for neglectful families and to reduce harm while keeping the children at home. The four main types of new planned interventions were: (1) professionals working in the family home; (2) groups for parents and children; (3) collaborations between schools, families, and social services; (4) supportive families. The program also aimed towards standardized family assessment.

These efforts have not yet yielded satisfactory results. Among the probable reasons for limited progress are insufficient education of workers, insufficient funding of the services, inefficient communication between clinical, child protection and justice services, and lack of efficient monitoring of the developmental pathways of children removed from the families. In other words, better training, better communication, and more money were needed.

In the absence of reliable data, ideologies clash in the public debate when single cases of children removed from the families make the news. For example, in response to the reaction to a 2019 scandal [43, 44], the Piemonte region approved in 2022 a regional law called "Zero separation: Interventions to support parenthood and norms to prevent separation from families of origin", which includes the provision of housing and financial support especially to marginalized groups. Such laws bring psychosocial priorities and legal constraints into greater agreement [45].

These laws are coherent with many of the recommendations in this paper, except the co-production principle. They appear to be "top-down" approaches to the problem, that are extremely progressive in principle, but may be slowed down or even halted by lack of cooperation from the workers who are not part of the origin of the programs. It might be necessary to ensure that professionals contribute to new programs so that they 'buy into' the solutions.

4. Tools to support alternatives to foster care based on family strengths

Most assessment is directed to parental deficits and child needs. To prevent parent-child separation, there needs to be a shift towards an assessment protocol that focuses on parents' strengths and readiness to learn.

4.1 Preventing foster placement by re-defining family problems

Defining family problems in terms of child maltreatment or parental psychopathology focuses professional attention on deficits, with current understanding of deficits being based on behavioral symptoms, not etiology. The efficacy of symptom-focused treatment is limited to a few studies, most of which are methodologically flawed, and provides only limited support for the interventions, e.g. for violence reduction [46]. Furthermore, group effects do not identify individual outcomes.

A framework for *functional* diagnosis is needed. It should seek to understand why particular behavioral symptoms develop and what purpose they serve for the functioning of each family. The *Dynamic-Maturational Model of Attachment and Adaptation* (DMM) [47] explains maladaptive behavior in terms of response to danger, i.e. adverse childhood events (ACEs) [48]. Danger is considered a normal part of life, and the human brain is seen as evolved to predict danger, cope with dangerous circumstances, and learn from dangerous experiences to protect self, partner, and progeny.

When children are unprotected and uncomforted from danger, they develop self-protective strategies to increase their safety and comfort. These strategies rely on quick 'rules' (psychological short-cuts) to make predictions. We propose that parents whose behavior does not protect and comfort their children often use outdated self-protective strategies that they learned as endangered children. In some cases, this is identified as maltreating behavior or symptoms of mental illness. We propose that teaching parents to better protect and comfort *themselves* in the present can free them from the psychological short-cuts, learned in the past, that lead to dangerous parenting behavior.

4.2 Preventing foster placement by assessing needs

Selecting interventions to enable parents to learn new self- and child-protective strategies is a difficult, but crucial, task. Learning occurs best when the gap between what has been learned already and what is to be learned next does not require a leap for which there is no bridge. The optimal gap is the Zone of Proximal Development. In cases of inadequate parental caregiving, the 'learner' is the parent and their ZPD determines which interventions will be most successful.

When children's needs are beyond parents' current ZPD and interventions are selected based solely on child needs, parents can be expected to fail to benefit from intervention. We propose that choosing services based on child needs can lead to repeated parental failure as one service is followed by another, and the goals of treatment are not met. A possible outcome is that both parents and professionals feel that change is impossible. When this happens, professionals sometimes seek foster care for the children. We think this mutually defeating process can be prevented by choosing interventions based on parents' ZPD and offering protective services while parents are learning.

We suggest evaluating parents' readiness to learn by framing family problems using a developmental and systemic perspective to understand both the array of specific problems that the family faces and a probable *critical cause* [49] of the problems. Addressing the critical cause can streamline the course of intervention by focusing action to create a cascade of changes that do not require additional interventions. Three increasingly detailed approaches are recommended:

4.2.1 Level of family functioning (LFF)

Level of Family Functioning (LFF) [33] is a global assessment completed by a family's social worker based on the case record, presenting problem, and 2–3 initial home visits. It places a family at one of five levels, each pointing to parents' intervention needs and likely period of needing managed services (see **Table 1**). Levels 3–5 (*Restorable, Supportable, and Needing New Services*) are relevant here. Knowing a family's LFF would promote better service planning by ordering appropriate services. Strikingly, parent education is most suitable for Levels 1 and 2 and least suitable at Levels 3–5. Ironically, it is often used first for everyone because it is inexpensive. Unfortunately, that wastes funds and adds to parent-professional friction when parents are not able to extract and use the self-relevant information. LFF 3–5 families need participatory interventions, practical household services, and sometimes psychotherapy for the parents. Using the LFF can reduce wasted services, wasted money, and parents' and professionals' experience of treatment failure.

4.2.2 Screening functional formulations (SFFs)

Screening Functional Formulations (SFFs) are quick screening procedures that ensure wide coverage of relevant, but often overlooked, topics. SSFs *c*onsist of 10 topics: (1) presenting problem, (2) the family structure, (3) the history of danger for the adults

I. Independent and Adequate
Families in this category are able to meet the needs of their children by combining their own skills, help from friends and relatives, and services which they seek and use. Such families, like all families, face problems and crises. It is their competence at resolving these problems which makes them adequate.
II. Vulnerable to Crisis
Families in this category need temporary, i.e., 6 months to a year, help resolving unusual problems; otherwise, the family functions independently and adequately. Examples of common precipitating crises include birth of a handicapped child, divorce, loss of employment, death of a family member, entry of a handicapped child into school, and sexual abuse in day care of a child. Because each of these crises could result in chronic problems, it is the nature of the family's response, not the nature of the crisis, that results in the classification.
III. Restorable
Families in this category are multi-problem families who need several types of training in specific skills or therapy around specific issues. Following intervention, it is expected that the family will function independently and adequately. The period of intervention can be expected to last 1–4 years and require active case management to organize the sequence of service delivery and to integrate the services.
IV. Supportable
There are no rehabilitative services which can be expected to enable these families to become independent and adequate. With specific on-going services, the family can meet the basic physical, intellectual, emotional, and economic needs of their children. Services, and management of those services, will be needed until all the children are grown. Examples of supportable families include those with a mentally retarded mother, a depressed mother, or a parent who abuses alcohol or drugs chronically.
V. Needing New Services
There are no existing services (in the family's locality) sufficient to enable these families to meet the basic needs of their children. New services should be tried or, if permanent injury or death are likely and imminent, permanent placement of the children in another family should be sought.

Table 1.
Levels of family functioning.

(ACEs), (4) unfulfilled family needs, using Maslow's Hierarchy of Needs (see **Figure 1**) [50], (5) somaticized expression of distress, (6) children's perspectives (considering their maturational level), (7) the use of sexuality by each family member (e.g., arousal regulation, self-comfort), (8) developmental transitions for each family member, (9) conflicting responsibilities of the adults, and (10) the appropriateness of specific interventions for family members (using the Gradient of Interventions (see **Figure 2**) [47]. In a written summary, the 10 topics are described in no more than 300 words by the family's primary worker. Then an intervention plan is made or, when a critical cause of the problem cannot be defined or too many important questions remain, a full *Family Functional Formulation* (FFF) is sought.

4.2.3 Family functional formulations

Family Functional Formulations [51, 52] use detailed diagnostic assessments of the entire family. FFFs are needed most often by those families at LFF 3 that have especially complex problems (most LFF 3 families do not require an FFF). FFFs use formal DMM *diagnostic* assessments for all family members and relationships. These attachment assessments are best evaluated by 'blinded' coders who are not biased by pre-existing information. A FFF can identify both the basic strategies used by family members, and the adaptiveness of the strategies in the current family context. A particular advantage of DMM diagnostic assessments is that they can identify active psychological traumas and losses as well as pervasive distorted states of mind, such as depression. These can derail a parent's usual strategic functioning and result in dangerous parenting behavior.

With good, detailed intake assessment, case workers can select interventions suited to adults' ZPD and provide services to keep the children safe until the parents have learned to care adequately for their children. Investment in early assessment can have profound long-term impacts by preventing foster care, reducing costs, reducing

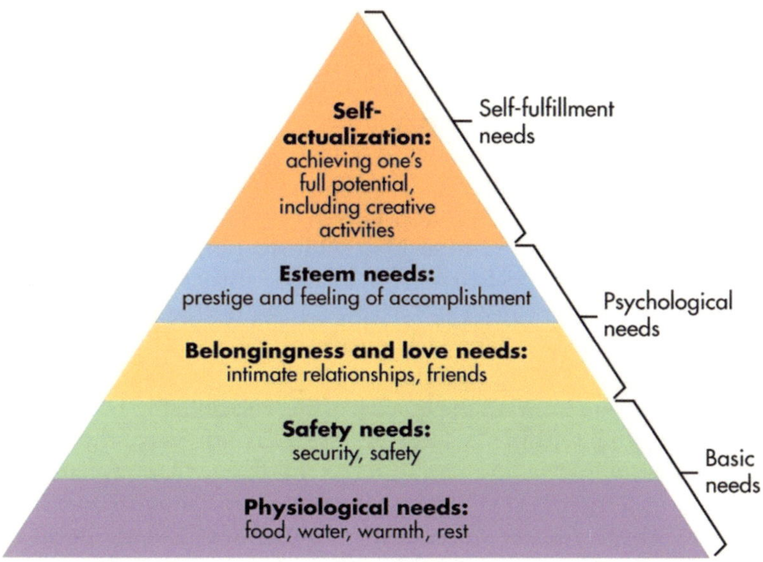

Figure 1.
Maslow's hierarchy of needs.

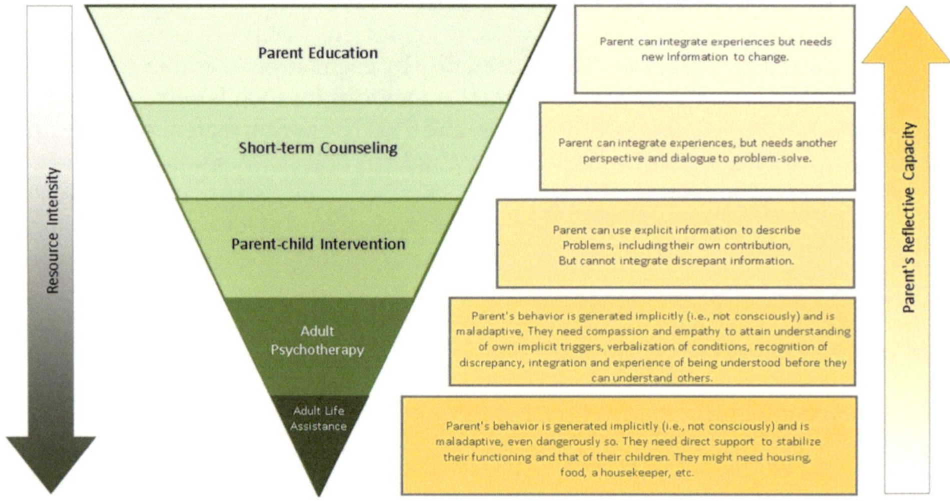

Figure 2.
Gradient of interventions.

professionals' distress, and, most important, protecting vulnerable children and their families. This is the opposite of the common practice of using inexpensive services first and assessing fully when all else fails.

5. Alternatives to placing children in care

In this section, we describe types of initiatives that have prevented the need for foster care. They are ordered from narrowly focused to broadly integrative.

5.1 Learning to observe and reflect

The *1-2-3* intervention was developed by Helen Johnson with Patricia Crittenden in response to a court request for an intervention to assess one mother's relationship with her child, prior to deciding whether to reunify them. Ms. Gotwel had resolved her addiction problems and sought reunification with her 3-year-old daughter Claire whom she had not cared for since infancy. This bespoke intervention was later named '1-2-3' and adapted for other families seeking reunification with their children. The central idea of 1-2-3 was to provide a personalized, sensitive response to each dyad's needs regarding their relationship. 1-2-3 used a 5-minute video-recorded interaction *Toddler CARE-Index* (TCI) [53]. The TCI consists of 3 minutes of play, 1 minute of parent-introduced frustration, and 1 minute of repair.

The 1-2-3 intervention built on the quality of the relationship between mother and daughter by working within Ms. Gotwel's ZPD, as opposed to the more usual approach of organizing intervention around the child's needs. The goals were to help Ms. Gotwel to (1) increase her awareness of her own thoughts and feelings, (2) explore her child's perspective, becoming aware of her likely thoughts and feelings (i.e., theory of mind work), and (3) lastly recognize what motivated her own behavior with her child (i.e., noticing when her behavior was self-protective versus child-protective). The structure of the TCI permitted the professional to begin by focusing on only the relatively positive play section, then move to the more challenging frustration and repair sections.

The professional replayed the TCI several times, sometimes in slow motion, asking Ms. Gotwel to describe what she saw. Step 1 was focused solely on identifying and naming hew own feelings, without any evaluation or approval/disapproval. Ms. Gotwel chose the moments to watch. Once saying how she felt became easy, the professional chose more challenging moments when Ms. Gotwel had negative feelings. This order is important for enabling parents to discover and accept negative feelings. Step 2 was to consider how Claire might have felt in the same moments. Step 3 was to consider whether Ms. Gotwel's actions had been self-protective or child protective. Self-protection was treated as a legitimate reason for acting, but one that a parent should be aware of.

After Step 3, Ms. Gotwel was ready to think about what she wished she had done. This enabled her to practice problem solving when things did not turn out quite as she had wanted, but to do so in a reflective manner and without Claire being present. These steps were repeated many times with new TCI videos taken by Ms. Gotwel.

The 1-2-3 intervention initially involved the professional establishing, as far as possible, a sense of safety in the parent-professional relationship so as to support the parent's capacity for reflection and exploration. This meant that Ms. Gotwel must not feel judged for negative feelings or behavior. To the contrary, she was praised for her recognition of these. This is especially important for birth parents seeking reunification because they all will have experienced negative evaluations and been judged to be inadequate.

To evaluate treatment efficacy, the professional observed (a) Ms. Gotwel's capacity for concrete reflection, (b) Claire's ability to play and explore with her mother without exaggeration or inhibition of negative affect, and (c) the degree of dyadic synchrony in their play. Because Ms. Gotwel did the filming on her mobile phone and the sessions took place over Zoom, this was a relatively low-cost intervention.

After 3 months, the court reunited Claire with her mother. One year later social services were discontinued.

It was crucial that Claire's foster parents were also involved. In this case, the foster parents were Ms. Gotwel's brother and his wife. They had cared for Claire since she was an infant and had expected to adopt her. They felt angry and betrayed by Ms. Gotwel seeking reunification and believed that she could not care adequately for Claire. It was vital for Claire's well-being that they did not pass their negative views to her, and that Claire maintained relationships with them.

Through listening and joint visits, the professional helped the foster parents to understand Ms. Gotwel's perspective and acknowledge the changes she had made. Conversely, Ms. Gotwel was able to see the importance for Claire of her relationship with her foster parents and Claire's need for it to be sustained. Although Claire's foster parents were family relatives, reducing the impact of separation on children and maintaining the relationship between children and foster parents are always important.

A similar, more structured, 10-week home visiting program in the United States is *Promoting First Relationships (PFR)* [54]. PFR is an attachment-based intervention that focuses on parents' reflective capacity using videorecorded observations of parent-child interaction. Every other week parents are videorecorded playing or interacting for 10 to 15 minutes with their child. The following week the parent and provider review the unedited video. PFR trains providers to use 'reflective' questions to help the parents pause and consider their own feelings and needs in the moment and the feelings and needs of their child. Reflection is particularly potent when the interaction is strained, or the child is displaying distress. Providers use parents' reflections to more deeply engage and support parents' insight and understanding of themselves and their child. PFR providers are also trained to provide strengths-based feedback to develop confidence and competence, beginning in the parent's ZPD. In a recent randomized clinical trial of PFR in a sample of reunited birth parents, one parent said:

> *I get it now! I get him! I want to think about him in a different way. It helped me to step back, take a breath, evaluate the situation and understand the situation, why is he acting this way? Is he scared? Is he stressed? Does he need me? It makes it a little more comforting in the situation--and for him, he is more happy and secure, knowing that mom gets what I'm saying or why I'm acting this way. I get him now ([55], p. 25).*

Five randomized control trials, two within child welfare populations, demonstrated that Promoting First Relationships improved parent-child relationships, increased parent's knowledge of child behavior and social-emotional development, regulated child stress physiology, and improved child behavior. Importantly, PFR also reduced foster care placements by 2.5 times and supported greater stability of foster care placements once they occurred [21, 55–58]. PFR had very high retention in child protection populations and high rates of satisfaction, because it is strengths based and supports parents in their ZPD. Such evidence is invaluable to buttress the argument that supporting parents in their capacity to safely reflect, in their ZPD, produces desirable outcomes including reduction of placement into foster care.

5.1.1 Commentary and variations

No intervention works for everyone. In this section, we describe the central features of an intervention, its limitations, and ways that it can be modified.

5.1.2 Video feedback

Video feedback is commonly used now, but it can be ineffective or even have undesirable effects. Play-based interventions involving professionals modeling positive interactions might undermine parents' sense of competence and are unlikely to address reflective integration and problem solving. Video-feedback using only the best moments between parents and children provides fewer opportunities for understanding negative emotions and motivations.

The 1-2-3 program was devised for a specific case because existing interventions did not appear helpful; it began with parents' understanding of themselves, following that with parents' understanding of the child and then more general reflection. The outcomes are anecdotal. PFR focuses more on reflection and has sound, wide-ranging evidence of positive outcomes.

Both 1-2-3 and Promoting First Relationships are tailored to each family. Both are simple, low-cost interventions that can be used when parents wish to improve their relationship with their child. They might not be suitable when parents do not want to change themselves and instead seek to change their child. Nor do they directly address tangible needs (food, safety, housing), but they can be combined with case management and other services.

5.2 Fostering families

Fostering Families in the UK is intended to implement ideas presented by Crittenden and Farnfield [59] to expand the definition of fostering to include long-term support to the *whole* family. The aims were to increase safety for children living with their biological family and prevent foster care with strangers. The project had three crucial components: (1) Whole family focus: parents and child's needs are not seen competing with one another; carers focus on strengths and connection; (2) Transitional attachment figures: long-term support by a single person allows carers to act in the interest of the whole family and be trusted by family members; and (3) Long-term support: many families require support for longer than stipulated by agencies. Fostering families is temporally open-ended. When the FFF indicates, support may be available until the children are grown.

Families referred to Fostering Families are under child protection supervision and assessed as either 'restorable' (LFF 3) or 'supportable' (LFF 4). Typically, they lack kin support. Carers are recruited, assessed, and supported like foster carers, including access to training and support groups; their families are also involved. Each carer is matched to one family in need. The carers' minimum commitment to families is 2 years for at least 15 hours per week, but often it becomes substantially more.

The activities vary to meet specific family needs, including travel to appointments, housework, and freeing parents to spend quality time with their children. The relationship is given time and space to develop as the two families merge, making it possible for the distressed family to experience a kinship connection with the fostering family.

5.2.1 A case example

Ms. Downs (19y) struggled with low mood, suicidal thoughts and managing day-to-day care of her children, Isla (3y) and Alfie (1y). The children's fathers were unknown and there was no other family support. Child Protection was concerned that the children were being neglected. In her own childhood, Ms. Downs had been separated from her birth family as an infant and placed in foster care; at 2 years of age, she was adopted by another family. When she was 12, she reported being abused by her adoptive parents and was placed in another foster home. She then had multiple different foster placements until she was 16 and became pregnant with Isla.

Initially, Ms. Downs was reluctant to accept a referral to Fostering Families. However, she wanted life to be different for her and her children. She wanted to enjoy spending time with them and have the patience to play with them. She wanted a tidier home and she wanted to feel more confident tackling daily tasks.

The Downs family were matched with an approved Fostering Families carer. Ms. Hopewell was 20 years older than Ms. Downs and had herself been a single mother. The 'click' between them was immediate and has lasted. During the first 6 months, radical change occurred for the whole family. Ms. Downs seemed happier and took better care of herself. She and Ms. Hopewell cleaned and organized the home, improved the children's nursery school attendance, and spent time together in the community. Ms. Hopewell invited the Downs family into her wider family, including family gatherings. Occasionally she offered overnight care to the children, so that Ms. Downs could have time to herself or with intimate partners.

After 2 years, there was no longer a plan to end Ms. Hopewell's involvement. Home conditions and school attendance fluctuated, depending on Ms. Downs's mental and physical health. Ms. Downs had several partners move into the home and leave again, usually following domestic altercations. At three and 5 years of age, life for Isla and Alife was in many ways just as, and sometimes more, challenging than it had been before Ms. Hopewell became involved. However, Ms. Hopewell remained in their life, offering time, care, love, and support to the whole family. This added the essential elements of safety and stability, enabling the children to stay with their mother. Ms. Downs sometimes did not accept specific practical elements of support, but she remained in almost daily contact with Ms. Hopewell. It seems important that compliance is not the criterion for success, as it often is when cases go to court. Ms. Hopewell offered to formally foster Isla and Alfie if that ever became needed.

Creating a safe network around a distressed family through the relationship between Ms. Hopewell and Ms. Downs and her children reduced the potential for repeated separations involving short-term foster placements with strangers, particularly strangers from a different social class or cultural group.

5.2.2 Costs

The cost differential between fostering a family in their home and fostering children outside the family is impressive. Two years of Fostering Families support for Ms. Downs's family cost £47,200 (~$60,000) whereas foster care for her two children would have cost £62,960 (~$80,000), plus the substantial cost of court proceedings.

5.2.3 Commentary and variations

Ten Fostering Families carers have been approved to provide long-term support to vulnerable families. Such families have an opportunity to remain together, unharmed by repeated separations. Child protection workers reported feeling hopeful and inspired by the opportunity to fulfill their values and principles of care which led them into their profession. There are increasing numbers of enquiries about Fostering Families as an effective and less expensive alternative to foster care. When applied to other families or by other localities, the details of training, intake, and contractual agreements can vary to fit needs.

5.3 Engaging distressed families with each other

The Mockingbird Society in the USA sought to improve the stability of foster care and reduce youth homelessness from placement breakdown or running away. To do so, it established 'extended families' of six to eight foster families supported by a 'hub home' of trained carers. The hub functioned a bit like an extended family, but with skill-based leadership.

The trained leaders, who were foster parents themselves, emphasized social networking, shared activities and 'normalizing foster care'. Preliminary findings suggested no differences in foster breakdown or running away for the Mockingbird children versus a comparison group. On the other hand, this program did support foster carers and the children found it easier to contact their birth parents and siblings than traditional foster care [60]. A cost-benefit analysis of the Mockingbird Program found no difference in costs.

5.3.1 Commentary and variations

The crucial question is whether this model can be adapted to support distressed *biological* parents with their children. The goals of social networking and shared activities might be more appropriate for troubled biological families than foster families (who have been selected partly based on their already having such skills). The hubs might promote both practical information and skills and a focus on relationships. The hub would create a network of connected families, rather like an extended family. Over time some 'graduate' biological parents could mentor families coming onto the network while other families might need support for a long time, even as long as childhood. This requires society's long-term commitment to children and their families, including a fundamental shift in power away from professionals towards skilled foster carers and biological families.

5.4 Family-centered social work

Love Barrow families (LBf) [30] is the most ambitious of the alternatives that we present. LBf is a community-based pilot service to 20 families living in a severely under-resourced neighborhood in the UK. Statutory service providers jointly funded intense service delivery for very troubled and complex families to test whether coordinated, strengths-based delivery of comprehensive and integrated services would have greater impact than multiple assessments and services delivered by different agencies. The families were deemed "complex" due to intergenerational involvement with mental health and social services.

5.4.1 Setting up a new service delivery process

Initially, a group of community families involved with local services worked with local service providers and executive directors in health and social services to co-design a different approach. Data from adult and child mental health services, child protection and child-in-need cases was reviewed and shared to identify 20 families with complex unresolved problems. Resources from the services were then pooled and reorganized to co-locate a team in the community to implement the top priorities identified by families:

1. *Compassion and understanding*: this underpinned everything, and without these, the other priorities would not be helpful.

2. *Teamwork:* A team that integrated child and parent services, providing 24-hour support when needed.

3. *Local input:* Services developed to meet local needs.

4. *Protecting families from removals:* The Team agreed not to take children away without first being open and clear about their concerns. Families was not to be afraid of having children taken away; they wanted honesty and clarity about professionals' concerns so that they could address them and not lose custody of their children.

5. *Transitional attachment figures:* A trusting relationship with one main professional, i.e., a transitional attachment figure for the parents who then also coordinated all other services.

The service reflected the National Health Service (NHS, UK) integration agenda at the time [61] and was intended as a catalyst for wider reform across the region.

5.4.2 Implementing the new service

The team included a lead social worker, a child and adolescent mental health professional, a systemic psychotherapist, and a consultant psychiatrist, in addition to a number of family workers. Families were assigned a qualified and trained key-worker (who functioned as a transitional attachment figure) based on the presenting issues and needs. Child protection social work, adult and child mental health services, and child-in-need social work were then managed through the project head (Robson) who was employed and managed by the NHS, i.e., within statutory services rather than outside of it.

An occupational therapist, family worker and community support worker were assigned to the team from the adult mental health service. They provided day-to-day support to families as part of the plan which was reviewed and adapted week-to-week to ensure that actions were within the parents' zone of proximal development, were implemented in small manageable steps, and met all statutory requirements.

The project developed one initial psychosocial assessment protocol, rather than the separate assessments used by mental health and social care. This prevented families from having to tell their story repeatedly and brought the information about adult and child functioning into one place. Alongside this were the DMM assessments of attachment which provided a FFF to guide the selection and sequencing of services.

Among the innovative approaches were access to staff during evenings and weekends, group indoor and outdoor activities. Because they have been strongly associated with good mental and physical health but are infrequently included in case planning [62]. A donated building in the neighborhood provided office space for the staff and a safe, accessible meeting space for families and group activities. When the family workers led walks for the parents and children, they hit the mental health jackpot: physical activity, outdoors, in a social context, with an attachment figure leading the group. If someone brought a snack to share, that person experienced the advantages of giving. Such activities aren't in the usual repertoire of mental health professionals, but they lay a basis for good mental health both during and long after the intervention.

The principles of co-production [63] were adhered to by the LBf team so that the service was collaborative and reciprocal - families' views were sought constantly and used to shape intervention and learning. Co-production principles also meant that parents wanted to contribute and knew that their skills were needed. They became volunteers, cooking, painting, organizing activities and giving visitors a warm welcome. They also offered practical support to one another when needed, changing lightbulbs, knitting baby clothes or being a listening ear. These forms of agency can transform a person from the object of professional attention to an important person who contributes to the well-being of others. Pride, based on performance, lends dignity to everyone, but is especially needed by distressed parents.

One of the outcomes that families described was the sense of belonging that they experienced. Parents who experienced this wanted to pass it on to others. One example was a father who went to a medical appointment and, when he saw another family struggling, he put a note on their car under the windscreen wiper with LBf's contact details. A further example of the ethos being enacted between one parent and another was the relationship that grew between two men, one younger who had been abstinent from alcohol for over a year and another older who was in ill health due to his drinking. When the older man lost his sight, he would come in with the letters from the children's home where his son lived and the younger man, knowing how precious these letters were to him, would sit with him and read them to him.

Eventually, two of the original parents were employed by Love Barrow families and became valued members of staff.

5.4.2.1 A case example

Ms. Seback (32y) and her three children were referred to LBf due to longstanding concerns of emotional abuse and neglect which had led to the threat of court proceedings and removal ([52], pp. 353–334). Ms. Seback herself had been in foster care when she was a child - as had her mother. Ms. Seback and her children reached a crisis when the eldest child threatened his mother and sister with a knife and was placed in foster care. All the children were subject to child protection plans which were transferred to and jointly managed by the LBf transitional attachment figure.

Ms. Seback's *DMM Adult Attachment Interview* (DMM-AAI) revealed a history of overwhelming abuse and psychological trauma leading to a disconnection from her feelings and a coping mechanism of "putting things into boxes". The DMM-AAI helped the team to understand Ms. Seback's terror at her son's behavior which ultimately required her to look at the memories that she had locked away. In an amazing moment, Ms. Seback was recalling her feelings about being in foster care when she suddenly wondered if that was how her son felt. That moment of empathy [64] changed the direction of therapy and of her behavior with her son. However, understanding and empathy alone are not enough. Alongside Ms. Seback's therapeutic support, the family also needed hands-on daily practical intervention in the home. The psychological understanding provided by the FFF was used to guide the practical interventions and ensure that they were within Ms. Seback's ZPD. A further consequence of this way of working was that the whole staff team benefitted from the understanding provided by the FFF which enabled them to understand why Ms. Seback and her children behaved as they did and supported them to manage risk meaningfully. After 9 months of intensive support, Ms. Seback's son was returned home and, 6 months later, the child protection cases were closed for all three children.

5.4.3 Outcomes and cost

An independent evaluation of LBf by the University of Northumbria outlined the reduced health and social care costs with this family and included a cost saving of £89,000 (~$113,000) for children's social care and a reduction in the number of agencies involved from nine to just two [33]. A further pertinent outcome was the reduction in mental health and physical health appointments for both Ms. Seback and her children. During the intervention, Ms. Seback had lost a significant amount of weight and was no longer reliant upon mental health medications. She expressed her view as to why she felt that the approach taken by LBf helped her when other interventions had not: "Well, I'm not text book, I am unique" [65].

LBf's evaluation evidenced that overall LBf prevented nine children from being placed in foster care, plus the reduced costs of eliminating child protection plans and other savings across services. In total, LBf cost £250,000 (~$316,000) per year, saving £100,000 (~$126,000) compared to standard service [65].

There was also an 85.3% drop in referrals to adult and child mental health services outside of the team and a 40% reduction in absences from school. There were reductions in the number of crises experienced in families including domestic violence, reduced crime and anti-social behavior, and the number of professionals involved with each family outside of the LBf team. There was also an increase in engagement with local community resources, volunteering, and employability. Volunteering was a surprise benefit; distressed families benefitted from being givers instead of only recipients. Child Protection knocking at your door is not only terrifying; takes away your dignity. Giving to someone else restores it. Families reported that the sense of belonging that they felt to the LBf team meant that they felt able to make changes and they all felt that the co-produced design of the project meant that the priorities identified at the outset were their own [65].

The savings in reduced suffering cannot be calculated and do not end when the program ends. Indeed, the real effects of LBf can already be seen in the next generation. Ms. Seback's daughter now has two children of her own, both of whom are thriving and not subject to any statutory intervention.

5.4.4 Commentary and variations

LBf came about largely through the enthusiasm and commitment of two social workers working with local families and professionals in the health and social services. Someone needs to show dedicated leadership for such programs to succeed. The evaluation attests to the success of co-production of the service and responsiveness of the service to individual needs, cutting across agency limitations and barriers. The challenge to localities and the NHS is to enable services like LBf to become mainstream and change the wider culture and to be less dependent on specific leaders. Given the need for service and general agreement that current service provision is unsustainable [12, 66]. LBf's success is important. LBf highlights the knowledge, passion, and commitment of both helping professionals and the families who come to them; it demonstrates what is possible when families and professionals work together to solve local problems.

5.5 Supporting families

5.5.1 Stuck in a double-bind

Even after years of work, some families continue to face serious problems that threaten their children's well-being. The reasons include generational cycles of family distress, poverty, and structural inequalities [12]. Persistent failure to find relief can block engagement with social services, but when families withdraw, professionals have less information to guide appropriate service referrals. This can result in a double bind of parental resistance and non-compliance eliciting more professional control that produces more resistance.

5.5.2 Breaking the bind

To break this cycle, *Rethinking Families,* a UK initiative (Ellis), re-conceptualized child protection as family support, including exploring the functional meaning of problems and choosing responses that fit parents' ZPDs, without triggering their self-protective strategies. The critical cause of change was providing key workers who built enduring and trusting relationships with parents, i.e. transitional attachment figures, while providing services that ranged from practical day-to-day support to therapeutic interventions. A psychiatrist and experts trained in DMM assessments were also available.

5.5.3 Assessment, service, and success

The referral criteria required that parents be willing to engage and try something different. Parents who misused substances, had intellectual disabilities, or sought to change others but not themselves were excluded. Fourteen families were identified as 'supportable' (LFF 4). These families had entrenched problems with the risk of foster care for the children. Using the Gradient of Interventions (see Appendix 2), most needed adult psychotherapy, indicating that they were not aware of their maladaptive behavior, nor the reasons for it. It was difficult for key workers to engage these parents in transitional attachment relationships because the parents feared the power of workers to remove their children. This threat had to be taken off the table. Daily worker support prevented potential threats from becoming critical.

The Petty family was subject to a Pre-Proceedings Protocol, with placement of the children under consideration because two children were involved in drug trafficking. The key worker's effort increased school attendance, improved parental mental health, and strengthened family relationships, resulting in the family being moved from the Pre-Proceedings Protocol to a 'Child in Need' (a less urgent category) plan. There continued to be fluctuations in progress around drug use, the parental relationship, financial support, and physical neglect; these became the focus of continuing work. Almost daily social work support prevented these threats from becoming critical.

The Painter family was also subject to the Pre-Proceedings Protocol, with plans to remove the four children. After 2 years of Rethinking Families, the mental health and emotional well-being of the mother and the youngest three children had improved such that they were no longer on the edge of care. The 13-year-old girl remained troubled. She self-harmed, but this improved when her artistic talent was discovered and fostered. This enabled her to express herself more fully. Notably, only an out-of-box program could identify and meet her needs. School attendance improved for all the children.

In the Newtry family, one of the children was formally placed with his grandmother, with the other three having Residence Orders. The basis was concerns about intergenerational trauma, child neglect and emotional harm. Foster care was expected; it would have augmented harm to the children [66]. With intensive support, the home conditions, physical care, and supervision of the children improved considerably. Family conflict diminished and the children attended school regularly. The family's status was upgraded to 'Child in Need', without expectation of foster care.

These results used key workers to meet unique family needs. The services were not time limited and were built on family strengths (like art lessons). Housekeeping, taking children to school, offering out-of-hours services, and small grants to cover urgent family needs are not typically offered by agencies. The parents' trust of the key worker signaled to the children that cooperation was safe, thus permitting them to make relationships. Change was a progressive and recursive process, achieved through small steps.

A financial analysis estimated savings of more than £3.5 million (~$4.4 million) from the 41 children remaining with their families after the 2-year pilot [67].

5.5.4 Discontinuing the service

After 2 years, Rethinking Families was discontinued. Understanding the reasons is important for planning future service. Four problems stood out. First was staff turnover. The emotional effort of working in such intensive ways took a toll, especially when workers had personal vulnerabilities. Relational continuity was considered a key factor for sustaining change, yet over time, it could not be provided. Many workers became more involved than the word 'transitional' attachment indicated. Ms. Hopewell provided a better model because she understood and accepted the limits to advising an adult child. Professionals more often expect compliance. Second, it was hard to recruit staff for service on evenings and weekends, when it was most needed. Third, it was very hard to bring a new model of practice to an embedded service structure with such a small pilot team. Only a few senior managers had a working knowledge of the DMM and were invested in the new service. Maybe applying the principle of co-creation from the start would have engaged them. Fourth, families were not included in the planning so neither senior management nor families were invested in the new service.

5.5.5 Commentary and variations

The primary strength of Rethinking Families was establishing trusting relationships with previously hard to reach families. This was the result of a non-judgmental, non-threatening approach backed by frequent contacts that fit families' needs. This enabled workers to challenge families' limitations in ways that showed empathy and demonstrated the process of interpersonal repair. Key workers felt satisfied about working with families in more meaningful and supportive ways. Team members thought that previous work in risk-averse, budget-led, and time-limited services had been detrimental to families.

Difficulties included the contradiction between selecting *Supportable* (LFF4) families and expecting change as if they were *Restorable* (LFF3); instead, stabilization with long-term services would have been a more appropriate goal for these families. This misplaced expectation impacted staff well-being and retention. The lack of a manager to liaise with higher management and to ensure on-going funding was another problem. The service was more expensive than standard service unless it was compared to the costs of court proceedings and foster care; long-term budgeting and dissemination of the advantages were needed. A means of providing an *on-call* service, such as doctors have, was needed for these families in which life-threatening conditions could occur suddenly. The DMM assessments were essential to individualized planning, but the funds and personnel for these assessments were insufficient. Even the notion of early and detailed assessment to *prevent* foster placement was different from ordinary practice—which tended to withhold expensive assessment until child protection needed to confirm the need for placement. Another problem was defining what was 'good enough' to allow children to live with their parents.

Rethinking Families defined care as good enough when the children are safe and access to intensive support is available for as long as there are children in the family. That challenged ordinary standards. Possibly less than 'just barely good enough' [52] should be the standard for separating children from their parents. This needed to be accepted by higher management for Rethinking Families to endure.

5.6 Repairing the damage of good intentions

A Norwegian case of reunification highlights some reasons to avoid foster care. It also demonstrates the successful application of the ideas in this chapter to repair the harm resulting from foster care [68]. Mr. and Mrs. Ibrahem fled Syria's civil war across the Mediterranean Sea through Greece to Norway where they hoped to find safety for themselves and their two young boys. Instead, they found life hard, but in unfamiliar ways that they did not know how to manage. They began arguing and sometimes the boys saw their father hitting their mother. Child Protection placed the boys in short-term foster care to protect them and to give their parents time to repair their marriage.

Instead, the marriage broke up. A year and a half after being placed in a Norwegian foster home, the boys were returned to their mother's care. They hardly knew her, having only seen her briefly and at long intervals, partly because she lived several hours away. She did not know them either; they had changed a lot in 18 months, and she had not been part of their development. Adding to their re-adjustment problems were that the boys now spoke Norwegian and no longer spoke Arabic, as Mrs. Ibrahem did. They had forgotten Arabic because they never heard their native language except during contact. This resulted in many misunderstandings between mother and sons. Plus, they were squeezed into a tiny apartment, the only one Mrs. Ibrahem could afford; in the middle class foster home, they had had their own bedrooms.

The boys did not settle easily, giving their mother the impression that they were unhappy with her. They protested her limits and rules, howling and screaming at her, saying she wasn't their mother. They punched her and swore. The older boy pointed his finger at her and said he wanted another mom. Mrs. Ibrahem's emotions overwhelmed her. At 5 years old, her son would not let her touch him while she desperately wanted to hold him. She wondered why he rejected her and blamed herself; she wasn't told that he had behaved similarly while in care. She was scared that, if child protection saw this, they would take her sons away again. So even though she was very distressed, she never showed or talked about it to anyone, no matter how she felt. That meant no one could help her.

It took an insightful professional (Karlsen) to imagine what Mrs. Ibrahem had not said and both help her to understand what was happening and reassure her that she would not lose her boys again (like LBf). That reassurance made it possible to help her. Together they arranged family meetings so that many family members got involved to help the family (like kincare). The professional helped her get back into motherhood with personalized work so she could become a safe caregiver for her children (like a transitional attachment figure). An immigrant family from Syria was found to help with childcare (like fostering families). The older boy was offered trauma treatment. In addition, the professional believed that the children should have the opportunity to meet with the foster parents to ensure that the children's lives were connected (like the Mockingbird program). The children saw that their mother and foster parents both loved them and could work together (like 1-2-3). That made all the loyalty issues disappear and Mrs. Ibrahem could begin to talk with her children about their experiences in the foster home. Together, they filled in the missing time when they had been apart. The professional helped the mother to understand that the children's challenging behavior was related to adverse experiences the children had had in their early years, as well as adaptation to a new family culture and the need to develop relationships with the foster family. She also helped the mother to distinguish between her own needs and feelings and those of her children, and to realize that the children needed her to "see the world" from their point of view (like 1-2-3 and PFR).

It wasn't easy because Mrs. Ibrahem had had unfortunate relationship experiences in her past. So had her husband; he was later diagnosed with PTSD. Child Protection workers had not understood that life in a war zone and the process of escaping it were so dangerous that psychological trauma was almost inevitable [69]. Mr. and Mrs. Ibrahem had tried to keep their children and themselves alive – and they had succeeded! As Crittenden and her colleagues state in "Staying Alive," keeping the children alive is the single most essential responsibility of a parent and Mr. and Mrs. Ibrahem succeeded in protecting their children through extreme dangers. They were less able to manage in a safe environment and could not meet Norwegian standards for middle class life. But all of that was known when they arrived in Norway as war refugees! Why could not support and individualized treatment have been offered before the family broke down? Why could not the professionals and court see how protective the parents were and understand their need for protection themselves as they tried to cope with moving from war-torn Syria to foreign Norway? Prevention saves so much suffering – and it costs much less money. It took a year, but now Mrs. Ibrahem and her sons function well. Their case has been closed - but their father is no longer in their family.

5.6.1 Prevention is better than repair

We think preventive service might have preserved the whole family and saved everyone, especially the two young boys, from intense suffering. Moreover, now that neuroscience has made clear that early experience shapes brain development [70], we should strive to ensure that children do not experience traumatizing separation from their parents – and a second separation from their foster parents. Such separations cause avoidable iatrogenic harm. We can reunify families, but we cannot completely undo the psychological effects of adverse experience on developing brains. Fostering the Ibrahem might have worked better than fostering their children.

Everything that the professional did to support reunification is listed in this chapter as an alternative to foster care: extended family support, fostering whole families by culturally similar families, individualized parenting guidance in the parents' ZPD, individual trauma treatment, joining biological and foster families for the children's experience of continuity, differentiating parent and child perspectives, and age-suitable talking within the family about the children's experiences and perspectives. Possibly most important was the shared planning between Mrs. Ibrahem and the professional who worked with her.

All these approaches could have been implemented before separating the children from their mother. All the harm that Crittenden and Spieker [4, 5] found was associated with separation happened to these two boys and their parents: broken parent-child bonds, discomfort with closeness, behavior problems, psychological trauma from separation and distrust of professionals. Why could not these painful outcomes have been avoided by offering alternatives to foster care first?

5.6.2 Commentary and variations

This case is uncomfortably reminiscent of the way Norway, Australia, Canada, and the USA treated their native peoples [5]. Some professionals might think that this case can be dismissed because the family were refugees from a war zone where everyone had suffered psychological trauma. Instead, a close look at the personal histories of maltreating parents [71, 72] and the neighborhoods in which they live [73, 74] indicates that they too live in cultures of danger and suffering that almost always interfere with meeting middle class standards for childrearing. Mrs. Ibrahem chose to share her experience in publication [68]; in doing so, she moved from being the recipient of unwanted services to using her own resources to help others. This is a powerful testimony to the success of collaborative work between parents and professionals.

We think this Norwegian case highlights the changes that are needed in the next generation of alternatives to foster care in many countries. We address these next.

6. Part 5: conclusion

The only person you can change is yourself. This truism highlights the paradox of helping professionals trying to help others to change. Our review of alternatives to foster care suggests several ways that direct service professionals, managers and supervisors, policy makers, judges, and legislators could act to reduce the harm done by foster care. A central advantage of these ideas is that all were generated and implemented by clinicians in their daily settings; these are not ivory-tower, university-based, theoretically structured ideas. Each was built to function in the real and messy world of day-to-day child protection in local settings. Strikingly, all were effective with children and families and all saved money compared to placing children in foster care. Most important, they all reduced the iatrogenic suffering caused by separating children from their caregivers. Children, families, and professionals were all protected by the alternative we offer.

Because none of these alternatives has been implemented widely, despite being more effective and less far less costly than foster care, we also consider limitations to these approaches and the possible reasons why professionals might not use them. We conclude with some specific recommendations for action.

6.1 Ideas to retain in future approaches

Interventions that protected children in economically efficient ways had several characteristics in common. We offer ten basic principles.

1. *Both-and solutions*: Most important is that these alternatives to foster care were what Crittenden and Spieker called 'both-and' solutions [4, 5]; they were not a single best solution, but instead a combination of successful solutions, each fine-tuned to local conditions.

2. *Co-created services*: The most successful approaches *valued parent input* from the beginning and throughout; this gave parents agency (a strong mental health benefit) and often improved the service itself. It was also crucial that professionals, at all levels of the service structure, participated in the planning for their locality; this provided a *'buy-in' across the professional bureaucracy and community*.

This was fundamentally different from professionals functioning as a top-down team of service providers, delivering preset or manualized programs, managing services, and separating family members when there was trouble.

3. *Whole family focus*: In every case, even 1-2-3, *whole families were the focus*. Indeed, most distressed parents have experienced the very sorts of developmental histories from which we wish to protect their children. For anyone in a family to thrive, everyone must thrive [52].

4. *Communication skills*: Learning how to communicate with various types of professionals enabled parents to better present their perspectives and receive the services that they needed. Families assessed and treated as 'supportable' (LFF4), felt supported.

5. *Expanding connections*: Successful approaches *expanded parents' support networks*, through professionals becoming *transitional attachment figures, engaging kin* networks, or *fostering the whole distressed family*.

6. *24/7 availability*: A crucial advantage was associated with *being available* when family problems were likely to occur, that is, *on evenings and weekends*.

7. *Reflective integration*: Another important characteristic of successful alternatives to foster placement was parents' opportunity to observe themselves and recognize, without evaluation, their feelings, especially negative feelings [75]. Having a trusted professional to support reflecting on these and imagining their children's perspectives elicited theory of mind in both parents and professionals. Imagining how the other person feels is crucial to attuned behavior.

8. *Respecting family culture*: *Respecting families' culture* was central to families' sense of safety; this included not placing children in homes unlike their parents' home in social class, religion, ethnicity, etc.

9. *University input: Affiliation with a university* ensured access to a breadth of ideas, sound design, precise assessment, and critical analysis that yielded evidence about the crucial processes and their outcomes. These could then be adapted for individual professionals and families.

10. *Promoting basic mental health*: The most successful programs *promoted basic mental health strategies* as part of the intervention (for example, social connections with friends and family, physical activity outdoors, and balanced and regular meals [62]). LBf's Saturday group walks did four of these in one easy activity: social engagement with exercise outdoors when parents were not at work.

Money is always a concern. *Redirecting money spent on foster care to preventive services* could be done without needing additional funds. Similarly *redirecting some welfare funds to prevention services* would both increase the probability of family competence and independence and also reduce the risk of parents becoming welfare dependent. In both cases, paying entry level workers, night and weekend workers, and experienced supervisors enough to retain and build their skills is crucial; *paying staff well* is essential to having skilled staff. At the legislative and policy levels, *preventive and supportive services should be given funding priority over foster care*. *Reducing supervisory positions* (possibly through attrition only) and *reducing record-keeping requirements* would change the balance of spending on services versus bureaucratic functions. Consideration should be given to *ending foster care*, leaving the choices of sustaining families or having their children adopted immediately and permanently. Doing this would stop the dreadful harm of multiple separations. All of these proposals rely on currently allocated funds and offer the possibility of reduced financial needs going forward.

Our final recommendation is to use local co-creation of services to allow *variation among services*. After several decades of developing (and selling) mandated programs, it might be time to empower the creativity of local communities (from parents to professionals) to address their own problems. Let us treasure variation in people, families, professionals, and programs, highlighting the best in each. Let us find everyone's unique up-side and build on it. *Programs built on principles* might be more effective than defined, manualized, and replicable programs that do not have on-going input from service users.

6.2 Improvements to make

Most of these ideas are not new and most are validated in research and clinical literature. It is important to understand why they worked in these situations but did not spawn extensions.

Several conditions might have impeded the acceptance of these alternatives to foster care. One is an implicit, unspoken feeling that parents who endanger their children do not deserve to raise the children or to receive special individualized services. However, most of these parents were once unprotected children, often in foster care themselves, who suffered then and suffer now, as they struggle to do better than their parents did. Unfortunately, the system continues to threaten them, often with very little compassion for their experience. Recognition that *today's distressed parents were yesterday's distressed children* whom we did not protect adequately might help to soften punitive attitudes. Taking parents' perspective when they receive a knock on the door by child protection might help. As Robson noted for LBf noted, compassion is the essential base upon which everything else is built.

Recognition that separating children from their parents (or threatening to do so) harms both the children and their parents is new and unfamiliar information. Rather than demonstrating that separation is the way to solve problems, the alternatives that we offer can help to prime children both neurologically and behaviorally to seek solutions with family and supportive people. *Knowing how much iatrogenic harm is caused by 'protective' foster care might change professionals' recommendations*.

Another barrier to reducing the use of foster care may be a societal emphasis on independence, leading to an assumption that meeting the needs of long-term care families (LFF3-5) leads to undesirable dependency. Acceptance that change can take more than one generation is important. It begins with stopping the harm.

The advantage of professionals taking the role of transitional attachment figures was sometimes accompanied by over-involvement and burnout. *Having professional support teams* [5] that emphasized the limits of professional possibility and responsibility might reduce this source of stress for professionals.

Senior managers and policy makers are crucial for dissemination of new ideas and yet the discussed programs depended more on front-line clinicians and middle managers. Robson (personal communication, January 10, 2024) noted that she was mentored and protected by someone high in the command chain. Political will and leadership are critical to systemic change, yet most leadership is removed from the day-to-day challenge of keeping children safe and families together. We conclude that *inclusive decision-making (from families through service providers, managers, local politicians, legislators, and attorneys and judges) generates the most effective programs and leaves no one with too much responsibility.*

There will always be children who must be protected from their parents. Because foster care, as opposed to adoption, involves two separations (thus increasing the detrimental traumatic effects on brain functioning), we suggest that foster care not be used at all. Instead, high frequency, even daily, service should be provided. Nevertheless, when the home is so dangerous that even daily home visits cannot protect the children from parental outbursts, permanent adoption should be sought immediately. Because that solution is so drastic, professionals will almost always find ways to help the biological family.

For most troubled families, alternatives will be more protective than foster care. Nevertheless, because no solution can be perfect 100% of the time, professionals must be protected from problems that they did not foresee. Doing so can make child- and family-protection more prominent than professional self-protection. Right now, failure to remove a child who is later seriously harmed can put professionals at risk; laws and protocols that acknowledge the impossibility of perfect prediction of risk and that protect professionals when seriously dangerous outcomes occur are needed. That is, professionals' need to protect themselves should not put children at greater risk. Including the emotional and neurological harm of foster care in the evaluation of the need for foster care might protect both children and professionals. Our hope is that having safe alternatives to foster care can shift the focus from protecting professionals from blame to protecting children with their families.

Finally, the goals of avoiding foster care must be clear. A central goal is to avoid the iatrogenic harm that professionals cause by separating children from their caregivers. This will also reduce multigeneration family breakdown. Preventing the iatrogenic harm from separation is easily understood. More subtle is that our best services might only maintain the safety of some families without freeing the family needing assistance (Supportable LFF4 families) and that this, too, is a worthy goal. Accepting that can be difficult for clinicians and policy makers who want families to change. Reframing such outcomes as preventing iatrogenic harm can highlight what was gained.

6.3 Limitations

Although we can demonstrate case-based successes and the cost benefits of these alternatives to foster care, we cannot claim that a program's effectiveness was supported by gold standard research methods. An exception is Promoting First Relationships (PFR). When PFR researchers accessed administrative child welfare data years after the intervention, they found that the PFR group experienced significantly fewer child removals to out of home care. Nevertheless, as encouraging as this finding is, it can only be described at the group level. We cannot determine which specific families will and will not benefit, or even be harmed by, PFR or any alternative to foster care included in this chapter.

The reason is that success was dependent upon individualization of a range of intervention components. Individualization in turn was dependent on the skill of the providers in assessing family needs and then selecting and delivering support.

Each technique or action had empirically supportive evidence, but no technique is ever 100% effective. Further, their combination in each family's intervention was unique. In this chapter, we highlight the value of sets of clinical case studies, in which each case is based on the foundational principles, but none intervenes in precisely the same manner as any other [76–78]. It is in the gap between generalized information and person- or family-specific needs that clinical expertise is needed. Research on the characteristics and experience of successful clinicians is necessary, but beyond the scope of this chapter.

6.4 A final idea

First do no harm. Sometimes a little knowledge is a dangerous thing. If you learn only the dangers of foster care and do not learn to replace it with safe alternatives, you will have left children and their families at risk. If you use an alternative to foster care, you will have switched from doing unforeseen harm to doing the good you intended all along. If you think of a new combination of sound ideas, your creativity can propel your work further than faithful replication of someone else's ideas. If you pass the word up your chain of command, you multiply the good you are doing. Protecting families, supporting professionals, and engaging communities creates a *win-win-win* situation in which everyone wins and society is strengthened.

This chapter is being completed in early 2024. Is there something you can do to protect children and their families from foster care this year? What will you offer instead?

Author details

Patricia Crittenden[1*], Steve Farnfield[2], Susan Spieker[3], Andrea Landini[1], Monica Oxford[4], Katrina Robson[5], Siw Karlsen[6], Helen Johnson[7], Vicki Ellis[8] and Zoe Ash[9]

1 Family Relations Institute, Reggio Emilia, Italy

2 University of Roehampton, UK

3 University of Washington, USA

4 Barnard Center for Infant and Early Childhood Mental Health, University of Washington, USA

5 Love Barrow Families Community Interest Company, England

6 Self-Employed Social Worker, Norway

7 Attachment Works, UK

8 SWIFT Specialist Family Services, East Sussex County Council, UK

9 Bath and North East Somerset Council, UK

*Address all correspondence to: pmcrittenden@gmail.com

References

[1] Paddock C, Waters-Roman D, Borja J. Child welfare: History and policy. Encyclopedia of Social Work. 2022. DOI: 10.1093/acrefore/9780199975839.013.530

[2] Bowlby J. Child Care and the Growth of Love. London: Pelican; 1953

[3] Wilkins D. Book review: Cornerstones of attachment research by Duschinsky Robbie. Journal of Social Work. 2022;**22**(2):584-587. DOI: 10.1177/14680173211061788

[4] Crittenden PM, Spieker SJ. The effects of separation from parents on children. In: Cameron KD, editor. Child Abuse and Neglect - Perspectives and Research. London, UK, London, UK: IntechOpen; 2023. p. Ch. 0. DOI: 10.5772/intechopen.1002940

[5] Crittenden PM, Spieker SJ. The Effects of Separation from Parents on Children. 2023. Available from: https://familyrelationsinstitute.org/wp-content/uploads/Separation-5-15-23.docx-2.pdf

[6] Ottaway H, Selwyn J. "No-One Told us it Was Going to be like this": Compassion Fatigue and Foster Carers. Research Gate Technical Report; 2016. Available from: https://www.researchgate.net/publication/310803273_No-one_told_us_it_was_going_to_be_like_this_compassion_fatigue_and_foster_carers

[7] Reamer FG. Moral injury in social work: Responses, prevention, and advocacy. Families in Society. 2022;**103**(3):257-268. DOI: 10.1177/10443894211051020

[8] Helfer RE, Kempe. The Battered Child. Chicago: University of Chicago Press; 1968

[9] 2022 AFCARS Report #29. In: U.S Department of Health and Human Services, Administration on Children, Youth and Families, Children's Bureau. 2023. Available from: https://www.acf.hhs.gov/sites/default/files/documents/cb/afcars-report-29.pdf

[10] Children's Bureau (Administration on Children Youth, and Families. Child Maltreatment 2021. Washington, DC; 2023. Available from: https://www.acf.hhs.gov/cb/data-research/child-maltreatment

[11] Bennett DL, Schluter DK, Melis G, Bywaters P, A, Barr B, et al. Child poverty and children entering care in England, 2015-20: A longitudinal ecological study at the local area level. The Lancet Public Health. 2022;**7**(6):e496-e503. Available from: https://www.ncbi.nlm.nih.gov/pubmed/35660211

[12] Gupta A. Poverty and child neglect – The elephant in the room? Families, Relationships, and Societies. 2017;**6**(1):21-36

[13] Polonko KA. Exploring assumptions about child neglect in relation to the broader field of child maltreatment. Journal of Health and Human Services Administration. 2006;**29**(3):260-284. Available from: https://www.jstor.org/stable/25790694

[14] Dettlaff AJ, Boyd R. Racial disproportionality and disparities in the child welfare system: Why do they exist, and what can be done to address them? Annals of the American Academy of Political and Social Science. 2020;**692**(1):253-274. DOI: 10.1177/0002716220980329

[15] GOV.UK. Children looked after in England including Adoptions. 2023. GOV.

UK. Children looked after in England including adoptions. 2023

[16] Brownell M, McMurty D. Huffington Post Canada. 2016. Available from: https://www.huffingtonpost.ca/marni-brownell/foster-care-in-canada_b_8491318.htm

[17] Roberts L, Meakings M, Forrester D, Smith A, Shelton K. Care-leavers and their children placed for adoption. Children and Youth Services Review. 2017;**79**:355-361. DOI: 10.1016/j.childyouth.2017.06.030

[18] Oakley M, Miscampbell G, Gregorian R. Looked After-Children: The Silent Crisis. London: The Social Market Foundation; 2018. Available from: https://www.smf.co.uk/wp-content/uploads/2018/08/Silent-Crisis-PDF.pdf

[19] Biehal N, Sinclair I, Wade J. Reunifying abused or neglected children: Decision-making and outcomes. Child Abuse & Neglect. 2015;**49**:107-118. Available from: https://www.ncbi.nlm.nih.gov/pubmed/25975846

[20] Rubin DM, O'Reilly AL, Luan X, Localio AR. The impact of placement stability on behavioral well-being for children in foster care. Pediatrics. 2007;**119**(2):336-344. Available from: http://www.ncbi.nlm.nih.gov/entrez/query.fcgi?cmd=Retrieve&db=PubMed&dopt=Citation&list_uids=17272624

[21] Spieker SJ, Oxford ML, Kelly JF, Nelson EM, Fleming CB. Promoting first relationships: Randomized trial of a relationship-based intervention for toddlers in child welfare. Child Maltreatment. 2012;**17**(4):271-286. Available from: https://www.ncbi.nlm.nih.gov/pubmed/22949743

[22] Chisholm K. A three year follow-up of attachment and indiscriminate friendliness in children adopted from Romanian orphanages. Child Development. 1998;**69**(4):1092-1106. Available from: https://www.ncbi.nlm.nih.gov/pubmed/9768488

[23] Font SA, Gershoff ET. An Introduction to Foster Care. Foster Care and Best Interests of the Child: Integrating Research, Policy, and Practice. Cham: Springer International Publishing; 2020. pp. 1-19. DOI: 10.1007/978-3-030-41146-6_1

[24] Marthinsen E, Skjefstad N, Juberg A, Garrett PM. Social Work and Neoliberalism. Oxfordshire, England, UK: Routledge; 2021. DOI: 10.4324/9781003142225

[25] Munro E. Munro review of child protection. Final report. A Child Centered System [Online]. Department for Education. 2011. Available from: https://assets.publishing.service.gov.uk/government/uploads/system/uploads/attachment_data/file/175391/Munro-Review.pdf

[26] Featherstone B, Gupta A. Protecting Children: A Social Model. Bristol, UK: Policy Press; 2018

[27] MacAlister J. The independent review of children's social care. Final report. In: Education Df, editor. London; 2022. Available from: https://hubble-live-assets.s3.amazonaws.com/birth-companions/file_asset/file/491/The-independent-review-of-childrens-social-care-Final-report.pdf

[28] Office for Standards in Education. Children's Services and Skills. Main Findings: Children's Social Care in England. Gov UK; 2023. Available from: https://www.gov.uk/government/publications/ofsted-annual-report-202122-education-childrens-services-and-skills

[29] Competition and Markets Authority. Children's social Care Market Study 2022. Available from: https://www.gov.uk/government/publications/childrens-social-care-market-study-final-report

[30] Robson K, Tooby A, Duschinsky R. Love Barrow Famlies: A case study of transforming public services. In: Vincent S, editor. Early Intervention: Supporting and Strengthening Families. Dunedin Edinburgh; 2015. pp. 84-98

[31] Vygotsky LS. Mind and Society: The Development of Higher Psychological Processes. Cambridge, MA: Harvard University Press; 1978

[32] Crittenden PM. Relationships at risk. In: Belsky J, Nezworski T, editors. Clinical Implications of Attachment. Hillsdale, NJ: Lawrence Erlbaum; 1988. pp. 136-174

[33] Crittenden PM. The social ecology of treatment: Case study of a service system for maltreated children. The American Journal of Orthopsychiatry. 1992;**62**(1):22-34. Available from: https://www.ncbi.nlm.nih.gov/pubmed/1546756

[34] Crittenden P. Strategies for changing parental behavior. APSAC Advisor. 1991:9

[35] Crittenden PM, DiLalla DL. Compulsive compliance: The development of an inhibitory coping strategy in infancy. Journal of Abnormal Child Psychology. Oct 1988;**16**:585-599. DOI: 10.1007/BF00914268

[36] Winokur M, Holtan A, Batchelder KE. Kinship care for the safety, permanency, and well-being of children removed from the home for maltreatment. Cochrane Database of Systematic Reviews. 2014;**1**:CD006546. Available from: https://www.ncbi.nlm.nih.gov/pubmed/24488572

[37] Taylor S, Blackshaw E, Lawrence H, Stern D, Gilbert L, Raghoo N. Randomised Control Trial of Family Group Conferencing at Pre-Proceedings Stage. London, UK: Coram, Foundations; 2023. Available from: https://foundations.org.uk/wp-content/uploads/2023/06/Randomised-controlled-trial-family-group-conferencing.pdf

[38] Coram BAAF. Statistics on Special Guardianship. 2023. Available from: https://corambaaf.org.uk/practice-areas/kinship-care/special-guardianship/statistics-special-guardianship

[39] Harwin J, Alrouh B, Broadhurst K, McQuarrie T, Golding L, Ryan M. Child and parent outcomes in the London family drug and alcohol court five years on: Building on international evidence. International Journal of Law, Policy and the Family. 2018;**32**(2):140-169

[40] Harwin J, Simmonds J, Broadhurst K, Brown R. Special Guradianship: A Review of the English Research Studies. 2019. Available from: https://www.nuffieldfjo.org.uk/wp-content/uploads/2021/05/Nuffield-FJO_Special-guardianship_English-research-studies_final.pdf

[41] Svanberg PO, Mennet L, Spieker S. Promoting a secure attachment: A primary prevention practice model. Clinical Child Psychology and Psychiatry. 2010;**15**(3):363-378. Available from: http://www.ncbi.nlm.nih.gov/pubmed/20603424

[42] Centro nazionale di documentazione e analisi per l'infanzia e l'adolescenza. Dipartimento per le politiche della famiglia, Presidenza del Consiglio dei Ministri. I Programma P.I.P.P.I. 2010. Available from: https://www.minori.gov.it/it/il-programma-pippi

[43] Arnaldi G. Bibbiano: cos'è successo, il caso dall'inizio. Gli arresti, i processi, le polemiche. E ora cosa succede? Corriere Della Sera. 2023. Available from: https://www.corriere.it/cronache/23_giugno_07/bibbiano-cos-successo-caso-dall-inizio-arresti-processi-polemiche-ora-cosa-succede-bab80086-0525-11ee-874a-78fbf24a95c4.shtml

[44] Regione Piemonte. Allontanamento zero. Interventi a sostegno della genitorialità e norme per la prevenzione degli allontanamenti dal nucleo familiare d'origine. Legge Regionale. 2022. p. 17. Available from: http://www.regione.piemonte.it/governo/bollettino/abbonati/2022/44/suppo2/00000001.htm

[45] Cubelli R La. Psicologia in tribunale: Le teorie non sono ricette [psychology in the courtroom: Theories are not recipes]. Psicologia Clinica dello Sviluppo. 2023;**27**;1

[46] Whitaker DJ, Gurbani A, Rao N. Interventions to prevent violence in the family. In: Sturmey P, editor. Violence in Families: Integrating Research into Practice. Switzerland AG: Springer Nature; 2023. pp. 201-225. DOI: 10.1007/978-3-031-31549-7_9

[47] Crittenden PM. Raising Parents: Attachment, Representation, and Treatment. second ed. London: Routledge; 2016

[48] Felitti VJ, Anda RF, Nordenberg D, Williamson DF, Spitz AM, Edwards V, et al. Relationship of childhood abuse and household dysfunction to many of the leading causes of death in adults. The adverse childhood experiences (ACE) study. American Journal of Preventive Medicine. 1998;**14**(4):245-258. Available from: https://www.ncbi.nlm.nih.gov/pubmed/9635069

[49] Crittenden PM, Ainsworth MDS. Child maltreatment and attachment theory. In: Cicchetti D, Carlson V, editors. Handbook of Child Maltreatment. New York: Cambridge University Press; 1989. pp. 432-463

[50] Maslow AH. Motivation and Personality. New York: Harper & Row; 1954

[51] Dallos R, Crittenden PM, Landini A, Vetere A. Family functional formulations as guides to psychological treatment. Contemporary Family Therapy. 2019;**42**:202-203. Available from: https://www.ncbi.nlm.nih.gov/pubmed/9635069

[52] Crittenden PM. The secret lives of children. Child Psychology and Psychiatry. 2017;**22**:345. DOI: 10.1177/1359104517715933

[53] Crittenden PM. CARE-Index: Toddlers Coding Manual. Unpublished manuscript, Miami, FL. Available from the author. 1992

[54] Kelly J, Sandoval D, Zuckerman TG, Buehlman K. Promoting First Relationships: A program for service providers to help parents and other caregivers nurture young children's social and emotional development. 2nd ed. Seattle, WA: University of Washington NCAST Programs; 2008

[55] Oxford M, Abrahamson-Richards T, O'Leary R, Booth-LaForce C, Spieker S, Rees J, et al. The Development of the Promoting First Relationships® Home Visiting Program and Caregivers' Comments about their Experiences across Four RCT Studies. Seattle, WA USA: University of Washington; 2024

[56] Booth-LaForce C, Oxford ML, O'Leary R, Buchwald DS. Promoting first relationships (R) for primary caregivers

and toddlers in a native community: A randomized controlled trial. Prevention Science. 2023;**24**(1):39-49. Available from: https://www.ncbi.nlm.nih.gov/pubmed/35997845

[57] Booth-LaForce C, Oxford ML, Barbosa-Leiker C, Burduli E, Buchwald DS. Randomized controlled trial of the promoting first relationships(R) preventive Interv ention for primary caregivers and toddlers in an American Indian community. Prevention Science. 2020;**21**(1):98-108. Available from: https://www.ncbi.nlm.nih.gov/pubmed/31754964

[58] Oxford ML, Hash JB, Lohr MJ, Bleil ME, Fleming CB, Unutzer J, et al. Randomized trial of promoting first relationships for new mothers who received community mental health services in pregnancy. Developmental Psychology. 2021;**57**(8):1228-1241. DOI: 10.1037/dev0001219

[59] Crittenden PM, Farnfield S. Fostering families: An integrative approach involving the biological and foster family systems. In: Lee RE, Whiting JB, editors. Handbook of Relational Therapy for Foster Children and their Families. Washington, D.C: Child Welfare League of America; 2007. pp. 227-250

[60] Ott E, McGrath-Lone L, Pinto V, Danders-Ellis D, Trivedi H. Mockingbird Programme: Evaluation Report, Assets Publishing. UK: Department of Education; 2020. Available from: https://assets.publishing.service.gov.uk/media/5fa412dfd3bf7f03a40fe598/Fostering_Network_Mockingbird.pdf

[61] Thistlethwaite P. Integrating Health and Social Care in Torbay. Improving the Care for Mrs Smith. London: The King's Fund; 2011. Available from: https://assets.kingsfund.org.uk/f/256914/x/4267f4f7fb/integrated_health_social_care_torbay_march_2011.pdf

[62] Gootman JA, Eccles J, editors. Community Programs to Promote Youth Development. Washington, DC: National Academies Press; 2002

[63] Boyle D, Harris M. The Challenge of co-Production. Vol. 56. London: New Economics Foundation; 2009. p. 18

[64] Zhang H, Gao X, Liang Y, Yao Q, Wei Q. Does child maltreatment reduce or increase empathy? A systematic review and meta-analysis. Trauma, Violence, & Abuse. 2024;**25**(1):166-182. Available from: https://journals.sagepub.com/doi/abs/10.1177/15248380221145734

[65] Vincent S. The Magic Is in the co-Production: Full Report from the Evaluation of the Love Barrow Families Project. University of Northumbria; 2017. Available from: https://www.lovebarrowfamilies.co.uk/wp-content/uploads/2018/02/Love-Barrow-families-Full-Evaluation-Report-2017.pdf

[66] Gao S, Assink M, Bi C, Chan KL. Child maltreatment as a risk factor for rejection sensitivity: A three-level meta-analytic review. Trauma, Violence, & Abuse. 2024;**25**(1):680-690. Available from: https://journals.sagepub.com/doi/abs/10.1177/15248380231162979

[67] Ellis V, Pratt C, Leigh J. Rethinking Families Evaluation April 2022. East Sussex, UK: East Sussex County Council; 2022

[68] Karlsen SL. Da barna kom hjem. Fontene. 2024

[69] Mowafi H, Hariri M, Alnahhas H, Ludwig E, Allodami T, Mahameed B, et al. Results of a Nationwide capacity survey of hospitals providing trauma Care in war-Affected Syria. JAMA

Surgery. 2016;**151**(9):815-822. Available from: https://www.ncbi.nlm.nih.gov/pubmed/27332144

[70] Galvan A. Adolescent brain development and contextual influences: A decade in review. Journal of Research on Adolescence. 2021;**31**(4):843-869. Available from: https://www.ncbi.nlm.nih.gov/pubmed/34820955

[71] Crittenden PM, Landini A, Spieker SJ, Grey B. Using parental attachment in family court proceedings: DMM theory about the adult attachment interview. Child Abuse Review. 2021;**30**(6):536-549. DOI: 10.1002/car.2730

[72] Spieker SJ, Crittenden PM, Landini A, Grey B. Using parental attachment in family court proceedings: An empirical study of the DMM-AAI. Child Abuse Review. 2021;**30**(6):550-564. DOI: 10.1002/car.2731

[73] Coulton CJ, Crampton DS, Irwin M, Spilsbury JC, Korbin JE. How neighborhoods influence child maltreatment: A review of the literature and alternative pathways. Child Abuse & Neglect. 1 Nov 2007;**31**(11-12):1117-1142

[74] Garbarino J, Sherman D. High-risk neighborhoods and high-risk families: The human ecology of child maltreatment. Child Development. Mar 1980:188-198. DOI: 10.2307/1129606

[75] Garon-Bissonnette J, Duguay G, Lemieux R, Dubois-Comtois K, Berthelot N. Maternal childhood abuse and neglect predicts offspring development in early childhood: The roles of reflective functioning and child sex. Child Abuse & Neglect. 2022;**128**:105030

[76] Crittenden PM. A developmental case methodology to address new clinical questions. Human Systems. 2024;**4**(1):50-55 DOI: 10.1177/26344041231213924

[77] Maxwell JA. The importance of qualitative research for investigating causation. Qualitative Psychology. 2021;**8**(3):378. DOI: 10.1037/qup0000219

[78] Yin RK. Case study research and applications. Thousand Oaks, CA: Sage; Jan 2018

Chapter 9

Conceptualizing Negative Peer Interactions: Models of Analyzing and Intervention

Ioana Darjan and Mihai Predescu

Abstract

As humans, our most essential and desirable goals involve social interactions, connectedness, and acceptance. However, social rejection or exclusion, perceived discrimination or humiliation, and loneliness can drastically impact our psychological well-being. Negative social behaviors like bullying and mobbing can be particularly damaging and highlight certain types of abusers. Effective interventions require a deep understanding of negative peer interactions' functions, motivations, and dynamics. This chapter examines these dimensions through a cognitive paradigm lens and the classification and characteristics of specific self-defeating behavioral patterns in the Life Space Crisis Intervention (LSCI) Model. We delve into the underlying psychological structure of both parties in a bullying situation, the different types of bullying relationships and patterns of interaction, and the primary directions for intervention.

Keywords: social interactions, aggressive behaviors, bullying, cognitive paradigm, LSCI method

1. Introduction

The goals of professional intervention in managing bullying relationships are to eliminate the bullying action and its effects and help those involved to learn appropriate behaviors. In order to achieve these objectives, it is crucial to have a thorough comprehension of the dynamics involved in bullying. Since bullying is such a complex social relation, there are different levels of analysis of existing data and different paths of action. This chapter analyzes bullying on different levels. We consider it worthwhile to analyze bullying on four levels: descriptive, diagnostic, predictive, and prescriptive.

At a descriptive level, we focus on the genesis of aggressive behavior, its neurophysiologic roots, functions, and variations. Professionals must understand that all behaviors, even aggressive behavior such as bullying, serve a purpose and fulfill specific needs. It is crucial to acknowledge the needs of the aggressive child and work toward finding positive ways to fulfill them. Utilizing a descriptive approach enables practitioners to identify and describe the behavior and its underlying functions.

It is crucial to deeply understand aggressive behavior and its functions and identify possible behavioral patterns in aggressive children (diagnostic level). The cognitive paradigm and Life Space Crisis Intervention (LSCI) techniques utilize conceptual models to understand aggressive behavior and conflict cycles, which help practitioners interpret behaviors and choose appropriate interventions.

Predictive analysis is employed when we make assumptions about the child's response to a specific intervention. Based on the prognostic level, we could build a hypothesis about how our intervention will model the behavior. It is important to remember that every model is merely an estimation of reality and that behavior involves a vast number of variables. Therefore, it is necessary to conduct interventions through experimentation. Usually, we test our assumptions by analyzing data and utilizing preexisting models.

In guiding our practice through case analysis, we rely on the prognostic level and data-driven approaches for successful interventions. It is essential to observe the transfer of newly acquired knowledge and skills to similar situations, as well as the restructuring of cognitive schemes, to determine the effectiveness of an intervention.

We need models, not recipes! The models are based on relevant, significant scientific theories/knowledge and empirically validated strategies and practices.

A profound, in-depth understanding of theories, scientific knowledge, and their logical explanatory and intervention models favor insights into problem-solving and sustain informed, justifiable, flexible, and efficient interventions.

Initial training and continuous professionalization should develop this assessment and diagnostic knowledge and skills, compulsory for informed, independent, autonomous, insightful, inspired, and flexible educational specialists.

2. The descriptive level: human behavior

Throughout our lives, each of us displays a wide range of emotional and behavioral reactions collectively known as human behavior. This subject is essential to many fields of study, including neurophysiology, psychology, sociology, and philosophy. Researchers in these areas have conducted extensive studies, observations, and experiments to develop theories about the factors that influence human behavior, the various stages of its development, and the different types of behaviors that we exhibit.

Understanding the reasons and motives behind the emergence and development of various behaviors is crucial, and there are several reasons why. First, this helps us identify the critical factors and circumstances that reinforce or eliminate a particular behavior. Second, by observing and deciphering behavioral patterns, we can gain insights into the human mind, including thoughts, emotions, attitudes, and values.

Behaviors are sorted into normal/abnormal, rational/irrational, accepted/unaccepted, and appropriate/inappropriate based on different criteria and perspectives. Although these categories are historically, culturally, and socially dependent, they remain relevant in education, rehabilitation, and psychotherapy. We employ these behavioral classifications as criteria in the diagnostic process and interventions.

Human behavior is complex and can take various forms, such as impulsive, automatic, emotional, controlled, rational, and mature. Developmental psychologist Perry [1] explains that these behaviors depend on the nervous system's development level. The nervous system is structured hierarchically. Lower structures like the subcortical, limbic, midbrain, brainstem, and autonomic systems generate diverse reactions, from reflexive responses in newborns to abstract reasoning in adolescents and young adults. This neurosequential approach to therapy highlights the significance of evaluating a child's developmental age, including their physical, emotional, social, cognitive, and behavioral levels. As a result, educational and therapeutic expectations and activities can be tailored accordingly [1].

The maturity of neurological structures plays a crucial role in children's emotional self-regulation and behavioral self-control. However, external factors like the child's environment and life experiences influence these abilities through social learning, modeling, and altering neurological structures and functions.

The situation's characteristics can significantly influence impulsive and automatic behavioral responses. In the face of perceived danger or threat, the body instinctively reacts with fight, flight, or freeze responses. These reactions have specific objectives, such as avoiding or escaping, seeking attention, asserting power, or seeking vengeance.

2.1 Aggressive behaviors: determinants, types, and functions

Human aggression and aggressive reactions are multifaceted [2], involving genetic and hereditary factors, predispositions, or acquired, learned responses to specific events. The explanatory theories on aggression range from extreme positions. The biological approach searches for evidence of genetic predispositions for aggression. The environmentalist approach presents crucial environmental factors predisposing to aggressive reactions.

According to the behavioral model proposed by Nietzel, Hasemann, and Lynam [3], four factors can contribute to developing aggressive behavior across an individual's lifespan. These factors include distal triggers of violence, early signs of a predisposition to violence during childhood, aggravating factors like traumatic events or stressful life experiences, and specific variables that can sustain aggressive behavior.

Bandura's social learning theory [4, 5] suggests that external reinforcement and internal factors, like emotions and thoughts, influence human behavior, such as aggression. Bandura highlights the importance of motivation in shaping and maintaining behavior. Meanwhile, Stoff and Cairns [6] take a developmental psychobiological approach to understanding aggression, examining both top-down and bottom-up factors contributing to such behavior.

At every stage of life, specific factors affect the likelihood of aggressive behavior. There are various types of aggressive behaviors with specific motivations and meanings. As humans develop biologically and neurologically during childhood and adolescence, their aggressive reactions undergo significant changes, primarily due to developments and changes in brain structure and function [1]. Environmental conditions, life events, personal beliefs, and personality also play a crucial role in shaping an individual's response to aggression [7]. Economic, psychological, and environmental stressors can further impact an individual's behavior [8, 9].

According to research cited in Tremblay et al. [10], childhood aggression can take various forms. These forms include instrumental aggression (aimed at obtaining or retrieving an object or situation), teasing aggression (which lacks a specific goal), defensive aggression (a reaction to an attack), and game aggression (stemming from rough-and-tumble play). Categorizing aggression is crucial for understanding the genetic, biological, and social factors influencing aggressive behavior. This understanding can help improve educational and therapeutic approaches.

2.2 Functions of the aggressive behaviors

Every behavior, including aggression, serves a purpose to fulfill a need. According to Maslow's theory of human needs [11], needs are arranged hierarchically, beginning with physiological needs and advancing to safety needs, love and belonging, self-esteem, self-actualization, and self-transcendence. This theory highlights the significance of meeting fundamental needs before pursuing higher ones, such as self-actualization and self-transcendence.

According to Max-Neef [12], the human needs for development should be viewed as a comprehensive and interconnected system, with no fixed order of importance, except for the essential need for subsistence. To establish a Human Scale Development, Max-Neef categorized human needs into two groups: existential (being, having, doing, and interacting) and axiological (subsistence, protection, affection, understanding, participation, creation, leisure, identity, and freedom). This matrix can be utilized for diagnostic purposes, planning, assessment, and evaluation.

The Circle of Courage [13] presents a practical framework for comprehending human needs and their significance in fostering resilient and successful individuals. This model, derived from the medicine wheel of North American tribal communities, symbolizes balance and harmony. It emphasizes the critical requirements for positive human development, namely belonging, mastery, independence, and generosity, which are essential after fulfilling basic needs such as food, water, and shelter. Psychologically, these needs translate to attachment, achievement, autonomy, and altruism.

Numerous theories [14–17] suggest that all human behaviors, whether reasonable or unreasonable, appropriate or inappropriate, are motivated by the need to fulfill an objective and satisfy a need. Every human behavior serves a crucial purpose, sometimes even vital to the individual. In the context of education, intervention, or therapy, it is unhelpful and inefficient to impede or reject the function of any behavior. Instead, we should strive to promote socially accepted, appropriate, and suitable ways of action.

According to Adler [14], as social beings, humans have an inherent need for acceptance and belonging, which drives their behavior toward achieving social approval. Dreikurs [15] believes all human behaviors are motivated by fulfilling significant needs, such as attention-seeking, power-seeking, revenge-seeking, and failure-avoiding. Building on Adler's work, Nelsen [16] identifies four primary goals of students: seeking attention, gaining power, seeking revenge for a perceived injustice, or avoiding failure.

2.3 Bullying—a special kind of aggression

Bullying is aggressive, harmful behavior that involves intentional and repetitive actions in which an individual who holds a position of power targets someone who is (perceived) less powerful [18]. An essential characteristic of this type of aggression is the imbalance of power on which it is based. Bullying perpetration describes aggression against someone [19, 20], while peer victimization refers to the subject of aggressive or abusive behavior.

Allowing oneself to be bullied is a form of passive acceptance, whereas bullying involves aggressive behavior to achieve one's goals. Passive and aggressive predispositions have genetic determinants, being connected with a person's temperament.

However, they are also learned through cultural values, societal norms, gender role expectations, family dynamics, and parenting styles. Assertiveness is a learned approach to communication, conflict resolution, and goal attainment that emphasizes balance [21].

There are different types of bullying perpetration: physical, verbal, or relational [22], either direct (overt) or indirect (covert) aggression [23], or, more recently, online bullying by using electronic means (cyberbullying, cyber harassment) [24, 25].

Frequently, the most common presupposition is that the bullies/perpetrators come from adverse life experiences (neglect and abuse), with a difficult upbringing in hostile or rejecting family environments, resulting in poorly developed self-concept, negative, self-denigrating beliefs, and negative beliefs and attitudes about others. Inflicted prosocial skills and possibly underdeveloped communication and problem-solving skills negatively impact the ability to interact and communicate efficiently with the surrounding environments [26]. Some explanatory theories connect bullying perpetration with insecure attachment [27], learned aggressiveness [28, 29], or weak social bonds [30].

Bullying perpetrators do not seem to have low self-esteem [31], except for female perpetrators [32, 33]. However, some findings suggest that bullying perpetrators usually have lower self-esteem than children without behavioral problems [34]. Positive correlations were found between low self-esteem and peer victimization [35].

These characteristics and variables explain most children's aggressive predispositions and actions, but not all bullying actions. Bullying is based on unbalanced power between the abuser and the victim. One or more unflattering or undesired traits of the victim become the subject and the motive for the repetitive, intentional attack. Bullying relies on discrimination. This explains, in part, the attitudes and actions of the rest of the crowd: the followers and henchmen, the supportive and the passive audience.

The bully gains popularity, support, admiration, and power when the witness agrees and allies with him or chooses not to intervene.

Many factors contribute to aggressive behavior in children, but not all cases of bullying can be explained by these variables. Bullying occurs when the perpetrator and victim have an unequal power dynamic. The bully repeatedly targets their victim based on one or more undesirable traits. Discrimination plays a role in bullying, and this can influence the attitudes and actions of bystanders. The bully gains social status and power when others support or fail to intervene in their behavior.

Research indicates that boys' physical aggression is more prevalent [36, 37], whereas girls tend to engage in relational aggression [38]. Verbal aggression, on the other hand, appears to be equally used by both genders [39].

Bullying increases progressively during childhood, peaks in early adolescence, and declines in late adolescence [40]. However, this abusive pattern of behavior might continue into adulthood (abusive couple relationships, bullying and mobbing at the workplace).

Fluck [41] sustains that the taxonomies of the bullying phenomenon are essential for two reasons: the rationale for operationalizing the construct and the building of a solid foundation for further, more elaborated research on the matter. We want to add a third important reason for the relevance and necessity of the bullying taxonomies: the intervention. Only conceptualizing, identifying, and clarifying the motives and the functions of the aggressive behavior/bullying (especially from the abuser's point of view) permits the identification of efficient arguments for change (both mindset through cognitive restructuring and, subsequently, behavioral modification through contingencies' manipulations), and maintains the determinations to adhere to new, alternative, and socially acceptable ways of attaining the objectives/satisfying the functions of the initial behaviors [42].

3. The diagnostic level: conceptual models of aggressive behaviors

3.1 The cognitive model

Cognitive theories focus on the mental processes that enable us to perceive, name, categorize, and understand our world and assist us in problem-solving.

The basic principle in cognitive psychology is that people react differently, emotionally and behaviorally, to the events they go through due to their cognitive schemas (a hierarchical structure of core beliefs, rules, assumptions, and attitudes). These cognitive schemas develop progressively during childhood and adolescence, are structured and influenced by internalized cultural norms and values and each person's life experiences. We are the survivors of our life history.

According to the cognitive paradigm [7, 43], an uncertain or stressful situation activates a particular system of beliefs, leading to a specific behavioral reaction. The perceived stimuli are then evaluated by assessing and interpreting the situation, resulting in an automatic thought or cognition. This thought generates an emotional state that triggers physiological reactions, leading to a specific behavioral response (**Figure 1**).

Our beliefs (core, intermediate, and, hence, subsequent automatic thoughts) are formed through our childhood and adolescent experiences. These beliefs help us

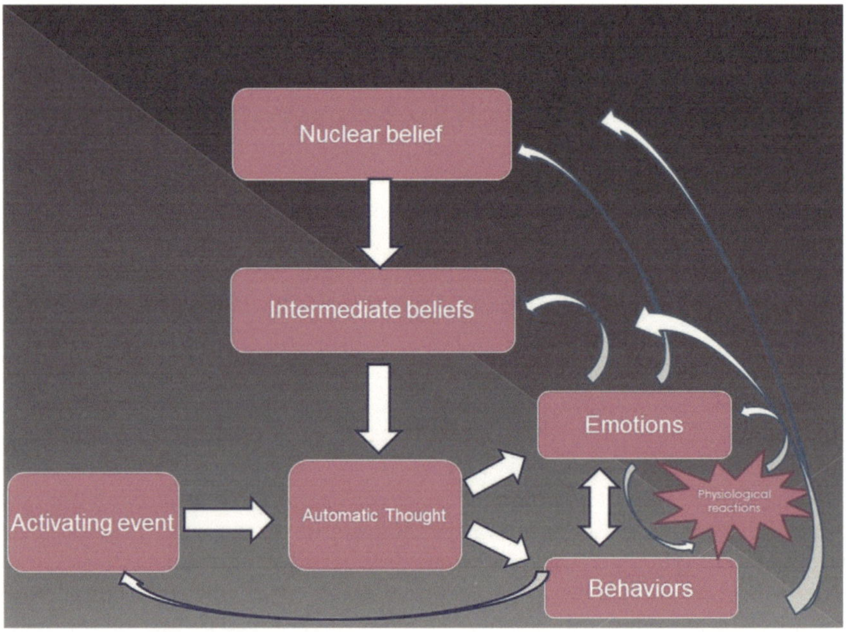

Figure 1.
The cognitive model of reaction to an activating event.

assess and categorize situations and react accordingly, allowing us to adapt to our environment.

However, certain circumstances exist where an individual's core beliefs, which are the most fundamental, can become irrational, rigid, and overgeneralized. These circumstances may include unique neurophysiological structures and functions, challenging upbringing conditions, or extreme and traumatic experiences. The structuration of these beliefs can involve cognitive distortions, resulting in inflexible and rigid emotional and behavioral responses to activating events. Consequently, such rigid ways of interpreting and thinking about life events can lead to undesirable behavioral patterns.

It is crucial to recognize how individuals perceive and interpret specific actions or events (known as automatic thoughts), as they can reveal fundamental beliefs, rules, assumptions, and attitudes that influence emotional and behavioral responses.

These cognitive schemes constitute a personal lens and perceptive prism of events. The particular perception generates a personal interpretation of the meaning of the perceived events (automatic thought); this interpretation depends on the emotional and behavioral reactions of the person.

Our cognitive schemes shape how we see and understand the world around us. They act like a lens through which we interpret events and generate automatic thoughts. This interpretation results from our unique personal perception, and the meaning assumed from what we perceive influences our emotional and behavioral reactions.

Emotional and behavioral issues are often caused by cognitive inflexibility and poorly structured irrational beliefs resulting from cognitive distortions.

Erikson [44] extends this approach and considers behavioral and emotional problems as the expression of identity crises, of inadequate solutions/responses to a series of existential dilemmas.

Jones [9] presents a theory of child development, marked by turning points and demands experienced by the child as developmental anxieties. She believes five general types of developmental anxieties involve complex interpersonal and intrapersonal processes from birth through adolescence. Themes of these developmental anxieties are abandonment, inadequacy, guilt, conflict, and personal identity. Identifying children's developmental anxieties provides a more explicit framework for understanding their behavioral responses in borderline, stressful situations [9].

Personal experiences causing stress can significantly impact the formation, structure, and function of various structures within the central nervous system. Trauma and abuse, in particular, can be sources of harmful stress.

When an individual experiences toxic stress, whether acute or continuous, it can result in the survival brain (which includes the hypothalamus and amygdala) being in a perpetual state of activation. This can cause the emotional brain to overwork, triggering the body's stress reactions of fight, flight, or freeze. As a result, the person develops a hyperalert pattern of brain functioning and body reaction, constantly perceiving the world as threatening and dangerous.

The particular modality in which an individual's beliefs are organized may significantly affect their responses in particular situations. In interrelations and communication, both parties (person 1 and person 2) come with personal systems of beliefs, values, rules, and attitudes. Person 1's behavior (the manifest and visible part of his or her thought-emotion-behavior path) becomes an activating event for the communication partner (**Figure 2**). The reaction (response) of the receiving partner (person 2) will depend on his mindset (system of beliefs).

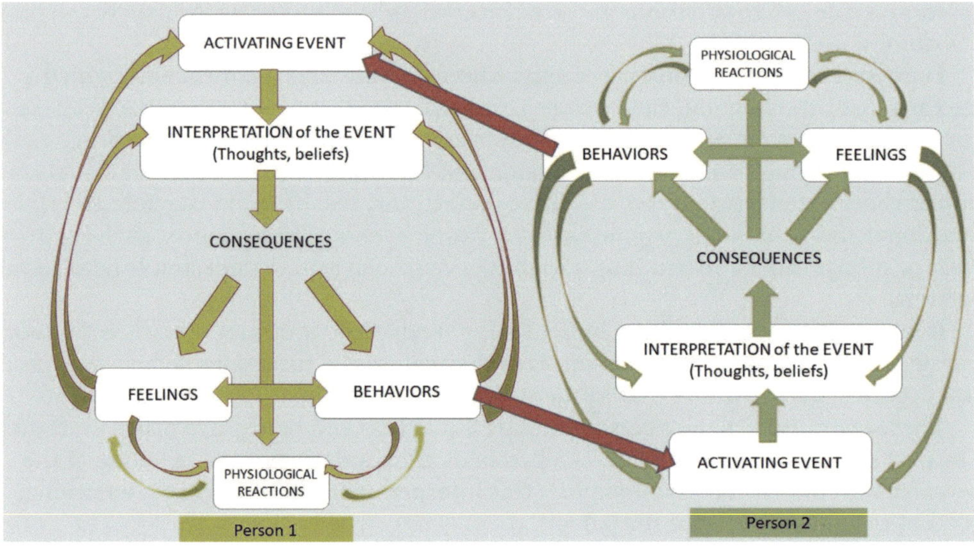

Figure 2.
A cognitive model of communication.

When beliefs become irrational and inflexible, it can lead to the formation of dysfunctional perspectives. This creates a rigid pattern of emotional and behavioral reactions that are difficult to adapt to different contexts, situations, or people/ relationships. This inflexibility can harm an individual's ability to adapt and function socially.

Understanding that this condition does not simply disappear as the child ages is essential. Their irrational beliefs and dysfunctional view of reality can persist into adulthood, potentially leading to disharmonious personality structures that have a pervasive impact on their life.

3.2 The conceptual model of the conflict—LSCI

The Life Space Crisis Intervention (LSCI) is an advanced therapeutic method that combines multiple theories, such as psychoanalytic, behavioral, cognitive, and practical, to identify repeating behavioral patterns in young individuals that hinder their personal development. This approach relies on theoretical and empirical data. It utilizes the Conflict Cycle model as its primary tool to illustrate how conflict communication is triggered and maintained, leading to a crisis [8, 9].

The Conflict Cycle sheds light on how the responses of others, such as adults and peers, can play a role in the escalation of conflicts (**Figure 3**). As in the cognitive model, one's behavior is an event perceived and interpreted by the dialog partner according to his system of beliefs. The reaction will depend on this interpretation. When the reaction is immature and impulsive, mirroring the other's aggressive behaviors, for example (anger generates counter-anger and aggression fuels counter-aggression), the conflictual communication evolves from an activating event to a critical incident. Eventually, it might escalate into a crisis (**Figure 3**). Reacting to negative actions rationally can help individuals regulate their emotions and impulses. This may result in less tension, displaying appropriate behavior and eventually putting an end to confrontational exchanges.

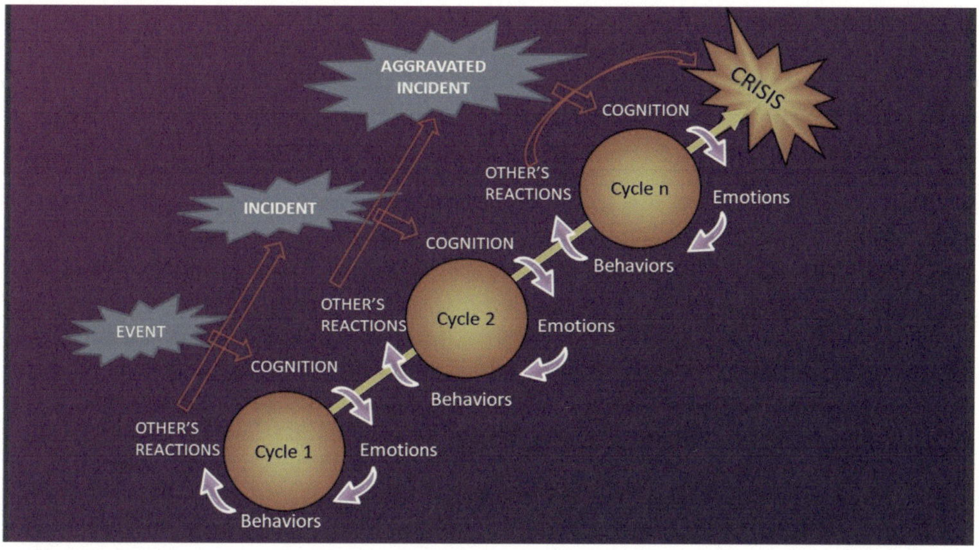

Figure 3.
The escalation of conflictual communication (the LSCI model).

Research has shown that uncontrolled emotions, particularly anger, can elicit a similar response in others, resulting in a cycle of aggression and retaliation [8]. This can escalate into a crisis as tension builds up [9]. This model can be applied in different environments, such as homes, schools, or workplaces, to identify the underlying problem and provide effective conflict resolution strategies.

The Reality Check Intervention is intended for children who may tend to misinterpret situations, be socially isolated, or make excuses to justify their actions. This program aims to provide a realistic perspective on life and help children overcome their challenges. These children may present symptoms of autism spectrum disorders, social (pragmatic) communication disorders, Attention Deficit/Hyperactivity Disorder (ADHD), low social and communication skills, and impulsivity.

The Red Flag Intervention concept illustrates how humans often use displacement as a defense mechanism. This means that when children experience distress, anger, pain, or frustration, they may discharge them toward someone who is not the actual cause of their feelings. The person who becomes the target of the outburst may be unrelated to past experiences and perceived as less threatening and available in a more secure context. This behavior can offer perpetrator relief, catharsis, and stress release, with fewer negative consequences. The main manifestations of these children are impulsivity and pain-based behaviors.

The Benign Confrontation Intervention is designed for children who have egocentric tendencies and believe they have the right to say or do anything to defend themselves or prove their superiority. They may often justify their actions and blame others, feeling emotionally detached from the victim and dismissing the impact of their behavior [9]. These behavior characteristics evoke behavioral disorders (oppositional defiant disorder and conduct disorder) and might develop into an antisocial personality disorder.

The Regulate and Restore Intervention is designed for children presenting self-abusive behaviors and self-denigrating comments. Usually, as victims of emotional, physical, and sexual abuse, they are overwhelmed by feelings of shame, unworthiness, inadequacy, and guilt and tend to have significant difficulties regulating their emotions and controlling their behaviors. The symptoms suggest emotional disorders, such as anxiety and depression, and bipolar personality disorders, converging to borderline personality disorders.

The New Tools Intervention is used for children presenting reduced (social) skills. They usually appear to have good intentions but lack the appropriate, socially accepted behaviors to pursue them. Usually, children with intellectual impairment, socio-emotional and communication immaturity, ADHD, autism spectrum disorders, and social (pragmatic) communication disorders access this inefficient behavioral pattern.

The final intervention, the Peer Manipulation Intervention, aims to expose problematic, unbalanced peer relations, either in false friendship (the manipulator and manipulated pairs) or in the form of set-up (the manipulator provoking a well-known impulsive and aggressive colleague). These dysfunctional relationships might occur due to the unhealthy and unfortunate meeting between children with externalized disorders (conduct disorder, oppositional defiant disorder) and children with internalized disorders (anxiety, depression, and bipolar personality disorder).

All these self-defeating behavioral patterns might determine, in particular situations, aggressive reactions, but their goals, cognitions, and emotions are quite different.

These patterns of self-defeating behaviors are interchangeable: a victim might become a bully, and a bully might find himself a victim in other circumstances and contexts. Bully behavior, like any other behavior, can be modeled and learned.

Prone to bully behaviors are children who appreciate the efficiency of this behavior in gaining and satisfying personal needs (attention/admiration/status, power, or revenge), and begin to justify it and detach emotionally from the victim.

The motives of followers reside in fear of association with the victim (when they could suffer the same treatment) or in need for appreciation and higher status (given to them if associated with the "popular" guy/girl or through reconnaissance of this popular guy if they obey him).

Based on the unequal power relationship assumption, bullying intentionally manipulates and exploits a victim's feelings and actions. While other patterns of inappropriate behavior might be explained mainly through specific cognitive or emotional determinants, bullying is based on social interaction and the need for one bully to control and push the emotional buttons of the victim to control his behavior.

In LSCI, the most illustrative pattern of bullying is Peer Manipulation. That is because bullying is based on an unequal power relationship. Peer Manipulation can take several forms. One of them is false friendship or frenemies.

In this pattern, we have a vulnerable child seeking appreciation and validation and a manipulative peer willing to fulfill those needs as long as the child acts as a puppet for him. In this unequal relationship, the manipulator persuades the vulnerable peer to misbehave. The manipulator's power resides in the victim's desperate need for affiliation and friendship, poor self-concept and self-confidence, fear of losing "the friend," and possible prestige and protection offered by this association. Usually, the manipulation act remains undetected and unreported, as the vulnerable child is trapped in this relationship and willing to pay for not losing it. The intervention should focus on clarifying the characteristics of a true friend, exposing the imbalance in the relationship, and developing the vulnerable child's assertiveness.

Another form of peer manipulation is The Set Up, a pattern that involves a vulnerable emotional child and a brilliant and passive-aggressive manipulator. The set-up works as the manipulator creates scenarios that reinforce the vulnerabilities of his peer and then triggers violent action by constantly pushing him to act. The bully has the satisfaction of manipulating the victim's emotions and actions. In this scenario, the aim is to teach the vulnerable child how to identify when his emotions are played and to learn to control his reactions.

Finally, the most aggressive pattern of peer manipulation is The Mastermind. This pattern is based on a power play in which the aggressive child manipulates others to demonstrate that he can do it for fun and his satisfaction. In this case, the intervention aims are common with benign confrontations and are addressed to the bully. We must build a secure relationship, openly confront the behaviors, and explore alternatives.

Although the sympathy and preoccupation go quickly and somehow naturally to the victim and the immediate interventions are addressed to her, we should stress the necessity of equally approaching the bully. First, just criticizing and punishing the misbehaviors of the bully do not change his mindset, beliefs, and attitudes. Thus, no fundamental, profound, sustainable behavioral and attitudinal changes will exist. More, these punishment-based interventions might confirm some irrational beliefs and reinforce misbehaviors. Second, the irrational beliefs sustaining misbehaviors might be rooted in personal pain and grief that must be acknowledged and addressed therapeutically.

4. The prescriptive and prognostic levels: implications for intervention

The cognitive paradigm works on the cognition-emotion-behavior model, explaining the differences in human reactions to the same stimuli through the differences in the cognitive system of beliefs. When considering modifying unhelpful behavioral patterns and strategies, an essential technique is cognitive restructuring. This means we must identify the underlying core beliefs and their potential cognitive distortions and expose, confront, and test them using cognitive techniques or behavioral experiments. Therapeutic intervention could also focus on behavioral modification (through contingencies manipulations) or emotion regulation. Any modification of one of these terms of the equation (thought, emotion, behavior) will trigger a change in the other two.

Our actions and behaviors are driven by the need to achieve our goals. Acknowledging these needs and prioritizing their fulfillment, especially as they play a significant role in our personal growth, is essential. It is crucial to identify their underlying motivations to understand their behaviors better and make effective interventions. Aggressive behavior, for instance, is a means of achieving a goal and should be addressed by educators and therapists by replacing it with more socially acceptable alternatives. Behaviors serve different functions, some of which are adaptive, reflective of our past experiences, and help us navigate different situations.

When someone experiences emotional and behavioral disorders, their undesirable behaviors may be a way to cope with their feelings and maintain a sense of predictability and control over situations. These behaviors serve as experiments to test their beliefs and fulfill them. Engaging in these actions, children may provoke unpleasant events to confirm their expectations of adverse outcomes. Unfortunately, this cycle reinforces harmful behaviors and confirms irrational beliefs.

We begin helping the student by challenging their expectations. We can distinguish between different diagnoses by accurately identifying the purpose of their negative behavior in the diagnostic process. For example, aggressive behavior may stem from fear, shame, inadequacy, anger, or pride [17]. The cause of aggression can be attributed to a specific way of perceiving things, personal beliefs, and emotional responses. Through assessment, we can determine the triggers and outcomes of the behavior and establish its intended purpose. The assessment result should provide a clear description of the behavior's characteristics.

In education or therapy, relying solely on observable behavior characteristics for intervention methods can be ineffective or even detrimental. It could reinforce negative behaviors, intensify negative emotions, and confirm irrational beliefs, leading to a self-fulfilling prophecy. The LSCI theory suggests that unprepared adults may react to disruptive behavior with inappropriate emotional and behavioral responses, such as counter-anger and retaliation, leading to a cycle of conflict.

According to Brendtro [9] and Tobias & Chapanar [45], a successful intervention should uncover the underlying purpose of behavior and address the hidden needs rather than just reacting to the problematic behavior itself.

The LSCI method offers six intervention strategies that address self-destructive behaviors frequently seen in school and family environments. These behaviors could be a sign of emotional or behavioral disorders, both internalized and externalized, and are customized to suit specific emotional and behavioral reactions to stressful circumstances. It is a comprehensive approach to helping individuals overcome such patterns [9].

Being a crisis-designed strategy, the LSCI method begins with the de-escalation stage. This stage (Drain off) responds to the emotional outburst/meltdown demands when the emotional brain (hypothalamus and amygdala) overwrites the rational brain (neocortex), and intense emotions control the reactions. The objective of this stage is to offer time and space for the person to calm down gradually as the stress hormones dissipate and the cortex regains control, expressed through restored rational thinking and superior psychological processing (e.g., language). In this stage, we allow the children to relieve stress and drain off the powerful emotions that hinder their irrational approach to the situation. Our goal is the de-escalation of emotion, creating a supportive relationship in a safe environment.

The following two diagnostic stages of the LSCI, like in the cognitive paradigm intervention, clarify the client's perspective and recollection of the event, identify the personal perceptive, thinking, and emotional and behavioral reactions (the Timeline stage), identify the main self-defeating behavioral pattern, and differentiate between transitory/circumstantial or habitual (patterns) responses (the Central Problem stage).

The second stage also helps to clarify the specific triggers, maintaining factors, and aggravating factors of the target behavior. We need to understand the event from the child's perspective. In this step, we encourage the child to express his understanding of the situation in a structured mode, allowing us to draw a timeline of events. Our goal in this stage is to understand the event from the child's point of view. By assessing the student's perception of the event, their feelings, and their reaction before, during, and after the event, we can identify the function of the behavior.

The third stage of the diagnostic phase (the Central Issue stage) concludes the diagnostic phase of the intervention. At this point, we try to identify the central issue: the specific pattern of self-defeating behavior. Although most behaviors could usually be framed in one of the six patterns described earlier in this chapter, there are always particularities of the situation and specific traits we must consider. We can make assumptions about the appropriate intervention and possible outcomes based on the identified patterns. The final goal is to assess whether the behavior fits a specific pattern and decide what intervention to employ.

The three diagnostic stages aim to facilitate an insightful understanding of the problem by the client, acknowledging the pattern used in coping with stressful content (the Insight stage), a guided process of finding new solving solutions (the New Tools stage), and implementation of these solutions in life space contexts (the Transfer of Learning stage).

The intervention phase has three stages: Insight stage, New Tools, and Transfer of Learning stage.

The Insight stage is the core of the intervention, as we try to help the children to gain a new understanding of the event and his/her behavior, including the consequences. This step is crucial for a successful intervention because it is the base for the child's intrinsic motivation for relevant and sustainable behavioral change, as he primarily acknowledges its benefits for himself. Our goal for this step is to guide the child into understanding the self-defeating effects of his current behavior and how the suggested change could improve his function and probability of success.

The New Tools stage is a learning process of new, acceptable, and efficient ways to respond positively to future stressful events. We aim to guide the child in a problem-solving approach to identify, practice, apply, and assess alternative reactions. This step promotes communication and social abilities' development.

The Transfer of Learning stage advocates and supports the attempts to implement and practice the newly achieved skills in similar future situations. Our goal is to prepare the children to return to their ecological environment and to assist them in practicing and improving the new, socially accepted, and efficient solving strategies.

The LSCIs follow the steps mentioned above in specific ways according to specific behavioral patterns. The first three steps (the diagnostic phase) are identical, but the other three are tailored to each type of identified behavioral pattern.

5. Conclusions

Understanding the function of a person's behavior is vital for the assessment, diagnosis, and intervention process. It helps to identify how he or she copes with threatening or stressful situations. When conceptualizing an undesirable behavior, it is essential to consider its antecedents, triggers, description, and consequences. This conceptualization should come from an unbiased interview with the client and be refined with additional information. Ultimately, the evaluation should aim to identify the function and goal of the behavior—what purpose does it serve? Even if two behaviors appear similar, their functions may be entirely different.

It is crucial to identify the function of a person's behavior to correctly diagnose and distinguish between different disorders or patterns of self-defeating behavior with similar symptoms. The intervention decisions and techniques should be based on a thorough assessment, or they may be ineffective or harmful, making inappropriate behavior worse. Understanding the behavior's purpose will also help select the most effective therapeutic approach and technique. Intervention strategies and techniques should acknowledge the behavior's identified function and focus on teaching alternative, socially acceptable behaviors that fulfill that function. Therefore, a successful intervention should be tailored to the individual's circumstances and needs at every stage, from conceptualization to strategy selection.

Author details

Ioana Darjan* and Mihai Predescu
West University of Timisoara, Timisoara, Romania

*Address all correspondence to: ioana.darjan@e-uvt.ro

References

[1] Perry B. Applying principles of neurodevelopment to clinical work with maltreated and traumatized children. The neurosequential model of therapeutics. In: Webb B, editor. Working with Youth in Child Welfare. New York: The Guilford Press; 2006

[2] Ramirez J. Human Aggression—A Multifaceted Phenomenon. Madrid: UCM Centreur; 2003

[3] Nietzel M, Hasemann D, Lynam, D. Behavioral perspective on violent behavior. In: Van Hasselt V, Hersen M. editors. Handbook of Psychological Approaches with Violent Offenders: Contemporary Strategies and Issues. New York: Kluwer Academic/Plenum Press; 1999.

[4] Bandura A. Social Learning Theory. Englewood Cliffs: Prentice-Hall; 1977

[5] Bandura A. Social Foundations of Thought and Action: A Social-Cognitive Theory. Englewood Cliffs: Prentice-Hall; 1986

[6] Stoff D, Susman E. Developmental Psychobiology of Aggression. Cambridge: Cambridge University Press; 2005

[7] Cognitive BJ, Therapy B. Basics and Beyond. New York: The Guilford Press; 2011

[8] Long N, Fecser F, Morse W, Newman R, Long J. Conflict in the Classroom. Austin: Pro-Ed; 2014

[9] Long N, Wood M, Fecser F, Whitson S. Taking with Students in Conflict. Life Space Crisis Intervention. Austin: PRO.ED, Inc.; 2021

[10] Tremblay R, Hartup W, Archer J. Developmental Origins of Aggression. New York: The Guilford Press; 2005

[11] Maslow A. Motivation and Personality. New York: Harper; 1954

[12] Max-Neef M. Human scale development. In: Conception, Application and Further Reflections. New York: The Apex Press; 1991

[13] Brendtro L, Brokenleg M, Van Bockern S. The circle of courage and positive psychology. Reclaiming Children and Youth. 2005;**14**(3):130-136

[14] Adler A. What Life Should Mean to You. New York: Capricorn; 1958

[15] Dreikurs R, Loren G. A New Approach to Discipline: Logical Consequences. New York: Hawthorn Books; 1968

[16] Nelsen J, Lott L, Glenn S. Positive Discipline in the Classroom. 3rd ed. Rocklin: Prirna Publishing; 2000

[17] Darjan I, Predescu M, Tomita M. Functions of aggressive behaviors – Implications for intervention. Journal of Psychological and Educational Research. 2017;**25**(1):74-91

[18] Olweus D. Bullying among schoolchildren: Intervention and prevention. In: Peters R, McMahon R, Quinsey P, editors. Aggression and Violence Throughout the Life Span. Newbury Park: Sage; 1992. pp. 100-125

[19] Chen J, Wei H. The impact of school violence on self-esteem and depression among Taiwanese junior high school students. Social Indicators Research. 2011;**100**:479-498

[20] Gendron B, Williams R, Guerra G. An analysis of bullying among students within schools: Estimating the effects of individual normative beliefs, self-esteem, and school climate. Journal of School Violence. 2011;**10**:150-164

[21] Dârjan I, Negru M, Ilie D. Self-esteem – The decisive difference between bullying and assertiveness in adolescence? Journal of Educational Sciences. 2020, 2020;**1**(41):19-34. DOI: 10.35923/JES.2020.1.02

[22] Crick N, Bigbee M. Relational and overt forms of peer victimization: A multi-informant approach. Journal of Consulting and Clinical Psychology. 1998;**66**:337-347

[23] Drennan J, Brown R, Mort S. Phone bullying: Impact on self-esteem and well-being. Young Consumers. 2011;**12**:295-309

[24] Hinduja S, Patchin J. Bullying Beyond the Schoolyard: Preventing and Responding to Cyberbullying. Thousand Oaks: Sage Publications; 2009

[25] Valkenburg P, Peter J, Schouten A. Friend networking sites and their relationship to adolescents' well-being and social self-esteem. Cyberpsychology & Behavior. 2006;**9**(5):584-590

[26] Cook C, Williams K, Guerra N. Predictors of bullying and victimization in childhood and adolescence: A meta-analytic investigation. School Psychology Quarterly. 2010;**25**:65-83

[27] Murphy T, Laible D, Augustine M. The influences of parent and peer attachment on bullying. Journal of Child and Family Studies. 2017;**26**(5):1388-1397. DOI: 10.1007/s10826-017-0663-2

[28] Aslan S. The analysis of the relationship between school bullying perceived parenting styles and self-esteem in adolescents. Procedia - Social and Behavioral Sciences. 2011;**30**:1798-1800. DOI: 10.1016/j.sbspro.2011.10.346

[29] Baldry A. Bullying in schools and exposure to domestic violence. Child Abuse & Neglect. 2003;**27**:713-732. DOI: 10.1016/s0145-2134(03)00114-5

[30] Chan H, Chui W. Social bonds and school bullying: A study of Macanese male adolescents on bullying perpetration and peer victimization. Child & Youth Care Forum. 2013;**42**:599-616. DOI: 10.1007/s10566-013-9221-2

[31] Pearce J, Thompson A. Practical approaches to reduce the impact of bullying. Archives of Disease Childhood. 1998;**79**:528-531. DOI: 10.1136/adc.79.6.528

[32] Rigby K, Cox I. The contribution of bullying at school and low self-esteem to acts of delinquency among Australian teenagers. Personality and Individual Differences. 1996;**21**:609-612. DOI: 10.1016/0191-8869(96)00105-5

[33] Slee P. Peer victimization and its relationship to depression among Australian primary school students. Personality and Individual Differences. 1995;**18**:57-62. DOI: 10.1016/0191-8869(94)00114-8

[34] O'Moore M, Kirkham C. Self-esteem and its relationship to bullying behavior. Aggressive Behavior. 2001;**27**:269-283. DOI: 10.1002/ab.1010

[35] Fredstrom B, Adams E, Gilman R. Electronic and school-based victimization: Unique contexts for adjustment difficulties during adolescence. Journal of Youth and Adolescence. 2011;**40**:405-415. DOI: 10.1007/s10964-010-9569-7

[36] Rosen N, Nofziger S. Boys, bullying, and gender roles: How hegemonic masculinity shapes bullying behavior. Gender Issues. 2019;**36**:295-318. DOI: 10.1007/s12147-018-9226-0

[37] Ploeg R, Steglich C, Veenstra R. The way bullying works: How new ties facilitate the mutual reinforcement of status and bullying in elementary schools. Social Networks. 2020;**60**:71-82. DOI: 10.1016/j.socnet.2018.12.006

[38] Eriksen I, Lyng S. Relational aggression among boys: Blind spots and hidden dramas. Gender and Education. 2018;**30**(3):396-409. DOI: 10.1080/09540253.2016.1214691

[39] Fares E, Ramirez J, Cabrera M, Lozano F, Salas F. Justification of physical and verbal aggression in Uruguayan children and adolescents. The Open Psychology Journal. 2011;**4**:45-54

[40] Nansel T, Overpeck M, Pilla R, Ruan W, Simons-Morton B, Scheidt P. Bullying behaviors among U.S. youth: Prevalence and association with psychosocial adjustment. Journal of the American Medical Association. 2001;**285**:2094-2100. DOI: 10.1001/jama.285.16.2094

[41] Fluck J. Why do students bully? An analysis of motives behind violence in schools. Youth & Society. 2014;**49**:1-21. DOI: 10.1177/0044118X14547876 Available from: http://yas.sagepub.com/content/early/2014/08/28/0044118X14547876

[42] Alstot A, Alstot C. Behavior management: Examining the functions of behavior. Journal of Physical Education, Recreation & Dance. 2015;**86**(2):22-28. DOI: 10.1080/07303084.2014.988373

[43] Ellis A. Reason and Emotion in Psychotherapy. New York: Lyle Stuart; 1962

[44] Erikson E, Joan M. The Life Cycle Completed: Extended Version. New York: W. W. Norton; 1997

[45] Tobias S, Chapanar T. Predicting resilience after cyberbully victimization among high school students. Journal of Psychological and Educational Research. 2016;**24**(1):7-25. Available from: http://www.marianjournals.com/files/JPER_articles/JPER_24_1_2016/Tobias_Chapanar_JPER_2016_24_1_7_25.pdf

Chapter 10

Effortless Attention Trainings: The Intersection of Attention and Mental Health in Children and Teenagers

Juan M. Guiote, Miguel Ángel Vallejo and Blanca Mas

Abstract

This chapter presents several effortless attention trainings—mindfulness, yoga, qigong, nature exposure and more especially, autogenic meditation—which not only improve attention but also facilitate stress reduction and emotional regulation. Cultivating serene attention is a relevant strategy to promote mental health and well-being in children and teenagers. Fostering serene attention plays a fundamental role in shaping life experience because part of the individual's identity and knowledge is founded on what they pay attention to—their conscious experience—. By training children and teenagers to focus and direct their attention from a calm state of mind, we allow them to mould their own conscious experiences, laying the foundation for a balanced and fulfilling life.

Keywords: effortless attention training, attention state training, attention balanced state, emotional regulation, mental health, autogenic meditation

1. Introduction

Attention is the interface of consciousness, and its education is a relevant aspect in the adaptation and mental health of the individual [1, 2]. Childhood and adolescence constitute a sensitive period for shaping its capacity [3, 4]. Science has generally assumed that attention training requires effort [5]. However, there is a set of effective approaches that train attention in a more effortless way and also show a positive impact on the emotional and behavioural sphere [1, 6].

It is well known that attention and emotion interact [7–9], suggesting that those who train their attention optimally can lay the foundation for a proper emotional management and a calmer lifestyle. This is not a trivial matter. In the twenty-first century, the rise of technology offers new generations a world of opportunities, such as the Internet, artificial intelligence and online omnipresence, although these opportunities come with potential dangers. Much of children's leisure time is spent between screens that constantly compete for their attentional resources. At the same time, today's society encourages a fast pace of life, which results in stressful school and extracurricular agendas, all against a worrying backdrop of serious ecological problems, wars and in some cases, violence at school and the family. Consequently, young people often exhaust their energy with little time to connect with themselves and cultivate a calm and conscious way of being.

When analysing the mental states of children and adolescents, it is pertinent to consider 'mind-wandering', a common phenomenon that involves the involuntary shift of attention from the immediate external context or any specific task to self-generated thoughts unrelated to the ongoing activity [10]. It is estimated that mind-wandering accounts for between 25 and 50% of mental activity during waking hours [11, 12]. This suggests that the typical state of the mind is not being present-focused. Such a tendency to wander is associated with the Default Mode Network (DMN), negative affect, reduced psychological well-being and diminished learning capacity, although some studies have also related it to creativity [11, 13–16].

In this regard, the sum of attentional states throughout life will reflect a trait or a way of being. An idea that William James himself reflected in the following way: 'The faculty of voluntarily bringing back a wandering attention, over and over again, is the very root of judgment, character, and will' ([17], p. 424). The education of attention is the key that opens the floodgate of the cognitive process and constitutes the seed of character in interaction with temperament. In individual counselling or training groups, we present this idea to children and adolescents with the following statement: 'You are what you pay attention to, even when you are not aware that you are paying attention'. Therefore, we propose to train this ability to improve cognitive performance, to react with equanimity to the flow of thoughts wandering through the mind and to improve self-control.

As can be seen, educating attention is a relevant issue and is postulated as a preventive mental health measure. The following sections outline the nature of attention and how to train it from the perspective of effortless attention training, presenting its key methods and preliminary evidence supporting its efficacy.

2. What is attention?

Since the dawn of scientific psychology, many definitions and theoretical models of attention have been put forward. William James, in 1890, outlined a pioneering definition, stating: 'Everyone knows what attention is. It is the taking possession by the mind, in clear and vivid form, of one out of what seem several simultaneously possible objects or trains of thought. Focalization, concentration, of consciousness are of their essence. It implies withdrawal from some things in order to deal effectively with others and is a condition which has a real opposite in the confused, dazed, scatterbrained state which in French is called distraction, and Zerstreutheit in German' ([17], pp. 403–404).

Today, the understanding of attention as a limited resource that requires selection and is intrinsically linked to consciousness continues to prevail. However, although the term is ubiquitous in everyday language, the ongoing scientific debate reveals discrepancies. Some argue that the concept of attention is elusive and that no one really knows what attention is [18–20]. This interpretation underlines the inherent complexity of its definition and makes it difficult to encapsulate it from a monolithic perspective. In contrast, the current contemporary alternative approaches the understanding of attention from a modular and multifaceted perspective. In this context, Rueda defines attention as: 'The optimal state of activation that allows the individual to select the stimulation he receives through his senses in order to process the most relevant information with priority and efficiency, and thus be able to voluntarily and consciously control his behaviour′ ([21], p. 20). This definition highlights three essential functions: activation, selection, and executive control. (1) Therefore, to achieve attentional efficiency, an optimal activation level is crucial, a concept supported by the Yerkes-Dobson law [22], which shows that performance improves with moderate activation levels. (2) Because humans receive an infinite number of stimuli and have many thoughts running through their minds, it is necessary to select what to pay attention to. This selection process can be exogenous, bottom-up, reacting to external stimuli or endogenous, top-down, based on intention [23]. (3) Finally, executive attention also known as control attention regulates endogenous attention persistence, distractor inhibition, and self-regulation of behaviour. This function is closely linked to consciousness.

The intellectual journey of attention has seen the emergence of several theoretical models. During the first half of the twentieth century, the behaviourist paradigm conceived attention from stimulus control of observable behaviour [24]. Attentional models of classical conditioning were formulated in the second half of the century with the arrival of the cognitive paradigm [25, 26]. In the field of human attention were postulated models of functioning as selection or filter systems, whether rigid [27], attenuated [28], delayed [29] or flexible [30]. The markedly structural character of these proposals, and the emphasis on processing from data and other constraints, gave rise to a resource-centred conception of attention, conceiving it as a mental effort that can be distributed across tasks [5, 31, 32]. However, these theories lacked explanations for adaptability in attentional demand, encapsulating it as fixed, and could not account for the effect of practice, so automaticity models emerged in response [33]. The predominantly passive nature of these models gave way to control models [34], emphasising the active nature of attention. Finally, the emergence of cognitive neuroscience is making it possible to study the neuroanatomical structures involved in the functions of attention.

Among the emerging neuroscientific models [23, 35, 36], the neurocognitive approach outlined by Posner and Petersen [37] is noteworthy. This model articulates the existence of three attentional networks: alertness, orienting and executive, interconnected, but with neuroanatomical and functional independence. The model has been reconfigured by incorporating additional subnetworks to the orienting and executive attention networks, to incorporate new evidence [38]. The alertness network is predominantly located in the right hemisphere, includes regions of the frontal and parietal cortex and is associated with the reticular system, particularly the locus coeruleus, with norepinephrine as its main neurotransmitter [39]. The orientation network is responsible for selection and prioritisation. While the original model argued for the importance of the pulvinar nucleus and superior colliculus [37], subsequent neuroimaging studies highlighted the relevance of the parietal and frontal regions of the cortex [38]. Two subnetworks are identified within this network: the dorsal frontoparietal, linked to endogenous orienting, and the ventral frontoparietal, associated with exogenous orienting [23]. Acetylcholine acts as its main neurotransmitter. The executive network responsible for voluntary control, inhibition, and planning extends predominantly through the dorsolateral prefrontal cortex, the dorsomedial prefrontal cortex, and the anterior cingulate cortex (ACC) [40]. The CCA shows functional specialisation in its dorsal and ventral divisions: the dorsal is activated in conflict situations devoid of emotional content, while the ventral responds to emotional conflict processes. The CCA is highly interconnected with different brain regions, with evidence pointing to the existence of two essential neural circuits that perform specific but coordinated functions: the cingulo-opercular network, responsible for processing goals and executing behaviours, and the frontoparietal network, responsible for selecting and adapting responses at any given moment [41, 42]. In the dynamics of the executive network, dopamine is the predominant neurotransmitter. This network is related to self-regulation or self-control, reflecting the ability to regulate one's emotions, cognitions and behaviours [6, 38, 43]. Within the framework of self-regulation, it is relevant to highlight the conceptual parallelism between executive attention and what the cognitive literature defines as Executive Functions (EFs). These functions, intrinsically associated with the dynamics of the executive network, encompass critical domains such as cognitive flexibility and inhibitory control. According to landmark studies in the field [44, 45], these domains comprise two of the three fundamental pillars of executive functions, the third being working memory.

Finally, it is important to note that attention is the result of a complex biological and ecological interaction. Comparative studies with monozygotic and dizygotic twins suggest a significant relationship between genetic heritability and the executive network and to a more subtle degree with the alertness network [46]. In regard to executive attention, through specific inhibitory control tasks, polymorphic variations in specific genes, such as DRD4 and DAT [47], as well as SLC6A3 and COMT [48, 49], have been shown to play a role in modulating dopamine levels in the prefrontal cortex. Likewise, a polymorphism in the CHRNA4 gene, involved in the modulation of cholinergic receptors, has been associated with selective visual attention [50]. Among environmental conditions, some studies indicate that socioeconomic status influences alertness and executive attention [51] and the performance of executive attention and other cognitive processes [52]. In parallel, factors such as parenting and attachment style also seem to play a relevant role. In this sense, as revealed by a longitudinal study, sensitivity to children's needs in the first years of life, but above all, a maternal educational style that promotes autonomy correlates with better performance in executive attention and EFs [53]. It is worth recalling the overlap between attention and most EFs. A meta-analysis of the influence of parental behaviour on the EFs of children aged zero to eight years revealed details of interest. Specifically, there is a stable relationship between positive behaviours such as sensitivity or warmth and negative behaviours such as control or detachment. In contrast, parental cognitive behaviours such as autonomy support are moderated by children's age, showing a stronger effect size in younger children [54].

The set of findings described suggests the neuroplasticity of attention. Indeed, attention is not a fixed entity, but is susceptible to malleability. A direct intervention in this capacity constitutes attentional training. In the following, traditional attentional training is explained succinctly and, in more detail, a set of emerging attentional trainings that require a lower level of attentional effort.

3. Attention trainings

Meta-analysis studies on attention training have confirmed its efficacy, showing a medium effect size. It has been shown that, although it is possible to train attention at any age, childhood and adolescence are particularly sensitive periods, representing a clear window of opportunity [3, 4]. The meta-analyses mentioned above index studies are based on the effort or cognitive control paradigm. Identifying attention with effort has established itself as the dominant current in the field. An essential reference for this topic is Kahneman's seminal work, entitled 'Attention and Effort' [5], which has been widely cited and has had a notable influence on the configuration of attentional training. These trainings usually use computer programs to train a specific attentional skill, where the subject, through continuous practice in increasing difficulty and with high cognitive effort, improves the trained ability [55, 56]. Effortful training engages the sympathetic nervous system and the frontoparietal network [6] with the disadvantage of inducing mental fatigue, due to the metabolic increase [5] needed to counteract mind-wandering and sustain cognitive effort.

The biunivocal identification between attention and effort, as postulated by Kahneman, is a widely accepted idea, not only in the cognitive academic tradition but also resonates in popular conception. However, Bruya and Tang have presented a critical discussion highlighting the shortcomings and biases of this approach [57]. They argue that the notion of effort is not clearly defined in Kahneman's work. Furthermore, they explain that Kahneman conceives of effort/attention as a particular case of sympathetic dominance of the autonomic nervous system leading to increased metabolic activity in the brain. However, current evidence questions the direct equivalence between attention and effort, indicating that attention is not necessarily linked to the consumption of metabolic resources directly, but to the priming of those resources. This preparation, under sympathetic dominance, may be perceived as effort. It is also noted that attention can also be exercised in a state of parasympathetic dominance. This is the case of less effortful or attentional state training [6, 58–60]. The particularity of this, it promotes a balanced attentional state between mental fatigue and mind-wandering, which constitutes an optimal relationship between the level of effort and attentional performance [59]. Some theoretical bases underlying this approach are found in the Yerkes-Dodson law [22] and attention restoration theory [61, 62]. It is relevant to note that these practices are not explicitly configured to train attention, but are oriented towards psychophysical well-being, and yet they improve the efficiency of attention. This training framework encompasses experiences such as exposure to nature and various meditation practices, including mindfulness, yoga, Qigong or autogenic meditation. These forms of experience promote a soft and flexible attentional state that favours emotional and behavioural self-regulation. The neurophysiological state that unfolds in addition to parasympathetic predominance involves the synergistic cooperation of the central and autonomic nervous systems [60] and involves specific brain regions such as the anterior and posterior cingulate cortex, insula or striatum [6]. A distinctive aspect is that these practices show both a stress reduction response and a non-stressful attentional state.

3.1 Exposure to nature

Nature seems to exert a revitalising influence on human well-being and health. Strolling through green landscapes and forests immerses us in a fascinating setting, where the symbiosis of plants and fresh air creates an atmosphere of harmony and serenity. In tune with this, the blue surroundings, with their vast sea horizons and melodious waves, offer a sonorous and visual spectacle that facilitates a state of contemplation. These and many other possible experiences are not limited to mere pleasurable sensory experiences, but review studies suggest the restorative potential of nature on health and well-being, as well as on the cognitive domain of attention [63]. It is timely to reflect on the influence of the environment on children and young people. Under this consideration, having natural spaces in front of or in conjunction with urban and digital environments, which seem to be the trend of the twenty-first century, could have advantageous consequences on their development. In the case of attention, the Attention Restoration Theory (ART) [61] argues that contemporary urban life demands more and more endogenous or top-down attentional resources, which can result in attentional exhaustion. In contrast, natural environments deploy exogenous or bottom-up attention, less effortful, which helps the recovery of endogenous or executive attention [64–66]. This view is complemented by Stress Reduction Theory, which postulates that natural spaces attenuate physiological responses, favouring recovery from cognitive fatigue and optimising attentional performance [67, 68].

A systematic review comprising thirty-one meta-analysis studies identifies that twenty-one of them empirically support ART, based on three objective measures of attention [66]. In the adult population, research using an experimental paradigm of comparing urban and natural environments, such as forest walks, park walks and viewing natural landscapes, demonstrates the benefit of green spaces on both mood and attentional performance [69, 70]. This evidence has also been documented in people diagnosed with depression [71]. However, there are also cases where exposure to nature does not show efficacy. Specifically, a study using this same paradigm, but with the variant photographic exposure in a sample of healthy long-lived adults did not reveal positive effects, compared to a control group of young individuals. This finding suggests that age may moderate the efficacy of nature exposure [72].

Upon reviewing the empirical evidence for children and young people, a positive effect is also found, characterised by the following findings. One study shows that walking in a forest or a small to medium-sized park improves the level of well-being and selective and sustained attention in all conditions compared to the urban context baseline [73]. Another study focusing on a child population using the natural vs. urban walking paradigm assessed executive attention. The results reflected that while the performance of both groups was comparable, the natural walk group exhibited a more stable and faster response rate. An additional measure of the study was gaze fixation which was indexed by recording eye movements during walks in both conditions. The results showed that the natural walk group fixated their gaze more on their environment than the urban walk group. This finding could explain the attentional restoration effect attributed to nature [74]. Following this line of research, an additional study with children and adolescents aged eight to fifteen years examined the differential effects of the natural vs. urban environment on two types of attention, specifically, endogenous and exogenous. This study revealed a significant improvement exclusively in endogenous attention following exposure to the natural environment. These findings, therefore, provide empirical support for the ART hypothesis, which posits an exclusive enhancement in voluntary or endogenous attention following interaction with nature [75].

Broadening the spectrum of analysis on exposure to nature and in line with the underlying stress reduction theory for ART, both direct interaction with natural environments and simple observation from the classroom have been identified as reducing cortisol levels and heart rate [76, 77]. This evidence supports the notion that nature facilitates a less effortful attentional focus, and its effects appear to be interconnected with the modulation of the stress response. Furthermore, it is relevant to note that there appears to be a minimum age at which exposure to nature works. Such is the case of research using the urban nature walk paradigm, comparing attentional performance in a group of four- to five-year-old preschoolers versus a group of seven- to eight-year-old school children. The results support that only the nature-walking group of school children significantly improves attentional performance [78]. This finding, in conjunction with previous evidence found in older adults [72], indicates the need to continue to explore the peculiarities of each age range in order for exposure to nature to be effective.

It is worth noting that a recent systematic review analysing the impact of green spaces in the school context on cognitive functioning in children and adolescents supports the efficacy of these interventions on selective and sustained attention and working memory. In parallel, the review credits the underlying mechanisms of ART as reducing stress and decreasing cognitive fatigue, and supports the state of well-being facilitated by nature [79]. This evidence, although preliminary, suggests the desirability of establishing green educational contexts, taking advantage of the benefits that nature classrooms can offer for young people's well-being and cognitive development. In line with these findings, one study found that the density of tree cover in the school environment is positively associated with the academic performance of adolescents. This finding reinforces the idea that not only general exposure to nature but also specific aspect of the natural environment, such as the presence of trees, can have a significant impact on young people's cognitive and academic development [80].

On the other hand, it is worth mentioning that interaction with nature has shown efficacy not only in typically developing children and adolescents but also in those on the psychopathological spectrum. Circumscribing the details of studies to the specific area of attention, it has been found that nature shows therapeutic potential in children with attention deficit disorder (ADD) and attention deficit hyperactivity disorder (ADHD). A pioneering study evaluated the impact of different activities performed by a sample of children aged seven to twelve years diagnosed with ADD after school and on weekends. Parents took responsibility for indexing and reporting their children's activities. This task included classifying the context of each activity into three categories: natural (e.g., fishing), unnatural (e.g., playing video games) and ambiguous (e.g., playing outside); in addition, they were to assess the children's level of functioning in these activities. The results showed that activities performed in natural contexts, compared to those performed in non-natural or ambiguous contexts, significantly reduced ADD symptoms and facilitated better functioning of the children. Notably, the non-nature context elicited an inverse response, characterised by increased symptoms and poorer functioning. In addition, the study shows that the higher the density of green areas in the play space, the more ADD symptoms were reduced [81]. A study on the effects of 49 activities on children and young people between the ages of five and eighteen years, in this case, diagnosed with ADHD, is along the same lines. The study supports that outdoor green environments significantly reduce symptoms compared to other environments, even when the activities were comparable across environments. This effect was shown across all age groups, irrespective of gender, socio-economic status, symptom severity level and other individual and residential characteristics [82]. In line with previous research is another study that conducted a direct assessment of children diagnosed with ADHD using an objective attention test. The results show significant improvements in attention after a twenty-minute dose of nature walking compared to the same amount of walking time in other urban settings. It is noted in the study that the effect size found is comparable to that reported for methylphenidate, suggesting that nature is an accessible, ecological and cost-effective alternative for children with ADHD [83].

3.2 Meditation training

Defining meditation is not a trivial matter, due to the diversity of ancient practices that converge in this concept. In essence, meditation is a tool for a deep understanding of human beings in their relationship with themselves and their surrounding universe. This experiential learning comprises four dimensions: a path to wisdom, a technique, a state and a trait. The path to wisdom is forged in the doctrine imparted by the various schools with millennia-old roots, encompassing dogmas, spiritual or religious beliefs and ethical conduct that guides the meditator towards values such as compassion and responsibility. The technique constitutes the vehicle or set of specific exercises with the aim of achieving its purpose. Through the practice of this technique, an expanded state of consciousness is induced that gradually integrates the bodily, emotional, cognitive, social and spiritual spheres of 'being'. This state is accompanied by multi-level neuropsychophysiological changes. The trait constitutes the transfer of the state—or, more precisely, set of states—and the accumulated experiential learning into everyday life.

It is pertinent to underline that the rules of original or 'pure' meditation transcend the logic and reason dominant in Western thought, and, thus, for a long time, remained on the fringes of scientific knowledge. However, in its quest for understanding, science made its way towards its study. Thus, arose contemplative science: the scientific analysis of meditation which, from a secular perspective, examines the underlying basis for the functioning of meditative technique or practice and subjects the efficacy of these in clinical and non-clinical applications to empirical scrutiny. This view overcomes the pitfalls of religious and spiritual dogmas or beliefs inherent in the term 'meditation'. Without entering into the profound debate whether it is possible or correct to detach the technique from its values or beliefs, it is undeniable that the emerging evidence provided by contemplative science supports its efficacy in both educational and mental health settings.

Contemplative science identifies two specific modes of attention that are exercised in the contemplative practice set: Focusing Attention Meditation (FAM) and Open Monitoring of attention (OM) [84, 85]. FAM is the ability to direct attention in a calm attitude in a selective and sustained manner towards a specific meditation object, such as the breath, a mantra, the beating of the heart or the flame of a candle. If a distraction occurs, it is prescribed to redirect the attention to the object of meditation. The peculiarity of FAM compared to the attentional focus of daily life is that, unlike the latter, which demands constant effort, FAM requires an initial effort, but with a relatively low dose of practice, this effort is significantly reduced. An illustrative example occurs when contemplating a campfire for one minute. The field of consciousness merges to such an extent with the object that what is called absorption occurs, drastically decreasing the activation of the sympathetic tone. This absorption and calming effect is well described in ancient practices such as samadhi [86] or samatha [87]. Nowadays, the set of meditative practices circumscribed to this ability is also called 'concentration meditation'. FAM deploys stable monitoring, or a constant flow of processing of the meditative object, as opposed to distraction and mind-wandering, which appear to be the default mode of the human mind states, highly associated with unhappiness in adults, as well as in children and adolescents [11, 88, 89]. OM is conceptualised as a meta-attention skill. The meditator performs an attentional registration of the continuous flow of experience in an attitude of equanimity. In contrast to FAM, he or she does not have to focus on any particular aspect or content, but deploys open and global attention [85, 90]. Rather than anchoring to a stimulus and identifying with its content, as in FAM, this modality monitors the vast ocean of consciousness in an unbiased way, welcoming the waves or fluctuations of thoughts, sensations and emotions. This open monitoring, in its highest expression, allows us to reconnect with the wonder and awe of everyday experience, but also confronts us with the inescapable reality of human suffering. One practice that deploys this mode of attention is vipassana meditation [91]. Practices that fall under this domain of deep understanding are called 'insight meditation'.

It is common for meditative protocols to begin with experiences that encompass FAM and evolve into OM, although it is possible for OM to emerge naturally. These meditative praxis produce states that transcend standard conditions of sensory consciousness and cognition. Such states have received multiple labels, such as altered, enhanced, exceptional or expanded [92–95]. The term 'expanded state of consciousness' reflects a more accurate encapsulation of experience. In addition to changes in consciousness and cognition, meditation has an impact on the emotional sphere of the individual. Notably, a review analysing the efficacy of a range of attentional trainings on emotional regulation concludes that meditative practice emerges as the most effective option [96].

One of the prevailing practices in the psychotherapeutic landscape and in contemporary society is mindfulness. The origin of this term dates back to 1881 when W. Rhys Davids translated the Pali word 'sati' [97]. Mindfulness-based interventions involve the practice of FAM on the breath as the preferred anchor of concentration, and often evolve into OM. There are multiple empirically supported mindfulness-based programmes and therapies [98, 99]. Recent meta-analyses indicate that mindfulness is an effective training for improving attention, particularity, sustained and executive attention, albeit with a small effect size [100, 101].

When examining the role of mindfulness in the child and adolescent population, it is remarkable that it has a wide acceptance. There is no school or child and adolescent psychology clinic in the world that is unaware of its knowledge and probably its practice. Does it work? The evidence supports that it does, although it is not a magic bullet. Regarding its effects on attention, a recent systematic review notes that mindfulness-based training and other meditative practices improve children's sustained attention or concentration to a greater extent than effortful cognitive training, for which no reliable improvement in attention is found. However, the review concludes that the level of evidence is preliminary [102].

When seeking to understand how mindfulness works, a pioneering study that addresses the intersection between mindfulness and the neuroscience of attention provides a clarifying answer. The research compares a mindfulness-based intervention with active control in terms of sustained attention in thirteen-year-old schoolchildren. In addition, the study looked at brain connectivity. Specifically, the relationship between the default mode network (DMN), linked to mental wandering, and the right dorsolateral prefrontal cortex (DLPFC), an epicentre of cognitive control, was recorded. The initial assessment showed that those students with better-sustained attention had a higher negative correlation between these two areas. After the intervention, the group that practised mindfulness improved their level of sustained attention and maintained this negative correlation. In contrast, the control group experienced a decrease in both sustained attention and the negative correlation between DMN and DLPFC. These results demonstrate that mindfulness-based training improves not only sustained attention but also influences how these critical brain regions interact with each other. Furthermore, the study is pioneering in crediting a causal connection between mindfulness training and both sustained attention and associated neural plasticity [103].

Importantly, mindfulness engages not only less effortful attention but is also linked to stress reduction. In concordance with this, a study analysed the efficacy of a mindfulness-based intervention versus a control group on selective and sustained attention and daily stress in adolescents. The results indicated a medium effect size for attention and a small effect size for stress [104]. Following this line of research, another mindfulness intervention of only six weeks examined attention and anxiety involving children aged six to thirteen years. Although the evidence of attentional improvement was subtle compared with the control, it is noteworthy that a decrease in trait anxiety was found. This latter finding denotes a stable and extensible change beyond the classroom in the children's anxiety response [105].

The field of meditation is vast and varied, ranging from techniques that require stillness to those that incorporate movement. Despite the popularity of mindfulness in its more static form, one cannot overlook dynamic practices such as Qigong. This form of meditation, rooted in the Chinese medical tradition, intertwines movement and breathing exercises, unfolding an expanded state of consciousness associated with the flow of qi or vital energy [106]. It has been shown that Qigong can mitigate stress [107, 108] and enhance attention. A study highlights this potential, in which a four-week Qigong programme significantly improved selective and sustained attention in adolescents compared to a sham Qigong placebo and a passive control [109].

In another vein, it is worth noting that the application of meditation extends its scope to child and adolescent psychopathology. In the field of attention-related disorder, it is crucial to describe the evidence in the field of ADHD. In this sense, systematic reviews indicate the efficacy of meditative practices, whether static such as mindfulness, or dynamic such as yoga or Tai Chi [110–112]. While the evidence may still be considered preliminary, it is remarkable that these interventions do not have the adverse side effects of conventional pharmacological therapy and, at the same time, promote an increase in well-being. Nevertheless, the 'status quo' in this second decade of the twenty-first century considers them as adjuvant therapy.

Further to this research topic, a study showed the benefits of a mindfulness intervention in female adolescents aged thirteen to sixteen with pronounced ADHD symptoms. Compared to a control group, the girls in the mindfulness group showed significant improvements in certain aspects of attention, such as resistance to interference (inhibition) and, to a lesser extent, attentional span, but not in others such as sustained attention. Crucially, after the intervention, only mindfulness participants showed a significant and large effect size increase in planning ability and emotional regulation in the facets of impulse control and emotional acceptance [113]. In concordance with the previous line of research, a study focusing on children aged seven to eleven years compared the effectiveness of a mindfulness-based intervention with an emotional education programme. The results showed significant improvements with a large effect size unique to participants in the mindfulness programme in the set of neuropsychological tests employed, including the assessment of sustained and executive attention. In addition, a significant reduction in ADHD symptoms was observed only in mindfulness programme participants [114].

Additionally, ADHD impacts not only the health of children and adolescents but also family dynamics. Therefore, interventions involving both children and parents are a crucial line of research. A study involving both parents and their adolescent children examined the efficacy of an eight-week mindfulness-based cognitive therapy (MBCT) programme. Comparisons between pre -and post-intervention assessments revealed a significant reduction in symptoms of inattention, learning disabilities and peer relationship problems, as measured by parental assessments on the Conners' 3 scales. Results of assessments implemented with adolescents revealed significant improvement in family relationships and internalising symptoms, particularly depression and anxiety. In terms of parenting stress, a significant decrease was identified in parents, especially in social isolation and life restrictions. In the area of family functioning, although time effects were reported, detailed comparisons did not reveal significant changes. It is essential to underline the increase in mindfulness in parents after the intervention and its inverse correlation with parental stress. In a follow-up evaluation six weeks later, the persistence of these improvements was confirmed, with additional benefits emerging in parental stress reduction [115]. Consistent with these findings, a similar result was obtained in a study involving children and their parents. Specifically, the intervention facilitated a significant reduction in children's ADHD symptoms as assessed by parents, which was not supported in the teachers' assessment. Additionally, a significant reduction in parental stress and reactive behaviour was evident [116]. The set of findings suggests the desirability of involving the family in mindfulness-based interventions implemented with children and adolescents with ADHD.

Other emerging evidence of therapeutic efficacy for ADHD is found in yoga. Yoga is derived from a set of meditative practices rooted in the Veda tradition, which, according to its doctrine, facilitates holistic mind-body-spirit union [117]. Among the neurophysiological effects associated with its practice is a modulation of the breathing pattern, which slows down and becomes abdominal. At the same time, it induces low-frequency brain waves, with a predominance of alpha waves during meditation, transitioning to theta waves at the end [118]. In addition, a significant reduction in cortisol and adrenocorticotropic hormone (ACTH) levels has been found [119]. In this context of stress reduction, a theoretical model is proposed in which yoga, by reducing sympathetic tone and enhancing parasympathetic tone, favours efficient emotional regulation [120].

In parallel, under this activation reduction approach, yoga promotes an expanded state of consciousness. The state of consciousness is intimately linked to attention, which makes it possible to propose that the practice of yoga improves attentional efficiency. In order to explore possible effective therapeutic alternatives for ADHD, a randomised controlled trial was conducted, contrasting yoga training with neurofeedback training, and also incorporating a wait-list control group. This study assessed sustained attention and attentional span in children diagnosed with ADHD, aged between seven and eleven years. The findings revealed that both alternatives produced a significant effect, with a large effect size on both attentional dimensions compared to the wait-list control [121]. The recommendation of yoga for children diagnosed with ADHD in school and out-of-school settings is the conclusion of a study crediting that the practice in ten-year-olds led to significant improvements in selective, sustained attention and resistance to distracting interference compared to a control group. These improvements were evident with medium to large effect sizes [122]. In a similar vein, another study in children aged six to eight years compares an eight-week yoga intervention with a control group. The results of the study show how the intervention significantly improves emotional regulation and ADHD symptoms in the experimental group compared to the control, which prevailed at the follow-up assessment [123].

In this chapter, we highlight the uniqueness and relevance of autogenic meditation. In contrast to other contemplative practices that have been adapted to fit into the Western worldview, this meditation emerges directly from the Western rational-scientific perspective. It is the legacy of Johannes Heinrich Schultz, a visionary German neuropsychiatrist, who in 1932 introduced the world to this methodology through his revelatory work 'Das Autogene Training-Konzentrative Selbstentspannung' (Autogenic Training-Concentrative Self-relaxation) [124]. Beyond presenting a secular meditative practice of a medical-scientific nature, this method lays the theoretical foundations for a new paradigm in twentieth-century psychotherapy, known as autogenic psychotherapy. In addition to standard and advanced autogenic meditation, autogenic psychotherapy includes a wide range of psychophysiologically oriented approaches. Unlike other medical or psychological forms of treatment, this therapeutic arsenal has the peculiarity of involving both mind and body simultaneously, with autogenic meditation as its core and starting point [125]. Clinical applications cover a broad spectrum, with particular relevance to stress disorders and psychosomatic conditions [125–129]. Non-clinical applications include the enhancement of well-being and psychophysical performance [126, 130].

The term 'autogenic', meaning self-generated, refers to two key therapeutic aspects. From a neuropsychophysiological point of view, it refers to the self-induced transition to the autogenic state that stimulates homeostatic, restorative and self-normalising self-regulatory processes [125]. From the locus of the control point of view, it emphasises the active role of the individual in his or her own training or treatment. Autogenic meditation comprises six exercises, formulas, or dual meditation anchors meticulously designed to access a specific expanded state of consciousness that activates self-regulatory technical keys not normally accessible to the non-practitioner. The exercises are: 1. Weight. 2. Warmth. 3. Cardiac regulation. 4. Breathing regulation. 5. Solar plexus regulation and 6. Fresh forehead. For a detailed explanation of the method, a protocol of autogenic group meditation, adapted for children and adolescents, is freely available [131]. In order to gain a better understanding of autogenic meditation, it is also recommended to read the work of González de Rivera [132].

It is essential to recognise that there are currently two predominant interpretations of the autogenic method: the autosuggestive and the meditative approaches. This is unsurprising, as both are the fundamental antecedents. These perspectives are relevant and effective. However, from its origin, the method is deeply anchored in meditative practice. For illustrative purposes and without entering into an interesting debate, two quotations from its creator are enough to support the tendency we are presenting here. Schultz affirmed: 'There is an approximation and even coincidence between many aspects of the mystical and millenary tradition of Buddhism and the scientific-organismic attitude represented by autogenic training' ([130], p. 213). He further emphasised that: 'We have repeatedly pointed out that our technique does not consist of measures of a suggestive nature, and that it consists primarily of an exercise of concentration. There is in no way a forced relationship between autosuggestion and autogenic training' ([130], p. 206). It is imperative to understand that while both approaches are valid, they involve different perspectives and instructions, which may result in variations in efficacy and effects. This issue is especially relevant in the education or training of attention at hand, where results may diverge.

Almost a century after the origin of autogenic training through concentrative relaxation, a contemporary explanation of the standard training, framed as autogenic meditation, is presented. It is important to note that under the original labels of 'passive concentration and passive acceptance', the practice of autogenic meditation involves the two attentional skills elucidated in current contemplative science: Focused Attention Meditation (FAM) and Open Monitoring of attention (OM) [2]. Autogenic meditation facilitates an expanded state of consciousness by exercising FAM or 'passive concentration' on six specific formulas or dual meditation objects. The uniqueness of FAM in autogenic meditation is that it combines in a single meditative act a meditation object that is simultaneously mental and bodily. The practitioner activates FAM by using subvocal repetition of the corresponding formula (e.g., my heart beats) while focusing attention on the mental meditation object (the idiosyncratic representation of the beating heart). Simultaneously, the practitioner focuses attention on the concurrent physiological-somatic sensations (heartbeat), the bodily object of meditation.

This process of conscious interaction allows a harmonious bridge between mind and body, integrating two perspectives of the same experience, the mental representations and their bodily correlates. Two information processing pathways converge: a semantic pathway that gives access to psychological or personal meaning and a somatic pathway that gives access to spatial information, the body schema and the proprioception of the internal physiology. This sign is unique, to the authors' knowledge, there is no dual meditation in six anchors. As practitioners hone their FAM skill on these synchronous dual objects, an Open Monitoring of attention (OM) capability surfaces. This favours a non-reactive meta-attention or an equanimous, 'passive acceptance' of the phenomena occurring in the field of consciousness, paving the way for meta-consciousness. It is interesting how this practice that begins with a dual perspective progressively leads to a unified state of consciousness. The meditator in his or her mind-body conscious attentional space transcends from a dual state to a non-dual state in harmony. Through autogenic meditation, the practitioner blurs and overcomes the intangible boundaries between mind and body, bringing about an awakening to the autogenic self. This is the essence of autogenic experiential learning. The autogenic meditation learning process is presented in **Table 1**.

Although the autogenic state is predominantly calm and pleasant and often confers a pronounced sense of egosyntonic peace, it possesses a singular phenomenon termed: 'discharge'. This allows the release of physical or psychological tensions. Such therapeutic effect is elicited by the self-regulating homeostatic processes activated by the brain during the autogenic state. Manifestations can range from muscle twitching, eyelid vibration, lacrimation and release of somatosensory or cognitive

Dual synchronous meditative attentional focusing		
Formulas: mind-body integration exercises	**Mental meditation object representation**	**Body meditation object awareness**
I. Weight	My arm-arms-neck-legs-body (is-are) heavy	Body mass
II. Warmth	My arm-arms-neck-legs-body (is-are) warm	Body temperature
III. Heart	My heart beats	Heartbeats
IV. Breathing	My breathing is	Respiratory flow
V. Solar plexus	My abdomen is pleasantly warm	Surrounding area of abdominal organs
VI. Forehead	My forehead is pleasantly fresh, and my mind is lucid	Frontal cephalic region

The representation of the mental meditation object is idiosyncratic and may be acoustic or visual, among other modalities. The body meditation object involves physiological-somatic awareness. Note 1: In addition to the dual meditative attentional focus (DMAF), as the process progresses, open monitoring of attention (OM) begins to develop progressively, which is usually noticeable from formula VI onwards. Note 2: In combination with each formula, the rest formula can be introduced: "I am calm", which represents a cross-sectional value of calm during meditation training. The recommended ratio is 6:1, i.e., six repetitions of the corresponding formula to one repetition of the rest formula.

Table 1.
Autogenic meditation learning process.

experiences, among others. These experiences, which are almost always neutralised naturally, are a sign of progression. Furthermore, if necessary, as the creator of autogenic therapy, Luhte, taught, an opportunity for psychotherapy arises from it by means of specific methods, which must inevitably be dealt with by a specialised psychologist or psychiatrist [125, 133, 134].

Once the autogenic meditation has been presented, it is relevant to frame it within the context of 'state training' or effortless attention training. These trainings develop a non-stressful attention state of parasympathetic dominance, facilitating an optimal level of attentional effort [6, 58–60]. The autogenic state has been defined in terms of 'relaxed alertness' [135], which simultaneously indicates a state of relaxation and optimal cognitive performance.

Neurophysiological changes accompanying the autogenic state include a reduction in heart rate, vagal tone and salivary amylase levels [136, 137], regulation of blood pressure [138] and an increase in muscle distension and peripheral vasodilatation [130, 139]. A reduction in reticulo-cortical and thalamo-cortical activity is also observed, as well as immediate changes in structures connected to the reticular formation, such as the hypothalamus, cerebellum and limbic system, among others [139]. Regarding the brain wave pattern, EEGs show a predominance of theta and alpha waves [140]. Furthermore, research has identified a synchronisation between cardiac coherence and alpha waves during the autogenic state, indicating a harmonisation between the heart and brain [141, 142]. Overall, the evidence shows a state of self-regulation involving synergistic cooperation between the autonomic and central nervous systems [2]. Regarding the autonomic nervous system, this complementary and reciprocal cooperation is predominantly manifested as an increase in parasympathetic activation and a decrease in sympathetic activation [143–145]. It is noteworthy to underline that autogenic meditation goes beyond relaxation, as it allows the exercise of voluntary control of involuntary functions of the autonomic nervous system.

The neurophysiological profile, characteristic of the autogenic state, decreases stress reactivity and facilitates an optimal level of response [144]. In agreement with this assessment, the renowned endocrinologist Hans Selye pointed out in the foreword of the manual: 'Introductory Workshop on Autogenic Therapy Methods' that autogenic meditation unfolds a response diametrically opposed to that provoked by stress [146], underlining its relevance for holistic well-being. This has been corroborated in meta-analysis studies and systematic reviews on the efficacy of autogenic meditation in regulating stress and anxiety in both clinical and non-clinical populations [126–128]. In addition, this research also highlights its potential for well-being [126], depressive symptomatology and increasing cardiac variability [127].

It is evident that the autogenic state achieved through a serene attention education based on FAM and OM skills fully coincides with that delineated for less effortful attentional training. However, despite theoretical postulations in specialised manuals for children and adult populations suggesting attentional improvement [130, 147], empirical research in this area remains limited.

One of the pioneering research studies in the field involves five experiments in different age cohorts [148]. The first study focused on schoolchildren between the ages of eight and ten. Subsequent studies, from the second to the fourth, included young university students with average ages between twenty-two and twenty-three years. Finally, the fifth study focused on older adults, with an average age of seventy-two years. The first experiment compared a group assigned to a single guided session based on some autogenic FAM anchors (weight, warmth, breath and calm) of ten minutes with another group with a silent break of equivalent duration. Subjects were tested pre- and immediately after the experiment finished on their attentional span, verbal fluency and general intelligence. Results indicated significant improvements with a large effect size in attentional span and verbal fluency, but no improvement in general intelligence in the guided meditation group and no significant change in the control. The second experiment, similar in design to the first, replaced the intelligence test with a measure of selective and sustained attention or concentration. The results showed a similar pattern to the previous experiment, with significant changes and large, though slightly attenuated, effect sizes. In addition, concentration improved significantly, with a quasi-large effect size. The third experiment also focused on university students but had a variation in design, as half of the participants had at least six months of experience in autogenic meditation. The same test battery was used as in the previous experiment, comparing efficacy with a control condition that rested for ten minutes. The results showed significant changes with large effect sizes on all measures exclusive to the autogenic meditation group. Notably, Cohen's d nearly doubled in magnitude from the previous experiment. The fourth experiment, which also involved university students and used the same test battery, had the peculiarity that, although all participants had experience in autogenic meditation, some were asked to practise just before the final assessment, and others were asked to listen to their favourite music selected beforehand. It is relevant to note that in the initial assessment, all participants obtained high scores compared to their normative groups. The results of the trial showed a significant improvement with large effect sizes in attentional span and concentration only for the group that practised autogenic meditation. This was not the case for verbal fluency; although the improvement was not significant in either group, it was better in the music rest group. Finally, the fifth experiment replicated the previous trial in older adults skilled in autogenic meditation and used relaxing music in the control condition. Although baseline scores on all tests were lower compared to undergraduates, those who meditated showed significant improvements in attentional span and concentration, with a medium effect size. In summary, the five experiments presented here show remarkable attentional change at different developmental stages due to autogenic meditation, highlighting childhood and youth as sensitive periods of attentional plasticity.

The following are several studies that, although they do not use an objective test of attention, require optimal attentional performance and have a transfer to academic performance. Following this line of research, the impact of autogenic meditation on the correction of spelling errors was examined. The trial included 399 schoolchildren with an average age of eleven years. The experimental task consisted of a classroom dictation followed by a correction phase. Those pupils who had been trained in abbreviated autogenic meditation (focusing on the first two formulas) practised meditation for four minutes. Simultaneously, the students in the control group rested with their eyes closed. At the end of this period, both groups had the opportunity to review and correct their dictations. This procedure was repeated on three different occasions during the course. The findings revealed that the autogenic meditation group showed significant improvements in error correction and obtained higher scores compared to the control group. Conversely, the control group also showed significantly fewer correct corrections and more incorrect revisions, with their academic performance worsening after the possibility of correction [149].

Expanding upon the previous line of research, a study analysed the efficacy of autogenic meditation in schoolchildren with reading disabilities. The efficacy of a specific intervention programme for this problem was compared with another programme that included an autogenic meditation module in addition to the programme. The duration of the interventions was one year. The findings highlighted that the participants in the combined programme showed a significant reduction in reading and writing errors, as well as in anxiety, neuroticism and increased extroversion compared to the standard intervention. The study attributes the efficacy to the increased concentration and decreased anxiety acquired with autogenic meditation [150].

More specifically, aligned with the central topic of this chapter—Effortless attention trainings and its intersection with mental health—the authors of this work and their team conducted a recent randomised controlled trial entitled: 'Autogenic meditation: a framework for promoting mental health and attention regulation in children' [2]. The uniqueness of this study lies in its multifaceted and comprehensive approach, investigating not only attention but also state and trait anxiety, and a screening of mental health. The study compared the efficacy of a 12-week autogenic meditation training programme with two controls, one active based on reading training and value orientation with equivalent duration and implementation, and one passive, wait-list condition. The findings were revealing. Following the interventions, participants in the meditation programme raised their selective and sustained attention prominently, manifesting significant changes with large effect sizes. Moreover, not only their state anxiety was significantly reduced, but also their trait anxiety, and in both cases with large effect sizes. These findings suggest in the first case that attention is exercised with a lower level of arousal, facilitating an optimal degree of effort, and in the second case it indicates that this capacity for anxiety regulation extends its reach to different situations of daily life, where children respond less reactively to life events, generating an upward state-trait spiral of calmness that promotes a disposition to be calm and attend serenely. The research also shows in mental health screening that meditators increased their ability to self-regulate emotionally, manage behavioural problems and regulate peer problems, as well as hyperactive-inattentive spectrum symptoms. All these significant changes were shown with large effect sizes. In contrast, controls showed no significant effects.

As can be seen, beyond attention, or more precisely in connection with it, autogenic meditation aims to be a multilevel self-regulation strategy: emotional, cognitive, behavioural and neurophysiological. It is a law of life that young people face challenges, cope with change and deal with stressors of various kinds. An important question is whether autogenic meditation is effective when these difficulties overwhelm their resources and break their psychophysical equilibrium. In this context of distress, one study evaluated the efficacy of autogenic meditation as a single treatment in a sample of adolescents aged seventeen years on average with a diagnosis of adjustment disorder (F 43.2, in accordance with ICD 10) [151]. Specifically, the aim of this research was to determine the therapeutic efficacy of an autogenic meditation training programme through biophysical and biochemical indicators assessed at baseline, completion and six-month follow-up. Results indicated a significant reduction in arterial systolic and diastolic blood pressure, brachial pulse rate, cortisol and blood cholesterol levels after completion of the training, which were maintained at the six-month follow-up assessment. The findings suggest that autogenic meditation is a potential resource for reducing distress, recovery and coping with adaptive challenges. In short, it is a strategy that is not only exclusively promotive but also therapeutic for psychophysical health.

The capacity for emotional and behavioural self-regulation was also explored in an intervention based on autogenic meditation lasting only four hours compared to passive control. The selected sample consisted of children and adolescents aged six to fifteen years with mild or subclinical internalising and some externalising symptoms such as aggression, impulsivity and attention deficit. Following the intervention, a significant decrease in symptoms was observed in the group that practised autogenic meditation. Although the effect size was small, the research concludes that even a minimal four-hour dose of this meditation has broad-spectrum mental health benefits and recommends its implementation in primary care for children and adolescents with subclinical mental health symptoms [152].

It is important to know whether autogenic meditation promotes, alongside emotional regulation, changes in character that can contribute to a balanced and healthy development in young people. This was the purpose of research that scrutinised two mind-body integration techniques. Specifically, the study compared the efficacy of an autogenic meditation intervention and a mindfulness-based meditation intervention, both with an equivalent implementation of eight weeks. The sample consisted of healthy young people with an average age of seventeen years. The study evaluated three-character traits as outlined by Cloninger's personality model—self-determination, cooperation and transcendence—and also incorporated a mental health screening. At the conclusion of the trainings, the results indicated a significant increase in the trait of self-determination only for the participants of the autogenic meditation programme. In addition, a significant increase in the trait of cooperativeness was observed for participants of both meditation practices. The mental health screening showed a significant increase in emotional self-regulation, which supported the efficacy of both meditation programmes. Emotional self-regulation, in turn, showed a correlation with cooperativeness [153]. What is most remarkable about the study is that there were changes in personality traits. That is, stable and consistent increases in self-determination, a trait linked to autonomy and trust exclusively in the autogenic meditation group. Also, cooperativeness, a trait that entails acceptance and compassion, improved for participants in both interventions.

The trait findings cited above, coupled with the observed increases in extroversion and reductions in neuroticism and trait anxiety [2, 150], suggest that autogenic meditation induces profound characterological modifications in an individual's personality structure essential for fostering adaptability and strengthening mental health. In tandem with these traits, the emerging body of evidence found in the sphere of emotional, cognitive and behavioural self-regulation highlights autogenic meditation as a tool that empowers children and young people towards a calm and fulfilling life, where the meditator is a proactive architect of his or her own well-being and mental health.

In addition, it is worth noting that autogenic meditation is one of the most convenient and simplest forms of meditation practice. Its secular nature, the ergonomics of its posture, its sequential learning, the dual focus of concentration on six easily or naturally accessible synchronous meditative anchors, the short periods of practice, its immediate calming effect and most importantly, the fact that only oneself is needed, are reasons that position it as a highly recommended choice. Considering that it is inherently anchored and supported by a psychotherapy approach, it is not only recommended for children and young people but also for mental health professionals who may find in its clinical practice and application an effective tool and response to mental health problems, even more profound than the one addressed in this preliminary instance. While the findings presented are encouraging, and reveal that autogenic meditation has the potential to be a shining beacon on the vast horizon of mental health, research must continue and further studies are needed to establish more robust conclusions in both clinical and paraclinical contexts.

4. Conclusion

In this chapter, it is concluded that emerging evidence supports the capacity of less effortful attentional training to enhance attentional performance and its concurrent role in the sphere of emotional, cognitive and behavioural self-regulation among child and adolescent populations. As highlighted in the introduction, the statement 'You are what you pay attention to' remains pertinent. This allegory is a profound truth about identity and existence. In the act of attending, the individual selects not only what to perceive but also what to be. The sum of attentional states will configure the future identity. Therefore, every act of attention is an opportunity to mould who we will be tomorrow. Attention is intimately linked to all cognitive processes, emotions and behaviour. It is in how one pays attention that the virtue of exercising the conscious self resides, so rather than proposing mere training, one should consider talking about educating attention. Educating attention in a serene and conscious state of mind favours self-regulation in the present and, as James rightly pointed out, sculpts the seed of future character. The preliminary evidence presented in this chapter on attention, anxiety, stress, well-being and personality traits supports this position, although future research should explore this topic further.

Focusing on the present day, one must not end this chapter without reflecting on our contemporary twenty-first century, its circumstances and the fundamental role of child and youth mental health. The influence of digital environments, multi-stimulant devices, online omnipresence and multitasking as predominant lifestyles must be given attention and a watchful eye. In addition to the above, we must consider that we live in a volatile, changing, complex, ambiguous and not always friendly world, so methods that empower children and young people in serenity, psychophysical balance and daily stress management are undoubtedly welcome. The confluence between attention and health is a novel topic that transcends the cognitive approach towards an educational and psychotherapeutic approach. Exposure to nature and meditative practice invites reflection on the appropriateness of mind-body integration in the mental health landscape. Hence, understanding the person and, therefore, children and young people from a holistic perspective is a challenge in the realm of health and well-being. The appropriateness of these less effortful attention approaches in the areas of education, psychotherapy and mental health opens up a new opportunity for the full development of children and young people who are at a peak period of attentional plasticity. Ultimately, this chapter highlights the relevance of educating attention to promote a more fulfilling childhood and adolescence. In the twenty-first century context, it's essential to emphasise that those who best educate their attention will be better prepared to face and successfully adapt to future challenges.

Conflict of interest

The authors declare no conflict of interest.

Author details

Juan M. Guiote[1,2,3]*, Miguel Ángel Vallejo[1] and Blanca Mas[1]

1 Department of Personality, Assessment, and Psychological Treatment, National University of Distance Education (UNED), Madrid, Spain

2 Psychological and Psycho-pedagogical Care Service, University of Granada (UGR), Granada, Spain

3 Inspire Psychology Center, Granada, Spain

*Address all correspondence to: jmguiote@baza.uned.es

References

[1] Tang YY, Posner MI. Attention training and attention state training. Trends in Cognitive Sciences. 2009;**13**(5):222-227. DOI: 10.1016/j.tics.2009.01.009

[2] Guiote JM, Lozano V, Vallejo MA, Mas B. Autogenic meditation training in a randomized controlled trial: A framework for promoting mental health and attention regulation in children. Revista de Psicodidáctica (English ed.). 2022;**27**(1):47-55. DOI: 10.1016/j.psicoe.2021.10.002

[3] Wass SV, Scerif G, Johnson MH. Training attentional control and working memory—Is younger, better? Developmental Review. 2012;**32**(4):360-387. DOI: 10.1016/j.dr.2012.07.001

[4] Peng P, Miller AC. Does attention training work? A selective meta-analysis to explore the effects of attention training and moderators. Learning and Individual Differences. 2016;**45**:77-87. DOI: 10.1016/j.lindif.2015.11.012

[5] Kahneman D. Attention and Effort. Englewood Cliffs, NJ: Prentice-Hall; 1973

[6] Tang YY, Tang R, Posner MI, Gross JJ. Effortless training of attention and self-control: Mechanisms and applications. Trends in Cognitive Sciences. 2022;**26**(7):567-577. DOI: 10.1016/j.tics.2022.04.006

[7] Taylor JG, Fragopanagos NF. The interaction of attention and emotion. Neural Networks. 2005;**18**(4):353-369. DOI: 10.1016/j.neunet.2005.03.005

[8] Raymond J. Interactions of attention, emotion and motivation. Progress in Brain Research. 2009;**176**:293-308. DOI: 10.1016/S0079-6123(09)17617-3

[9] Hartikainen KM. Emotion-attention interaction in the right hemisphere. Brain Sciences. 2021;**11**(8):1006. DOI: 10.3390/brainsci11081006

[10] Smallwood J, Schooler JW. The science of mind wandering: Empirically navigating the stream of consciousness. Annual Review of Psychology. 2015;**66**:487-518. DOI: 10.1146/annurev-psych-010814-015331

[11] Killingsworth MA, Gilbert DT. A wandering mind is an unhappy mind. Science. 2010;**330**(6006):932-932. DOI: 10.1146/science.1192439

[12] Kane MJ, Brown LH, McVay JC, Silvia PJ, Myin-Germeys I, Kwapil TR. For whom the mind wanders, and when: An experience-sampling study of working memory and executive control in daily life. Psychological Science. 2007;**18**(7):614-621. DOI: 10.1111/j.1467-9280.2007.01948.x

[13] Webb CA, Israel ES, Belleau E, Appleman L, Forbes EE, Pizzagalli DA. Mind-wandering in adolescents predicts worse affect and is linked to aberrant default mode network-salience network connectivity. Journal of the American Academy of Child and Adolescent Psychiatry. 2021;**60**(3):377-387. DOI: 10.1016/j.jaac.2020.03.010

[14] Mrazek MD, Phillips DT, Franklin MS, Broadway JM, Schooler JW. Young and restless: Validation of the mind-wandering questionnaire (MWQ) reveals disruptive impact of mind-wandering for youth. Frontiers in Psychology. 2013;**4**:560. DOI: 10.3389/fpsyg.2013.00560

[15] Cherry J, McCormack T, Graham AJ. The link between mind wandering

and learning in children. Journal of Experimental Child Psychology. 2022;**217**:105367. DOI: 10.1016/j.jecp.2021.105367

[16] Baird B, Smallwood J, Mrazek MD, Kam JWY, Franklin MS, Schooler JW. Inspired by distraction: Mind wandering facilitates creative incubation. Psychological Science. 2012;**23**(10):1117-1122. DOI: 10.1177/0956797612446024

[17] James W. The Principles of Psychology. Vol. 1. New York: Henry Holt and Company; 1890. 689 p

[18] Di Lollo V. Attention is a sterile concept; iterative reentry is a fertile substitute. Consciousness and Cognition. 2018;**64**:45-49. DOI: 10.1016/j.concog.2018.02.00

[19] Hommel B, Chapman CS, Cisek P, Neyedli HF, Song J-H, Welsh TN. No one knows what attention is. Attention, Perception, & Psychophysics. 2019;**81**(7):2288-2303. DOI: 10.3758/s13414-019-01846-w

[20] Hommel B, Colzato LS. Learning from history: The need for a synthetic approach to human cognition. Frontiers in Psychology. 2015;**6**:1-4. DOI: 10.3389/fpsyg.2015.01435

[21] Rueda MR. Educar la atención Con Cerebro [Educating Attention with Brain]. Madrid: Alianza Editorial; 2021. 414 p

[22] Yerkes RM, Dodson JD. The relation of strength of stimulus to rapidity of habit-formation. Journal of Comparative Neurology and Psychology. 1908;**18**(5):459-482. DOI: 10.1002/cne.920180503

[23] Corbetta M, Shulman GL. Control of goal-directed and stimulus-driven attention in the brain. Nature Reviews. Neuroscience. 2002;**3**(3):201-215. DOI: 10.1038/nrn755

[24] Skinner BF. About Behaviorism. New York: Vintage Books; 1976. 304 p

[25] Mackintosh NJ. A theory of attention: Variations in the associability of stimuli with reinforcement. Psychological Review. 1975;**82**(4):276-298. DOI: 10.1037/h0076778

[26] Mas B, de Puga RPS. Modelos atencionales del condicionamiento clásico [Attentional models of classical conditioning]. 3ª ed., 13th reprint ed. Madrid: Universidad Nacional de Educación a Distancia; 2009. 125 p

[27] Broadbent BF. Perception and Communication. London: Pergamon Press; 1958. 338 p [Online]. Available from: http://www.communicationcache.com/uploads/1/0/8/8/10887248/d_e._broadbent_-_perception_and_communication_1958.pdf

[28] Treisman AM. Selective attention in man. British Medical Bulletin. 1964;**20**(1):12-16

[29] Deutsch JA, Deutsch D. Attention: Some theoretical considerations. Psychological Review. 1963;**70**(1):80-90

[30] Johnston WA, Heinz SP. Flexibility and capacity demands of attention. Journal of Experimental Psychology. General. 1978;**107**(4):420-435. DOI: 10.1037/0096-3445.107.4.420

[31] Norman DA, Bobrow DG. On data-limited and resource-limited processes. Cognitive Psychology. 1975;**7**(1):44-64. DOI: 10.1016/0010-0285(75)90004-3

[32] Navon D, Gopher D. On the economy of the human-processing system. Psychological Review. 1979;**86**(3):214-255. DOI: 10.1037/0033-295X.86.3.214

[33] Shiffrin RM, Schneider W. Controlled and automatic human information processing: II. Perceptual learning, automatic attending and a general theory. Psychological Review. 1977;**84**(2):127-190. DOI: 10.1037/0033-295X.84.2.127

[34] Norman DA, Shallice T. Attention to action. In: Davidson RJ, Schwartz GE, Shapiro D, editors. Consciousness and Self-Regulation. Boston, MA: Springer; 1986. DOI: 10.1007/978-1-4757-0629-1_1

[35] Mesulam MM. Large-scale neurocognitive networks and distributed processing for attention, language, and memory. Annals of Neurology. 1990;**28**(5):597-613. DOI: 10.1002/ANA.410280502

[36] Miller EK. The prefrontal cortex and cognitive control. Nature Reviews. Neuroscience. 2000;**1**(1):59-65. DOI: 10.1038/35036228

[37] Posner MI, Petersen SE. The attention system of the human brain. Annual Review of Neuroscience. 1990;**13**:25-42. DOI: 10.1146/annurev.ne.13.030190.000325

[38] Petersen SE, Posner MI. The attention system of the human brain: 20 years after. Annual Review of Neuroscience. 2012;**35**:73-89. DOI: 10.1146/annurev-neuro-062111-150525

[39] Aston-Jones G, Cohen JD. An integrative theory of locus coeruleus-norepinephrine function: Adaptive gain and optimal performance. Annual Review of Neuroscience. 2005;**28**:403-450. DOI: 10.1146/annurev.neuro.28.061604.135709

[40] Bush G, Luu P, Posner MI. Cognitive and emotional influences in anterior cingulate cortex. Trends in Cognitive Sciences. 2000;**4**(6):215-222. DOI: 10.1016/s1364-6613(00)01483-2

[41] Dosenbach NU, Fair DA, Miezin FM, Cohen AL, Wenger KK, Dosenbach RA, et al. Distinct brain networks for adaptive and stable task control in humans. Proceedings of the National Academy of Sciences of the United States of America. 2007;**104**(26):11073-11078. DOI: 10.1073/pnas.0704320104

[42] Dosenbach NU, Fair DA, Cohen AL, Schlaggar BL, Petersen SE. A dual-networks architecture of top-down control. Trends in Cognitive Sciences. 2008;**12**(3):99-105. DOI: 10.1016/j.tics.2008.01.001

[43] Posner MI, Rothbart MK. Genetic and experiential factors in brain development: The example of executive attention and self-regulation. In: Houdé O, Borst G, editors. The Cambridge Handbook of Cognitive Development. Cambridge: Cambridge University Press; 2022. pp. 105-121

[44] Diamond A. Executive functions. Annual Review of Psychology. 2013;**64**:135-168. DOI: 10.1146/annurev-psych-113011-143750

[45] Miyake A, Friedman NP, Emerson MJ, Witzki AH, Howerter A, Wager TD. The unity and diversity of executive functions and their contributions to complex "frontal lobe" tasks: A latent variable analysis. Cognitive Psychology. 2000;**41**(1):49-100. DOI: 10.1006/cogp.1999.0734

[46] Fan J, Wu Y, Fossella JA, Posner MI. Assessing the heritability of attentional networks. BMC Neuroscience. 2001;**2**(14):1-7. DOI: 10.1186/1471-2202-2-14

[47] Congdon E, Lesch KP, Canli T. Analysis of DRD4 and DAT

polymorphisms and behavioral inhibition in healthy adults: Implications for impulsivity. American Journal of Medical Genetics Part B. 2008;**147**:27-32. DOI: 10.1002/ajmg.b.30557

[48] Congdon E, Constable RT, Lesch KP, Canli T. Influence of SLC6A3 and COMT variation on neural activation during response inhibition. Biological Psychology. 2009;**81**(3):144-152. DOI: 10.1016/j.biopsycho.2009.03.005

[49] Kuc K, Bielecki M, Racicka-Pawlukiewicz E, Czerwinski MB, Cybulska-Klosowicz A. The SLC6A3 gene polymorphism is related to the development of attentional functions but not to ADHD. Scientific Reports. 2020;**10**(1):6176. DOI: 10.1038/s41598-020-63296-x

[50] Greenwood PM, Parasuraman R, Espeseth T. A cognitive phenotype for a polymorphism in the nicotinic receptor gene CHRNA4. Neuroscience and Biobehavioral Reviews. 2012;**36**(4):1331-1341. DOI: 10.1016/j.neubiorev.2012.02.010

[51] Mezzacappa E. Alerting, orienting, and executive attention: Developmental properties and sociodemographic correlates in an epidemiological sample of young, urban children. Child Development. 2004;**75**(5):1373-1386. DOI: 10.1111/j.1467-8624.2004.00746.x

[52] Noble KG, McCandliss BD, Farah MJ. Socioeconomic gradients predict individual differences in neurocognitive abilities. Developmental Science. 2007;**10**(4):464-480. DOI: 10.1111/j.1467-7687.2007.00600.x

[53] Bernier A, Carlson SM, Whipple N. From external regulation to self-regulation: Early parenting precursors of young children's executive functioning. Child Development. 2010;**81**(1):326-339. DOI: 10.1111/j.1467-8624.2009.01397.x

[54] Valcan DS, Davis H, Pino-Pasternak D. Parental behaviours predicting early childhood executive functions: A meta-analysis. Educational Psychology Review. 2018;**30**:607-649. DOI: 10.1007/s10648-017-9411-9

[55] Kirk HE, Spencer-Smith M, Wiley JF, Cornish KM. Gamified attention training in the primary School classroom: A cluster-randomized controlled trial. Journal of Attention Disorders. 2021;**25**(8):1146-1159. DOI: 10.1177/1087054719887435

[56] Rueda MR, Checa P, Combita LM. Enhanced efficiency of the executive attention network after training in preschool children: Immediate changes and effects after two months. Developmental Cognitive Neuroscience. 2012;**2**:S192-S204. DOI: 10.1016/j.dcn.2011.09.004

[57] Bruya B, Tang YY. Is attention really effort? Revisiting Daniel Kahneman's influential 1973 book attention and effort. Frontiers in Psychology. 2018;**9**:1133. DOI: 10.3389/fpsyg.2018.01133

[58] Posner MI, Rothbart MK, Tang Y-Y. Enhancing attention through training. Current Opinion in Behavioral Sciences. 2015;**4**:1-5. DOI: 10.1016/j.cobeha.2014.12.008

[59] Tang Y-Y, Posner MI. Attention training and attention state training. Trends in Cognitive Sciences. 2009;**13**(5):222-227. DOI: 10.1016/j.tics.2009.01.009

[60] Tang Y-Y, Posner MI. Training brain networks and states. Trends in Cognitive Sciences. 2014;**18**(7):345-350. DOI: 10.1016/j.tics.2014.04.002

[61] Kaplan S. The restorative benefits of nature: Toward an integrative framework. Journal of Environmental Psychology. 1995;**15**(3):169-182. DOI: 10.1016/0272-4944(95)90001-2

[62] Kaplan S. Meditation, restoration, and the management of mental fatigue. Environment and Behavior. 2001;**33**(4):480-506. DOI: 10.1177/00139160121973106

[63] Bowler DE, Buyung-Ali LM, Knight TM, Pullin AS. A systematic review of evidence for the added benefits to health of exposure to natural environments. BMC Public Health. 2010;**10**(1):1-10. DOI: 10.1186/1471-2458-10-456

[64] Bernardes M, Vergara LGL. Aprendiendo entre la naturaleza: Una revisión de los beneficios de los espacios verdes en el ambiente escolar [Learning among nature: A review of the benefits of green spaces in the school environment]. Arquitecturas del Sur. 2017;**35**(52):96-103. DOI: 10.22320/07196466.2017.35.052.09

[65] Kaplan S, Berman MG. Directed attention as a common resource for executive functioning and self-regulation. Perspectives on Psychological Science. 2010;5:43-57. DOI: 10.1177/17456916093567

[66] Ohly H, White MP, Wheeler BW, Bethel A, Ukoumunne OC, Nikolaou V, et al. Attention restoration theory: A systematic review of the attention restoration potential of exposure to natural environments. Journal of Toxicology & Environmental Health Part B: Critical Reviews. 2016;**19**(7):305-343. DOI: 10.1080/10937404.2016.1196155

[67] Ulrich RS. Aesthetic and affective response to natural environment. In: Altman I, Wohlwill JF, editors. Behavior and the Natural Environment, Human Behavior and Environment. Vol. 6. Boston, MA: Springer; 1983. pp. 85-125. DOI: 10.1007/978-1-4613-3539-9_4

[68] Ulrich RS, Simons RF, Losito BD, Fiorito E, Miles MA, Zelson M. Stress recovery during exposure to natural and urban environments. Journal of Environmental Psychology. 1991;**11**(3):201-230. DOI: 10.1016/S0272-4944(05)80184-7

[69] Shin WS, Shin CS, Yeoun PS, Kim JJ. The influence of interaction with forest on cognitive function. Scandinavian Journal of Forest Research. 2011;**26**(6):595-598. DOI: 10.1080/02827581.2011.585996

[70] Berman MG, Jonides J, Kaplan S. The cognitive benefits of interacting with nature. Psychological Science. 2008;**19**(12):1207-1212. DOI: 10.1111/j.1467-9280.2008.02225.x

[71] Berman MG, Kross E, Krpan KM, Askren MK, Burson A, Deldin PJ, et al. Interacting with nature improves cognition and affect for individuals with depression. Journal of Affective Disorders. 2012;**140**(3):300-305. DOI: 10.1016/j.jad.2012.03.012

[72] Cassarino M, Tuohy IC, Setti A. Sometimes nature doesn't work: Absence of attention restoration in older adults exposed to environmental scenes. Experimental Aging Research. 2019;**45**(4):372-385. DOI: 10.1080/0361073X.2019.1627497

[73] Wallner P, Kundi M, Arnberger A, Eder R, Allex B, Weitensfelder L, et al. Reloading pupils' batteries: Impact of green spaces on cognition and wellbeing. International Journal of Environmental Research and Public Health. 2018;**15**(6):1205. DOI: 10.3390/ijerph15061205

[74] Stevenson MP, Dewhurst R, Schilhab T, Bentsen P. Cognitive restoration in children following exposure to nature: Evidence from the attention network task and mobile eye tracking. Frontiers in Psychology. 2019;**10**:42. DOI: 10.3389/fpsyg.2019.00042

[75] Johnson SA, Snow S, Lawrence MA, Rainham DGC. Quasi-randomized trial of contact with nature and effects on attention in children. Frontiers in Psychology. 2019;**10**:2652. DOI: 10.3389/fpsyg.2019.02652

[76] Dettweiler U, Becker C, Auestad BH, Simon P, Kirsch P, Stress in School. Some empirical hints on the circadian cortisol rhythm of children in outdoor and indoor classes. International Journal of Environmental Research and Public Health. 2017;**14**(5):475. DOI: 10.3390/ijerph14050475

[77] Li D, Sullivan WC. Impact of views to school landscapes on recovery from stress and mental fatigue. Landscape Urban Plan. 2016;**148**:149-158. DOI: 10.1016/j.landurbplan.2015.12.015

[78] Schutte AR, Torquati JC, Beattie HL. Impact of urban nature on executive functioning in early and middle childhood. Environment and Behavior. 2017;**49**(1):3-30. DOI: 10.1177/0013916515603095

[79] Vella-Brodrick DA, Gilowska K. Effects of nature (greenspace) on cognitive functioning in school children and adolescents: A systematic review. Educational Psychology Review. 2022;**34**(3):1217-1254. DOI: 10.1007/s10648-022-09658-5

[80] Li D, Chiang YC, Sang H, Sullivan WC. Beyond the school grounds: Links between density of tree cover in school surroundings and high school academic performance. Urban Forestry & Urban Greening. 2019;**38**:42-53. DOI: 10.1016/j.ufug.2018.11.001

[81] Taylor AF, Kuo FE, Sullivan WC. Coping with ADD: The surprising connection to green play settings. Environment and Behavior. 2001;**33**(1):54-77. DOI: 10.1177/00139160121972864

[82] Kuo FE, Taylor AF. A potential natural treatment for attention-deficit/hyperactivity disorder: Evidence from a national study. American Journal of Public Health. 2004;**94**:1580-1586. DOI: 10.2105/AJPH.94.9.1580

[83] Taylor AF, Kuo FE. Children with attention deficits concentrate better after walk in the park. Journal of Attention Disorders. 2009;**12**(5):402-409. DOI: 10.1177/1087054708323000

[84] Lippelt DP, Hommel B, Colzato LS. Focused attention, open monitoring and loving kindness meditation: Effects on attention, conflict monitoring, and creativity—A review. Frontiers in Psychology. 2014;**5**:1083. DOI: 10.3389/fpsyg.2014.01083

[85] Lutz A, Slagter HA, Dunne JD, Davidson RJ. Attention regulation and monitoring in meditation. Trends in Cognitive Sciences. 2008;**12**(4):163-169. DOI: 10.1016/j.tics.2008.01.005

[86] Yamashiro J. Brain basis of samadhi: The neuroscience of meditative absorption. New School Psychology Bulletin. 2015;**13**(1):1-10. Available from: https://www.nspb.net/index.php/nspb/article/view/260

[87] Kalsang T. Shi-gnas (Samatha) meditation. The Tibet Journal. 1977;**2**(4):43-49. Available from: http://www.jstor.org/stable/43299886

[88] Hobbiss MH, Lavie N. Sustained selective attention in adolescence: Cognitive development and predictors of distractibility at school. Journal of Experimental Child Psychology. 2024;**238**:105784. DOI: 10.1016/j.jecp.2023.105784

[89] Hobbiss MH, Fairnie J, Jafari K, Lavie N. Attention, mindwandering, and mood. Consciousness and Cognition. 2019;**72**:1-18. DOI: 10.1016/j.concog.2019.04.007

[90] Vago DR, Silbersweig DA. Self-awareness, self-regulation, and self-transcendence (S-ART): A framework for understanding the neurobiological mechanisms of mindfulness. Frontiers in Human Neuroscience. 2012;**6**:296. DOI: 10.3389/fnhum.2012.00296

[91] Ahir DC. Vipassana: A Universal Buddhist Meditation Technique. Delhi: Sri Satguru Publications; 1999. 202 p

[92] Shapiro DH, Giber D. Meditation and psychotherapeutic effects: Self-regulation strategy and altered state of consciousness. Archives of General Psychiatry. 1978;**35**(3):294-302. DOI: 10.1001/archpsyc.1978.01770270044003

[93] Nash JD, Newberg A, Awasthi B. Toward a unifying taxonomy and definition for meditation. Frontiers in Psychology. 2013;**4**:806. DOI: 10.3389/fpsyg.2013.00806

[94] Alexander CN, Langer EJ, Newman RI, Chandler HM, Davies JL. Transcendental meditation, mindfulness, and longevity: An experimental study with the elderly. Journal of Personality and Social Psychology. 1989;**57**(6):950-964. DOI: 10.1037//0022-3514.57.6.950

[95] Reavley N, Pallant JF. Development of a scale to assess the meditation experience. Personality and Individual Differences. 2009;**47**(6):547-552. DOI: 10.1016/j.paid.2009.05.007

[96] Wadlinger HA, Isaacowitz DM. Fixing our focus: Training attention to regulate emotion. Personality and Social Psychology Review. 2011;**15**(1):75-102. DOI: 10.1177/1088868310365565

[97] Gethin R. On some definitions of mindfulness. Contemporary Buddhism. 2011;**12**:263-279. DOI: 10.1080/14639947.2011.564843

[98] Kabat-Zinn J. Full Catastrophe Living: Using the Wisdom of your Body and Mind to Face Stress, Pain, and Illness. New York: Dell Publishing; 1990

[99] Segal ZV, Williams JMG, Teasdale JD. Mindfulness-Based Cognitive Therapy for Depression: A New Approach to Preventing Relapse. New York: Guilford Press; 2002

[100] Verhaeghen P. Mindfulness as attention training: Meta-analyses on the links between attention performance and mindfulness interventions, long-term meditation practice, and trait mindfulness. Mindfulness. 2021;**12**(3):564-581. DOI: 10.1007/s12671-020-01532-1

[101] Yakobi O, Smilek D, Danckert J. The effects of mindfulness meditation on attention, executive control and working memory in healthy adults: A meta-analysis of randomized controlled trials. Cognitive Therapy and Research. 2021;**45**(4):543-560. DOI: 10.1007/s10608-020-10177-2

[102] Slattery EJ, O'Callaghan E, Ryan P, Fortune DG, McAvinue LP. Popular interventions to enhance sustained attention in children and adolescents: A critical systematic review. Neuroscience and Biobehavioral Reviews. 2022;**137**:104633. DOI: 10.1016/j.neubiorev.2022.104633

[103] Bauer CCC, Rozenkrantz L, Caballero C, Nieto-Castanon A, Scherer E, West MR, et al. Mindfulness training preserves sustained attention and resting state anticorrelation between default-mode network and dorsolateral prefrontal cortex: A randomized controlled trial. Human Brain Mapping. 2020;**41**(18):5356-5369. DOI: 10.1002/hbm.25197

[104] Baena-Extremera A, del Mar O-CM, Marfil-Sánchez AM, Granero-Gallegos A. Improvement of attention and stress levels in students through a mindfulness intervention program. Revista de Psicodidáctica. 2021;**26**(2):132-142. DOI: 10.1016/j.psicoe.2020.12.002

[105] Ricarte JJ, Ros L, Latorre JM, Beltrán MT. Mindfulness-based intervention in a rural primary school: Effects on attention, concentration and mood. International Journal of Cognitive Therapy. 2015;**8**(3):258-270. DOI: 10.1521/ijct_2015_8_03

[106] Greten J. Kursbuch Traditionelle Chinesische Medizin: TCM Verstehen und Richtig Anwenden. Stuttgart: Georg Thieme Verlag; 2007. 507 p

[107] Jouper J, Hassmén P. Intrinsically motivated qigong exercisers are more concentrated and less stressful. The American Journal of Chinese Medicine. 2008;**36**(06):1051-1060. DOI: 10.1142/S0192415X08006557

[108] Skoglund L, Jansson E. Qigong reduces stress in computer operators. Complementary Therapies in Clinical Practice. 2007;**13**(2):78-84. DOI: 10.1016/j.ctcp.2006.09.003

[109] Duarte L, Gonçalves M, Mendes P, Matos LC, Greten HJ, Machado J. Can qigong improve attention in adolescents? A prospective randomised controlled trial. Journal of Bodywork and Movement Therapies. 2020;**24**(1):175-181. DOI: 10.1016/j.jbmt.2019.05.005

[110] Gonzalez NA, Sakhamuri N, Athiyaman S, Randhi B, Gutlapalli SD, Pu J, et al. A systematic review of yoga and meditation for attention-deficit/hyperactivity disorder in children. Cureus. 2023;**15**(3):e36143. DOI: 10.7759/cureus.36143

[111] Barranco-Ruiz Y, Esturo Etxabe B, Ramírez-Vélez R, Villa-González E. Interventions based on Mind–Body therapies for the improvement of Attention-Deficit/Hyperactivity Disorder symptoms in youth: A systematic review. Medicina. 2019;**55**(7):325. DOI: 10.3390/medicina55070325

[112] Herbert A, Esparham A. Mind–body therapy for children with attention-deficit/hyperactivity disorder. Children. 2017;**4**(5):31. DOI: 10.3390/children4050031

[113] Kiani B, Hadianfard H, Mitchell JT. The impact of mindfulness meditation training on executive functions and emotion dysregulation in an Iranian sample of female adolescents with elevated attention-deficit/hyperactivity disorder symptoms. Australian Journal of Psychology. 2017;**69**(4):273-282. DOI: 10.1111/ajpy.12148

[114] Santonastaso O, Zaccari V, Crescentini C, Fabbro F, Capurso V, Vicari S, et al. Clinical application of mindfulness-oriented meditation: A preliminary study in children with ADHD. International Journal of Environmental Research and Public Health. 2020;**17**(18):6916. DOI: 10.3390/ijerph17186916

[115] Haydicky J, Shecter C, Wiener J, Ducharme JM. Evaluation of MBCT for adolescents with ADHD and their parents: Impact on individual and family

functioning. Journal of Child and Family Studies. 2015;**24**:76-94. DOI: 10.1007/s10826-013-9815-1

[116] Van der Oord S, Bögels SM, Peijnenburg D. The effectiveness of mindfulness training for children with ADHD and mindful parenting for their parents. Journal of Child and Family Studies. 2012;**21**(1):139-147. DOI: 10.1007/s10826-011-9457-0

[117] White DG. Introduction: Yoga, brief history of an idea. In: White DG, editor. Yoga in Practice. Princeton: Princeton University Press; 2012. pp. 1-23

[118] Arambula P, Peper E, Kawakami M, Gibney KH. The physiological correlates of kundalini yoga meditation: A study of a yoga master. Applied Psychophysiology and Biofeedback. 2001;**26**(2):147-153. DOI: 10.1023/a:1011343307783

[119] Pal R, Singh SN, Chatterjee A, Saha M. Age-related changes in cardiovascular system, autonomic functions, and levels of BDNF of healthy active males: Role of yogic practice. Age (Dordrecht, Netherlands). 2014;**36**(4):9683. DOI: 10.1007/s11357-014-9683-7

[120] Streeter CC, Gerbarg PL, Saper RB, Ciraulo DA, Brown RP. Effects of yoga on the autonomic nervous system, gamma-aminobutyric-acid, and allostasis in epilepsy, depression, and post-traumatic stress disorder. Medical Hypotheses. 2012;**78**(5):571-579. DOI: 10.1016/j.mehy.2012.01.021

[121] Rezaei M, Kamarzard TS, Razavi MN. The effects of neurofeedback, yoga interventions on memory and cognitive activity in children with attention deficit/hyperactivity disorder: A randomized controlled trial. Annals of Applied Sport Science. 2018;**6**(4):17-27. DOI: 10.29252/aassjournal.6.4.17

[122] Chou CC, Huang CJ. Effects of an 8-week yoga program on sustained attention and discrimination function in children with attention deficit hyperactivity disorder. PeerJ. 2017;**5**:e2883. DOI: 10.7717/peerj.2883

[123] Wang S. Yoga for emotional control in children with adhd. Revista Brasileira de Medicina do Esporte. 2023;**29**:e2022_0391. DOI: 10.1590/1517-8692202329012022_0391

[124] Schultz JH. Das Autogene Training: Konzentrative Selbstentspannung. Leipzig: Georg Thieme Verlag; 1932. 305 p

[125] Luthe W, Schultz JH. Autogenic Therapy: Vol.1. Autogenic Method. New York: Grune & Stratton; 1969. 255 p

[126] Yumkhaibam AH, Farooque S, Bhowmik SK. Effectiveness of autogenic training on reducing anxiety disorders: A comprehensive review and meta-analysis. European Journal of Physical Education and Sport Science. 2023;**10**(3):124-141. DOI: 10.46827/ejpe.v10i3.5059

[127] Seo E, Kim S. Effect of autogenic training for stress response: A systematic review and meta-analysis. Journal of Korean Academy of Nursing. 2019;**49**(4):361-374. DOI: 10.4040/jkan.2019.49.4.361

[128] Ernst E, Kanji N. Autogenic training for stress and anxiety: A systematic review. Complementary Therapies in Medicine. 2000;**8**(2):106-110. DOI: 10.1054/ctim.2000.0354

[129] Stetter F, Kupper S. Autogenic training: A meta-analysis of clinical outcome studies. Applied Psychophysiology and

Biofeedback. 2002;**27**(1):45-98. DOI: 10.1023/a:1014576505223

[130] Schultz JH. El entrenamiento autógeno: Autorrelajación concentrativa. Exposición clínico-práctica [Autogenic training: Concentrative self-relaxation. Clinical-practical exposition]. Barcelona: Científico Médica; 1969. 235 p

[131] Guiote JM, Lozano V, Vallejo MA, Mas B. Autogenic meditation training in a randomized controlled trial: A framework for promoting mental health and attention regulation in children [dataset]. e-cienciaDatos; 2021. Detailed protocol of the procedure with each group.pdf [fileName]. DOI: 10.21950/SVZ860

[132] de Rivera JL. Autogenic 3.0 the New Way to Mindfulness and Meditation. Madrid: ICAT; 2017. 238 p

[133] Luthe W. Autogenic Therapy: Vol. 5. Dynamics of Autogenic Neutralization. New York: Grune & Stratton; 1970. 344 p

[134] Luthe W. Autogenic Therapy: Vol. 6. Treatment with Autogenic Neutralization. New York: Grune & Stratton; 1973. 441 p

[135] Ikemi A. Psychophysiological effects of self-regulation method: EEG frequency analysis and contingent negative variations. Psychotherapy and Psychosomatics. 1988;**49**(3-4):230-239. DOI: 10.1159/000288088

[136] Kiba T, Abe T, Kanbara K, Kato F, Kawashima S, Saka Y, et al. The relationship between salivary amylase and the physical and psychological changes elicited by continuation of autogenic training in patients with functional somatic syndrome. BioPsychoSocial Medicine. 2017;**11**:17. DOI: 10.1186/s13030-017-0103-y

[137] Miu AC, Heilman RM, Miclea M. Reduced heart rate variability and vagal tone in anxiety: Trait versus state, and the effects of autogenic training. Autonomic Neuroscience. 2009;**145**(1-2):99-103. DOI: 10.1016/j.autneu.2008.11.010

[138] Watanabe Y, Cornélissen G, Watanabe M, Watanabe F, Otsuka K, Ohkawa S, et al. Effects of autogenic training and antihypertensive agents on circadian and circaseptan variation of blood pressure. Clinical and Experimental Hypertension. 2003;**25**(7):405-412. DOI: 10.1081/CEH-120024984

[139] Luthe W, Jus A, Geissmann P. Autogenic state and autogenic shift: Psychophysiologic and neurophysiologic aspects. Psychotherapy and Psychosomatics. 1963;**11**(1):1-13. DOI: 10.1159/000285660

[140] Lee JY, Lim CH. Prefrontal activation in the EEG biofeedback training using a general-purpose brainwave meter. Indian Journal of Public Health Research & Development. 2018;**9**(3):622-628. DOI: 10.5958/0976-5506.2018.00359.5

[141] Kim D-K, Lee K-M, Kim J, Whang M-C, Kang SW. Dynamic correlations between heart and brain rhythm during autogenic meditation. Frontiers in Human Neuroscience. 2013;**7**:414. DOI: 10.3389/fnhum.2013.00414

[142] Kim D-K, Rhee J-H, Kang SW. Reorganization of the brain and heart rhythm during autogenic meditation. Frontiers in Integrative Neuroscience. 2014;**7**:109. DOI: 10.3389/fnint.2013.00109

[143] Mitani S, Fujita M, Sakamoto S, Shirakawa T. Effect of autogenic training on cardiac autonomic nervous activity in high-risk fire service workers

for posttraumatic stress disorder. Journal of Psychosomatic Research. 2006;**60**(5):439-444. DOI: 10.1016/j.jpsychores.2005.09.005

[144] Cowings PS, Toscano WB, Reschke MF, Tsehay A. Psychophysiological assessment and correction of spatial disorientation during simulated Orion spacecraft re-entry. International Journal of Psychophysiology. 2018;**131**:102-112. DOI: 10.1016/j.ijpsycho.2018.03.001

[145] Mas B, Mas J, Ortego MJ. El entrenamiento autógeno [Autogenic Training]. In: Mas B, Mas J, Ortego MJ, editors. Hacia una vida más tranquila: Textos de educación permanente. Madrid: UNED; 2005. pp. 55-85

[146] Luthe W. In: De Rivera JL, editor. Introductory Workshop to the Methods of Autogenic Therapy. Madrid: ICAT; 2015. 185 p. (Original work published 1977)

[147] Kemmler R. Relajación para niños y adolescentes: El entrenamiento autógeno [Relaxation for children and adolescents: Autogenic training]. Madrid: TEA ediciones; 2009. 108 p

[148] Krampen G. Promotion of creativity (divergent productions) and convergent productions by systematic-relaxation exercises: Empirical evidence from five experimental studies with children, young adults, and elderly. European Journal of Personality. 1997;**11**(2):83-99. DOI: 10.1002/(SICI)1099-0984(199706)11:2<83::AID-PER280>3.0.CO;2-5

[149] Krampen G. Improvement of orthography test performance by relaxation exercises: Results of a controlled field experiment in basic secondary education. Educational Psychologist. 2010;**30**(5):533-546. DOI: 10.1080/01443410.2010

[150] Frey H. Improving the performance of poor readers through autogenic relaxation training. The Reading Teacher. 1980;**33**(8):928-932. Available from: http://www.jstor.org/stable/20195149

[151] Jojić BR, Leposavić LM. Autogenic training as a therapy for adjustment disorder in adolescents. Srpski Arhiv za Celokupno Lekarstvo. 2005;**133**(9-10):424-428. DOI: 10.2298/sarh0510424j

[152] Goldbeck L, Schmid K. Effectiveness of autogenic relaxation training on children and adolescents with behavioral and emotional problems. Journal of the American Academy of Child and Adolescent Psychiatry. 2003;**42**(9):1046-1054. DOI: 10.1097/01.CHI.0000070244.24125.F

[153] Feruglio S, Pascut S, Matiz A, Paschetto A, Crescentini C. Effects of mind-body interventions on adolescents' cooperativeness and emotional symptoms. Behavioral Sciences. 2022;**12**(2):33. DOI: 10.3390/bs12020033

Chapter 11

Perspective Chapter: Mind the Gap – Young People's Mental Health and Equine Assisted Interventions

S. Kezia Sullivan and Ann Hemingway

Abstract

Increasing numbers of adolescents are experiencing poor mental health, whether struggling with diagnosed conditions such as anxiety and depression, or simply suffering from poor wellbeing. Many have attributed this to changes experienced during the COVID-19 pandemic; however, it is likely that there are other factors which are also leading to difficulty maintaining positive mental health. A growing number of Equine Assisted Services (EAS) are being developed to meet needs for mental health support, ranging from therapeutic riding to equine assisted psychotherapy. This chapter will focus on non-riding interventions and include research primarily from equine assisted learning and equine assisted therapy programs. The authors acknowledge that there are differences between the two, but also that these modalities share several similarities which are relevant to discuss here. Four key aspects of EAS which could be supporting the development of positive mental health will be examined; the culture of EAS, key features of EAS, experiential learning of emotional skills, and common outcomes of EAS, followed by the limitations and a discussion of the current research in the area. This will indicate factors which might be missing from the lives of adolescents which could have implications for broader wellbeing and mental health programs.

Keywords: equine assisted, mental health, adolescent, wellbeing, equine facilitated

1. Introduction

1.1 What is positive mental health?

Mental health is comprised of many factors; the World Health Organization defines positive mental health as "a state of well-being in which the individual realizes his or her own abilities, can cope with the normal stresses of life, can work productively and fruitfully, and is able to make a contribution to his or her community" [1]. This definition encompasses a range of factors, which are themselves determined by other factors across many different life circumstances and skillsets. Circumstances such as family background, personal emotional regulation skills, and social support can all impact mental health and wellbeing, with Fusar-Poli et al. [2] suggesting the following core domains:

"(i) mental health literacy, (ii) attitude towards mental disorders, (iii) self-perceptions and values, (iv) cognitive skills, (v) academic/occupational performance, (vi) emotions, (vii) behaviours, (viii) self-management strategies, (ix) social skills, (x) family and significant relationships (xi) physical health, (xii) sexual health, (xiii) meaning of life, (xiv) and quality of life" [2].

Further discussions around wellbeing describe a state of "flourishing", defined as when both hedonic and eudaemonic wellbeing are satisfied. A study [3] found that subjective wellbeing was increased by striving towards eudaemonic (meaning & purpose), but not hedonic (pleasure) goals. The connection between flourishing and positive mental health was supported by a large-scale longitudinal study [4] in which it was found that participants with flourishing mental health at one time point were less likely to develop both first incidence and recurrent mood disorders and anxiety disorders during the following 3 years. Given the close relationship between types of wellbeing and the development and maintenance of positive mental health, this chapter will discuss factors which support both mental health and wellbeing when considering the impact of EAS on developing and maintaining adolescent's mental health.

1.2 What can support the development and maintenance of adolescent mental health?

The mental health of adolescents is particularly vulnerable to external factors, as they often lack the agency of adults in terms of making choices such as who to live with and what to do in their day-to-day life. A study [5] found that positive family relationships support both academic performance and health; in contrast, the development of mental health disorders such as depression [6] and social anxiety [7, 8] can be impacted by family factors. The relationship between adolescent's mental health and their family environments can therefore be either supportive or detrimental to their wellbeing, as is also evidenced by the efficacy of family-focussed programs for common mental health disorders [9].

As adolescents have little control over their family environment, learning skills such as emotional regulation, healthy communication and resilience can help to support wellbeing throughout the teen years. It is often expected that such skills can be learned in family environments through social modeling [10]. However, where this is not possible, for example in families where parents themselves are struggling, young people may not easily form behaviors and mindsets which contribute to positive mental health, such as adaptive emotional regulation strategies – for example, self-compassion [11]. This can be caused by a wide range of factors, including parents/carers who struggle to accept negative emotions [12], or a lack of coaching around managing negative emotions [13]. Where this is the case, it is important that adolescents are able to learn strategies for developing and maintaining positive mental health elsewhere.

Another area where young people may learn to develop positive mental health is through the education system – however, this relies on a supportive cohort of students and skilled teachers, who are themselves educated and able to educate others around positive mental health. A study [14] found that that positive mental health and resilience can be increased through a school-based social-emotional learning program, indicating that these factors, often viewed as invariant within an individual, can be improved through learning. A meta-analysis also found that social and emotional education programs in schools are effective across a variety of factors in the short term (up to 6 months) – but maintenance over the long-term tended to be poor [15].

In addition, in the UK the Child & Adolescent Mental Health Services (CAMHS) are struggling and in most areas overwhelmed by need and therefore often not able to see young people for 6–12 months after referral [16].

With the potential for these gaps in mental health education and support, many adolescents are struggling. A systematic literature review [17] following the effect of the COVID-19 pandemic on adolescent mental health found that loneliness, anxiety and depression were common mental health impacts. Young people with mental health difficulties are often referred to services for support, such as CAMHS, with rates of referrals for psychiatric assessment almost doubling between 2020 and 2021 [18]. However, in some cases, mainstream therapies such as Cognitive Behavioral Therapy (CBT) or psychotherapy are rejected by the young people, leading to dropout [19], thereby reducing efficacy of treatment delivery [20]. It is these participants who are often referred to Equine Assisted Services (EAS) due to refusal to engage with anything else; bonding with the horses appears to act as an intrinsic motivator for many participants [21].

1.3 What can the efficacy of equine assisted services reveal about adolescent mental health needs?

This chapter will compare observations from equine assisted programs with research surrounding factors which positively and negatively influence mental health. This will reveal ways in which EAS could be acting as a space for adolescents to develop socio-emotional skills which may otherwise be overlooked in home circumstances or school environments. Where research exists which specifically investigates delivery factors within equine assisted learning programs, it will be cited; otherwise, studies from adjacent areas of research such as social work, psychology and public health will indicate likely efficacy.

In this way, the needs of young people which may be unmet within other societal structures in the twenty-first century may be revealed, highlighting features which could be integrated into broader settings (such as school, or extra-curricular activities) to support the mental health of young people.

These needs will be divided into four groups; firstly, the EAS program culture, which often holds similarities across programs and provides key social learning opportunities through modeling positive behaviors and group facilitation. Secondly, features of the activities themselves will be examined, as spending time around horses takes place in a specific setting, with specific aspects of interactions with the horse contributing to improved wellbeing. Experiential learning of emotional skills will also be examined, as a core feature which could be leading to positive changes for participants within EAS. And finally, common outcomes of EAS programs will be discussed in terms of their contribution to positive mental health, as many act indirectly to support mental health outside of programs.

1.4 What are equine-assisted services?

Equine assisted services (EAS) are offered in many ways; some focus on therapeutic riding which may mean different things in an international context and may engage with individuals living with disability or individuals living with a specific physical or psychological problem. Others offer equine therapy or psychotherapy with each session including a registered therapist (psychotherapist, occupational therapist, or physiotherapist) and a horse most commonly either at liberty or with the horse on a lead rope. While another group focus on learning horse care, developing the wellbeing of the participants through taking part in the associated activities.

The largest growing group in the UK offer quine assisted learning (EAL), with learning to communicate with the horse being the focus. Participants also learn about the horse as a prey animal and their behavior and habits as a key part of programs which may also include some general horse care. There are growing groups within EAS, two of which are international; HETI, Horses in Education and Therapy International and PATH International. Both these groups are moving towards offering membership for equine practitioners and education on how to provide EAS.

2. How do equine assisted services improve adolescent mental health?

2.1 The culture of equine-assisted services

Equine-Assisted Services (EAS) aim to develop participants wellbeing through experiential learning in relation with the horse, facilitators, and other participants – depending on the format of the intervention. This relational approach to personal growth and learning can underpin transformative change for both individuals and communities [22] and creates a culture of emotional safety in which to learn. A qualitative study [23] operationalized components of emotional safety within an EAS program through a series of interviews with participants of an EAL program for at-risk youth. Four categories of emotional safety were identified:

Self-esteem: Having a self-perception which is positive, e.g., capable, kind

Personal security: A feeling of relaxation & safety

Connectivity: Ability to trust the horses and develop relationships

Respect: Learning to respect, and be respected with the horses.

Each of these aspects have been individually shown to improve wellbeing, from self-esteem to feeling safe, connected, or mutual respect. Further, a lack of these qualities within a person's environment are implicated in negative mental health, such as poor self-esteem and depression [24], indicating that interventions which provide an opportunity to experience connection and positive self-esteem could drive positive mental health. Participants of a study [25] into the impact of an EAL program described feeling as though the program offered a safe space to grow – supporting the idea that a culture of emotional safety is important for personal development to occur.

The emotional safety experienced by participants within EAS is not facilitated by interactions with the horse alone, or the specific actions of facilitators, but by the general culture of EAS organizations. A compassionate approach is taken to working with the horses, with many organizations preferring to use elements of natural horsemanship, or otherwise recognizing the horse as a sentient being with experiences worthy of consideration. By learning to provide this safe space for the horse, participants feel safe to explore their own experiences - for example, recognizing when they may feel overwhelmed and require a time out, or need to engage in an energetic activity before feeling calmer [26]. In this way, learning to have compassion for the horse translates to learning to have compassion for themselves – an important factor in developing and maintaining positive mental health [27].

Hamington argues that developing meaningful relationships with specific animals, as is often encouraged within EAS, can be a trigger for developing imaginative care and empathy - in other words, an ethical foundation for social behavior [28].

The ideas of philosopher Merleau-Ponty are cited; that empathy is essentially an embodied experience, as experiences of others are felt within the self [29]. The bidirectionality experienced within the EAS settings could be an important component of EAS cultures as participants both experience receiving empathy and compassion from the facilitator's whist learning to apply it to themselves and to the horses they interact with. In this way, empathy is no longer imaginative but also an embodied state to be reached, engaged with and developed throughout the course of programs. This can then be applied across interpersonal relationships, interspecies relationships, and practical activities such as grooming, whilst being positively reinforced by the facilitators and improved relationships with the horses.

The simple act of recognizing emotions in general as real, valid, and worthwhile to engage with can represent a learning experience for participants who may have adopted maladaptive strategies for managing emotions. These could include suppression [30], which is known to contribute to poor mental health and social outcomes, or externalization which can contribute to challenging behaviors such as aggression or substance abuse [31]. By consistently providing experiences of safely navigating difficult emotions, EAS helps participants to learn self-regulation strategies which work for them, within a positive environment. Working with horses can also provide enough desirable difficulty to facilitate greater retention of learning [32] to cause participants to stretch their emotional resilience, for example by completing tasks they are slightly afraid of (such as picking out hooves) or managing fluctuations in the horse's emotional state by staying calm themselves.

It can often be difficult to motivate learners to engage with tasks which include desirable difficulty, as they are, by nature, difficult. Zepeda et al. acknowledged this difficulty and proposed strategies to help learners to engage with desirably difficult tasks [33]. These included setting appropriate challenges, or where this is not possible, altering the self-perception of learners using positive affirmations. For participants who may have additional learning needs or struggle to regulate their emotions, introducing desirable difficulty at the correct level is particularly important, and something many EAS providers do particularly well.

In many programs, facilitators are experts at recognizing and celebrating achievements consistently throughout sessions – using specific positive terms to reinforce positive personal characteristics, such as "kind", "calm", or "brave". The specificity of these valenced terms could be helping participants to develop a positive self-concept beyond simply good or bad, instead helping them to develop a nuanced understanding of their own personal strengths. Weaknesses are intentionally not referenced here as the majority of programs adopt a strength-based approach [34] focusing on how participants abilities can help them to overcome challenges.

Working within a strengths-based approach helps participants to feel that they are worth knowing, understanding and caring about [35]. This can be an important step for some participants, as their self-concept may be otherwise dominated by weaknesses as they view themselves reflected in difficulties attending school, making friends, or staying out of trouble. Positive moral self-concept can predict prosocial behavior [36]; EAS programs help participants to relax into a positive experience of both the external environment and themselves by offering a space in which participants can achieve personal goals which are set flexibly according to their motivation and ability in the moment.

Negative self-concept has been found to predict the severity of adolescent depression, whilst those with fewer symptoms of depression were found to have a more positive self-concept [37]. The shifting self-concept as determined by the interplay between external circumstances and internal beliefs [38] has potential to be a strong driver of healing within a secure, positive environment such as that provided by EAS programs.

2.2 Features of EAS

In this section, features of EAS which have been shown to drive positive mental health impacts in any setting will be examined within the context of equine assisted services. There is a relative lack of literature examining specific features of EAS programs compared with other programs – therefore research will be generalized to EAS from other research around program or lifestyle factors which contribute to positive mental health.

Equine assisted services tend to take place outdoors, in a natural or semi-natural setting (such as an arena set amongst fields, or activities which take place in farm buildings). Time spent in these settings is likely to hold benefits, even without features of EAS such as facilitator skill or interactions with the horses. A study [39] found that time spent amongst nature for urban adolescents positively correlated with their mood, whilst another found that access to urban green space is associated with reduced distress [40]. These findings support the idea that the setting of EAS is conducive to positive mental wellbeing for adolescents without clinical conditions, but who may simply require some support to build and maintain positive mental health – for example during transitional periods or challenges.

Other studies have found reductions in symptoms for participants diagnosed with conditions which may impact their mental health or lead to behavioral concerns. For young people diagnosed with ADHD, playing in green spaces rather than indoors or outdoors play areas was associated with milder symptoms in one study [41] – and that hyperactive participants benefited from green spaces which were more open. Similarly, a study using structural equation modeling [42] suggested that sensory over-responsivity could be a driver of anxiety for people with high levels of autistic traits and suggested that neutral environments could help to prevent and manage anxiety. EAS programs are often conducted between stable-yards and arenas, which are usually neutral spaces without loud noises or bright lights (partly due to the innate sensitivity of horses). These may be helping to calm participants with hypersensitivity, as they are able to focus on tasks or simply enjoy being in a peaceful environment.

Whilst participants are in these settings, the variety of activities offered tend to be gently aerobic, such as grooming, mucking out, and leading horses. A systematic review [43] found a positive relationship between physical activity and dopamine, implying that physical activity is a valuable component of programs aiming to improve mental health. Dopamine also plays a role in reinforcement learning [44], meaning that activities which increase dopamine could help to prime participants to learn and retain new skills, such as self-regulation strategies, more effectively.

Another aspect of EAS which lends itself to enhanced learning outcomes is the precise application of desirable difficulty employed by facilitators, and available within the environment. The nature of working around horses means that tasks can often be modified to help participants feel comfortable, for example a participant who is unable to engage with horses at all may be able to complete tasks such as mucking out or talking about relationships between horses in a field. Conversely, a participant who is non-verbal might be perfectly able to engage with connective activities such as grooming or leading the horses. It is also frequently found by facilitators that a participants' desire to connect the horses sparks intrinsic motivation for participants who may struggle to engage with other programs.

Participants [45] reported several ways in which their connection with the horses helped them, with all participants describing their experience with the horse in positive terms. The relationship with the horse was described as key to emotional changes and shifts in self-perception such as feeling trusted and accepted and having more faith in themselves. The unspoken communication between horse and handler can create a bond described as parallel to a therapeutic alliance, which has been shown to mediate change across therapeutic programs [46] and is felt to contribute to recovery from trauma and associated mental health issues in an equine assisted setting [47].

Although the mechanism of action of EAS is still under study, it is generally accepted amongst practitioners that the relationship with the horses is a key contributor to the efficacy of programs. This is supported by findings in a qualitative study [48] which found that children involved in an EAS program were more likely to describe their experiences with the horses than the facilitators, indicating that the horses are primary agents of change. Another relationship-oriented feature programs which could be facilitating change is that EAS programs often work with rescue horses. Facilitators of such programs refer anecdotally to the backgrounds of the horses as a key feature which inspires positive changes in the participants, for example by discovering that it is possible to recover trust, even after mistreatment. A study [49] found that vicarious resilience is commonly developed amongst professionals working with trauma survivors. It is likely that in some cases, participants of EAS develop resilience and hope through a similar mechanism, drawing inspiration from the stories and responses of the horses.

Skin conductivity responses of participants involved with an equine assisted learning program were analyzed by Hemingway et al. [50], concluding that the opportunity to experience positive outcomes following emotional events could be a contributing factor which leads to change for participants. A description of the experience of "bringing up life" through and during interactions with horses by Smith gives a qualitative account which supports this idea – describing intense interactions which spark inter-affectivity [51]; the basis for primary empathy [52]. This flow of non-verbal communication in which participants feel both accepted and understood, as well as motivated to accept and understand another (the horse) is a feature commonly described by participants and facilitators as an important feature of EAS which differentiates it from other animal assisted therapies.

Facilitators often support this interspecies communication by compassionately interpreting horses' responses to participants and suggesting ways participants can alter their behavior in order to elicit a more positive response from the horse [26, 53]. Participants are then able to experiment with a new way of being and acting, which frequently leads to improved responses from the horse as they respond in the moment [26, 51]. Participants then have clear examples and embodied experiences of choosing to behave differently across different situations - for example, deciding to take a deep breath and try again when something is difficult, then succeeding.

These small successes, repeated across the duration of a program, with each acknowledged and celebrated by facilitators, help participants to build confidence and self-esteem [54], as well as to understand their own problem-solving processes with the support of facilitators. Participants are also able to practice nuances in embodied communication, such as the difference between being assertive and aggressive – receiving feedback without judgment. This kind of differentiation is an important skill to develop for effective communication and conflict [55] and can be difficult to practice in a way which is both authentic and safe.

The intentional practice of clear non-verbal communication is a key feature of many equine assisted services [26, 53] which enables participants to understand their physiological responses across different states, for example the raised heartbeat of anxiety or the slowing down which is characteristic of depression [56]. Helping participants understand how to navigate different emotional states in an equine assisted setting could be helping them generalize these learnings to other settings, enhancing their emotional regulation skills and giving them a greater degree of behavioral options when faced with stressful circumstances.

However, there is an important balance when working with horses and participants in order to ensure that equine welfare is not compromised. Horses often respond strongly to participants, thereby offering participants insight into their own behavior and current state – however, there is a need to consider the ethical implications of this for both horses and participants [57]. There are many ways in which this can be achieved (such as using a consent-based model and setting clear expectations for participants) – and there is growing recognition that it is a critical step in the development of the EAS industry.

2.3 Experiential learning of emotional skills

Temple Grandin, an animal scientist who has written extensively of her experiences as a person with autism, writes "To have feelings of gentleness, one must experience gentle bodily comfort... It was difficult for me to understand the feeling of kindness until I had been soothed myself" [58]. Many participants referred to EAS have had Adverse Childhood Experiences (ACES), which without being addressed can lead to long-term stress, poorer educational outcomes, and even chronic illness [59]. Grandin's account of experiential learning demonstrates the power that positive experiences of emotional regulation can have, in terms of helping to understand what is required for personal relationships in an embodied way.

Working with horses requires extensive and specific access to sensory information, resulting in a closely embodied experience for participants [60]. For some who have experienced trauma or Adverse Childhood Experiences (ACES), conscious embodiment may be missing from their daily lives, with dissociative tendencies because of trauma found to be reflected in neural changes [61]. However, this can be a double-bind; although re-accessing bodily awareness is a potential path to healing [62], it can be a difficult process, rife with triggers [63] – making it unappealing and even unsafe for young people who may still be living in difficult environments.

Controlled access to emotions and experiences is therefore an important skillset. Working with horses requires participants to access and manage emotions – rather than suppress or become overwhelmed by them. Grooming is a task commonly used within EAS, which is likely to produce oxytocin, similarly, to stroking a pet [64]. Oxytocin can help participants to share emotions around stressful life events [65], or to simply co-regulate with the horse, leading to a more relaxed state [57]. As described by Grandin, without prior experience within an emotional state, it is difficult to understand what it might be or how to reach it – however, once participants have learned to be calm and connected, they may be able to access it at other times outside of the intervention.

This is described by participants at EAS interventions, with some using alliterative terms formed through their activities with horses to describe how they reach desired states of embodiment outside of the program – for example, using their Polly Power Walk to feel confident, or Benji Breaths to calm down. Other older participants describe a different intervention as "what gets them through the week", as they visualize reaching their safe space during times of stress. The power of providing participants with lived experiences of positive, relaxed states is likely to be underestimated; for people who have always held a sense of safety or security, the precarious sensation of living without it is unimaginable, as is the sense of relief upon finding it.

This sense of relief may account for the frequent descriptions of tearful exchanges described within both EAS [66] and horse training styles which take account of both horse and human emotions [67]. Barbara K. Rector writes that following the centering and attunement exercise which takes place at the beginning of the AIA (Adventures in Awareness) program, many report "significant emotions rising to the surface" [66]. These are permitted and encouraged to be shared without judgment, then released. "Letting go" of attachment to experiences outside of the present is a powerful tool for wellbeing encouraged by Buddhist practices [68], with emotional breakthrough often acting as a catalyst for positive psychological change [69]. The sense of safety created by facilitators and horses within EAS [25] can help to provide space to manage, respond to and release negative emotions. This is likely to both improve adolescent mental health in the moment, as well as teaching skills for management of mental health outside of the program.

Rashid offers an account of how the honest reflection offered by horses can motivate people towards emotional honesty and "taking a hard look" at their lives [67] – as well as indicate areas where they may be hiding or holding onto unhelpful emotions. The lack of judgment and immediate biofeedback can help bring awareness to participants without triggering defensiveness and help them to make positive changes in a relatively short period of time. This experiential learning of emotional skills through interactions with the horses and facilitators represents both a key feature of many programs, and a core outcome.

2.4 Outcomes of equine assisted services

EAS has been found to have many outcomes across a variety of studies and participant groups, with a recent survey of equine assisted practitioners in the southwest of England finding over 88 common outcomes across programs. Many of these can be broadly categorized in alignment with the factors of the Strengths and Difficulties questionnaire [70] and will be examined in these categories during this chapter for the purpose of clarity.

2.4.1 Emotional symptoms

The first and potentially most important outcome is emotional symptoms, which are likely to moderate several other areas of behavior such as conduct problems and peer relationship problems. Research has [71] found a strong link between affect and personality; that is, the way we feel is strongly linked to who we are. It follows that helping participants learn to feel better is likely also to help them behave better, whether that's a young child learning to be calm in a classroom, or a teenager managing their frustration in a family setting. Whilst other therapies seek to help participants understand their emotions, and common interventions such as CBT help people to manage their thoughts [72], EAS provides a non-judgmental environment to develop emotional skills in practice.

A key emotional skill is the ability to calm down in times of stress; to return to baseline. The soothing impact of EAS has been described above, with several studies finding that improved emotional regulation and calmness are achieved by equine assisted services [73, 74]. Consistent with this, many programs find that reduced anxiety is a common outcome of EAS as participants learn to use adaptive strategies to calm themselves down [75]. There is some anecdotal evidence suggesting that this ability generalizes across contexts, with participants reporting thinking about their experiences at the services in times of stress, which helps them use strategies they have learned to calm down.

2.4.2 Conduct problems

Although conduct problems often stem from emotional dysregulation, a large proportion of participants are referred to equine assisted services for conduct problems, with emotional concerns either secondary or unrecognized. Therefore, alleviating or resolving conduct problems represents an important outcome measure, particularly as conduct problems are often the basis for funding EAS programs. Conduct problems can include fighting with other young people or family members, lying, stealing, refusing to attend school, and suffering from tantrums or other maladaptive behaviors.

A study with young offenders by Hemingway et al. found that a majority of participants improved in behavioral areas such as the ability to focus, communicate, and plan realistically [73]. It was suggested that the opportunity to rehearse calmness during communication with others, whether horse or human, helped them to make these behavioral changes which referrers reported as generalizing to other settings.

2.4.3 Hyperactivity/inattention

The access to calmness described above is also likely to help helps participants who may struggle to self-regulate and focus. A series of case studies [76] with institutionalized children found that an EAL program with a psychomotor intervention had a positive impact on participants ability to self-regulate, as well as improved appropriateness and intentionality of actions. This study involved a very small number of participants – though a meta-analysis of the effect of EAS for participants with autism also found significant reductions in hyperactivity [77]. Taken together, these findings imply that access to repeated experiences of embodied calmness via EAS is likely to reduce problematic hyperactivity for participants.

2.4.4 Peer relationships

EAS programs are often provided in a group setting, with some programs actively supporting participants to socialize and get to know each other. There is some preliminary evidence that social modeling by facilitators helps participants to develop the necessary confidence and skillsets to interact with peers. A study of an EAS program found improved social competence within the participant group following an 11-week equine facilitated learning program [78], which included social topics such as trust, mutual respect, and boundaries. These topics are frequently included in programs which work with horses, as they are qualities necessary to understand in order to safely spend time with large, flighty prey animals.

By creating a situation in which these core social skills become highly relevant for personal safety, EAS can simulate common potential relationship strains such as setting appropriate boundaries without becoming aggressive or afraid. This is similar to the idea put forward by Safran et al. that learning to repair ruptures within a therapeutic alliance is a key process for personal change within psychotherapy [79]. Learning to negotiate boundaries through common handling procedures with horses can help create scenarios for participants to experience a range of emotions (such as frustration, fear, or compassion) which can then be explored and understood with their implications for peer-to-peer relationships, or simply experienced and moved through – depending on the approach of the particular program.

In this way, participants may gain emotional stability by becoming comfortable with emotional experiences, understanding that they do not always need to act immediately based on emotion, but can instead choose their response. This ability to moderate their emotional reactivity is like that often achieved by mindfulness practices [80] and can lead to greater social competence. A series of studies [81] found that emotional intelligence improves social outcomes across a range of factors, from empathic perspective taking to having cooperative responses. As social competence is associated with the ability to behave well in relation to other people [82], programs which improve social competence are highly likely to improve peer-to-peer relationships.

2.4.5 Prosocial behavior

Much of the literature is focused on alleviating negative behavioral symptoms, such as reducing hyperactivity or conduct difficulties. However, the majority of EAS programs take a strengths-based approach, offering participants an environment to succeed at the level they can achieve at. EAS activities tend to be oriented around the care of horses, for example mucking them out, feeding and grooming them, and exercising them. This practice of other-directed care with the horse as intrinsic motivation could be helping participants learn to care for another through direct experience, resulting in increased likelihood of prosocial behavior outside the program. It has been found that pet arrival may trigger prosocial behaviors such as sharing with others and comforting others for people with autism [83], possibly due to the increased opportunities to learn such behaviors in a non-stressful environment.

It is possible that visiting the horses could have a similar impact for several participant groups. A study by Pelyva et al. found significantly improved prosocial behavior of adolescents involved with an equine assisted activity compared with a group who were not involved with horses [84]. Hauge et al. also investigated social dynamics for adolescents who took part in an equine assisted intervention (EAI), finding that perceived social support increased for participants who took part in the EAI [85]. Qualitative studies have described the importance of perceived connection with the horses [86], and participants are generally encouraged to see the horses as social agents, therefore it is likely that some of this perceived support is received via interactions with the horse. This could lead to a sense of reciprocity being experienced in the relationship, which is likely to support and motivate developing reciprocal relationships outside of EAS for participants.

2.5 Limitations

Although this chapter has used multiple research studies and reflections from the authors work and others, it is still worthwhile to consider what the limitations are in the field of research focused on equine assisted services overall. When considering the evidence base in this area from the perspective of the hierarchy of evidence [87], most published research sits within the mid-range of quality between expert opinion and randomized controlled trials and systematic reviews. In addition, studies often have small numbers and poorly describe exactly what the equine assisted service being evaluated consisted of. It is also important to note that the hierarchy of evidence itself has limitations for the equine sector as interventions may receive referrals for a very wide range of problems such as:

Anxiety
Depression
ADHD
Suicidal
Eating disorders
Anger management
Violence
Bullying
Being bullied
PTSD
Autism
OCD
Drug dependency
Alcohol dependency
Emotional dysregulation
Victim of crime
Victim of abuse
Witnessing abuse
Domestic violence

Standard practice for RCTs is to focus on one specific cohort and recruit and randomize participants to the intervention under study and `treatment as usual` and compare outcomes. An individual charity offering equine assisted services may see hundreds of individuals over a year with a whole range of issues, so recruiting enough participants with one specific issue to provide a large enough cohort for an RCT is challenging. In addition, often the equine assisted service is being used with individuals for whom other interventions such as talk based services are not working, so finding a comparable `treatment as usual` group is also a challenge [73].

2.6 Discussion

Emerging literature on EAS acknowledges that the nature of the horse as a prey animal and the skills required to successfully interact and learn with such an animal may be the key distinctive quality which helps humans to control their behavior. It may be that learning about prey animal behavior and that we as predators need to modify our behavior to enable calmness in the horse helps enable and motivate the human involved to practice being calm during the intervention. This motivation and the resulting positive calm response from the horse may help the human recognize what it is to be calm and learn the benefits [88]. Further research is required however, to see whether, for instance, dogs (as another predator) or other animals can achieve similar results in the humans they interact with.

Learning to be calm is becoming a common focus for interventions such as meditation, mindfulness and contact with nature. Enabling and experiencing calmness and teaching it as a skill seems to be a theme across EAS interventions. However, it is important to note that many of the individuals who are referred or who choose to attend EAS sessions are those for whom other interventions such as talk, or group or education-based interventions are not working or are not engaging them to complete the program. The unconditional positive regard and positive role modeling which occurs on EAS programs as a consistent quality may also be an important element or context for the experience with horses. Importantly the horse is not looked down on during the EAS programs for being afraid at times; it is seen as part of their nature and indeed of our nature as humans, and a useful response to some parts of life which are indeed dangerous for us and horses.

Is the presence of the horse the factor which motivates us, is it the opportunity to engage with another beautiful charismatic species or the understanding that this animal is prey and behaves as such? These prey animal characteristics (hypervigilance, vulnerability, claustrophobia, the strong need to be part of a group, and the desire to run from danger) in the research we have carried out to date seem to strike a chord with those who themselves feel vulnerable and preyed upon in our human groups, communities, and society.

Experiencing and achieving calmness in our bodies and our minds to be safely and calmly with a horse may be the main motivator and outcomes from these EAS programs. So little of our world now is experienced through our bodies primarily, and few experiences engage us so completely in the moment, enabling us to not focus on the future or the past but be completely in the present. Very few learning opportunities enable us to feel 'powerful', 'happy' and experience feelings of 'love' (in the words of some of our participants). Our pilot work suggests that asking a powerful mammal to do something with us is an emotional experience for the human. Learning to be emotionally aroused and achieve a positive calm outcome from that may truly be a way to interrupt previous destructive patterns of behavior in other parts of our lives [73, 74]. Through EAS interventions this may be achievable without recourse to medication or the need for prolonged examination of negative aspects of our lives.

2.7 Conclusions

In this chapter we have examined many aspects of EAS which could be leading to positive changes in adolescent mental health and well-being. **Table 1** shows which of Fusar-Poli et al's [2] core domains of wellbeing have been discussed in this chapter [2]:

This chapter has focused on emotional regulation in relationship with others, which includes both facilitators and horses working together with participants across a range of activities but always returning to calmness. Without this ability to return to calmness, participants are likely to be subject to chronic stress which can lead to behavioral, physical, social and mental health symptoms. It is as-yet unclear to what extent equine assisted interventions are differentiated from other animal assisted interventions or alternative well-being programs, but the existing literature is beginning to indicate that equine assisted interventions are an option for treatment and prevention of poor adolescent well-being by facilitating improvements to the domains above.

From our analysis, equine assisted interventions are bridging the connection gap which many adolescents have been suffering further to the COVID-19 pandemic, by finding a space to be accepted for being themselves. It is hoped that this will help them learn to provide such a space for others, thereby improving their relationships and the mental health of those around them. They are also finding opportunities to achieve personal success, whether that is mustering the courage to touch a horse for the first time, learning to communicate nonverbally, or developing the ability to set boundaries kindly and calmly. Critically, they are also finding a place where they feel safe and can practice emotional skills - building tolerance for quiet moments and

Wellbeing domain	EAS impact	Relevant literature
Mental health literacy	Compassion for the horse, understanding of fear & anxiety in themselves and others	Inwood & Ferrari [27]*
Attitude towards mental disorders	Not specifically covered	
Self-perceptions and values	Confidence building, developing prosocial behaviors	Fagan et al. [54]*
Cognitive skills	Not specifically covered	
Academic/occupational performance	Often improves attendance at school, or leads to vocational training & employment	Hemingway [73]
Emotions	Improves emotional regulation	Hemingway et al. [50]
Behaviors	Reduces conduct problems, increases prosocial behavior	Hemingway et al. [74]; Pelyva et al. [84]
Self-management strategies	Improves emotional regulation	Hemingway et al. [50]
Social skills	Increases prosocial behavior	Pelyva et al. [84]
Family and significant relationships	Improves emotional regulation and prosocial behavior	Grandgeorge et al. [83]*; Pelyva et al. [84]
Physical health	Often includes aerobic activity	Marques et al. [43]*
Sexual health	Practicing setting boundaries, improving social competence	Pendry and Roeter [78]
Meaning of life	Connection with the horses helps participants to feel that they are of value	Waite & Bourke [45]
Quality of life	Enhanced life chances via the skills above	

**Studies from broader psychological literature – not EAS-specific.*

Table 1.
Core domains of wellbeing [2] which may be impacted by EAS.

exploring their own emotions, or physically projecting their energy to prevent a pony from crowding them during an activity.

By experiencing themselves mirrored back via the responses of horses, whilst being compassionately coached by facilitators to make positive changes, young people are also able to learn how to develop themselves with kindness, accepting where they are and moving forwards. Participants can experience mastery of skills for perhaps the first time, whilst having early attempts honored and celebrated by facilitators and those around them. Within the broad range of new experiences offered by EAS is the opportunity for participants to experience and express a wide range of emotions, learning to manage them without shame or judgment. These experiences can form a foundation for maintaining mental health in other contexts, as well as for supporting others in their lives.

The changes made within EAS are supported by the skilled compassion of facilitators placed within the accuracy of the horse's responses, as participant's emotional and behavioral tendencies are amplified and resolved. Horseman Nahshon Cook describes the relationship between the horsemanship teacher and the student as like that of the student and the horse; imbued with the responsibility of creating safety [89]. This dynamic reveals how EAS are truly participant-centric, offering participants the opportunity to be both supported and supportive through changing their behavior to enable them to communicate and be with horses. In this way, the core domains of mental health and wellbeing are developed through a foundation of calmness first – creating potential for further growth.

Author details

S. Kezia Sullivan[1] and Ann Hemingway[2]*

1 Independent Researcher, London, UK

2 BU Centre for Public Health Lead, Bournemouth University, UK

*Address all correspondence to: ahemingway@bournemouth.ac.uk

References

[1] World Health Organization. The World Health Report 2001: Mental Health: New Understanding, New Hope. Geneva, Switzerland: WHO; 2001

[2] Fusar-Poli P, de Pablo GS, De Micheli A, Nieman DH, Correll CU, Kessing LV, et al. What is good mental health? A scoping review. European Neuropsychopharmacology. 2020;**31**:33-46

[3] Sheldon KM, Corcoran M, Prentice M. Pursuing eudaimonic functioning versus pursuing hedonic well-being: The first goal succeeds in its aim, whereas the second does not. Journal of Happiness Studies. 2019;**20**:919-933

[4] Schotanus-Dijkstra M, Ten Have M, Lamers SM, de Graaf R, Bohlmeijer ET. The longitudinal relationship between flourishing mental health and incident mood, anxiety and substance use disorders. The European Journal of Public Health. 2017;**27**(3):563-568

[5] Guevara RM, Moral-García JE, Urchaga JD, López-García S. Relevant factors in adolescent well-being: Family and parental relationships. International Journal of Environmental Research and Public Health. 2021;**18**(14):7666

[6] Jaffee SR, Moffitt TE, Caspi A, Fombonne E, Poulton R, Martin J. Differences in early childhood risk factors for juvenile-onset and adult-onset depression. Archives of General Psychiatry. 2002;**59**(3):215-222

[7] Luebbe AM, Bell DJ. Positive and negative family emotional climate differentially predict youth anxiety and depression via distinct affective pathways. Journal of Abnormal Child Psychology. 2014;**42**:897-911

[8] Brook CA, Schmidt LA. Social anxiety disorder: A review of environmental risk factors. Neuropsychiatric Disease and Treatment. 2008;**4**(1):123-143

[9] Pedersen GA, Smallegange E, Coetzee A, Hartog K, Turner J, Jordans MJ, et al. A systematic review of the evidence for family and parenting interventions in low-and middle-income countries: Child and youth mental health outcomes. Journal of Child and Family Studies. 2019;**28**:2036-2055

[10] Morris AS, Silk JS, Steinberg L, Myers SS, Robinson LR. The role of the family context in the development of emotion regulation. Social Development. 2007;**16**(2):361-388

[11] Trompetter HR, De Kleine E, Bohlmeijer ET. Why does positive mental health buffer against psychopathology? An exploratory study on self-compassion as a resilience mechanism and adaptive emotion regulation strategy. Cognitive Therapy and Research. 2017;**41**:459-468

[12] Meyer S, Raikes HA, Virmani EA, Waters S, Thompson RA. Parent emotion representations and the socialization of emotion regulation in the family. International Journal of Behavioral Development. 2014;**38**(2):164-173

[13] Katz LF, Windecker-Nelson B. Domestic violence, emotion coaching, and child adjustment. Journal of Family Psychology. 2006;**20**(1):56

[14] LaBelle B. Positive outcomes of a social-emotional learning program to promote student resiliency and address

mental health. Contemporary School Psychology. 2023;**27**(1):1-7

[15] Diekstra RF, Gravesteijn C. Effectiveness of school-based social and emotional education programmes worldwide. In: Social and Emotional Education: An International Analysis. Santender, Spain: Fundacion Marcelino Botin; 2008. pp. 255-312

[16] Campbell D. Swamped NHS mental health services turning away children, say GPs [Internet]. The Guardian. 2022. Available from: https://www.theguardian.com/society/2022/apr/03/swamped-nhs-mental-health-services-turning-away-children-say-doctors [Accessed: 17 Oct 2023]

[17] Theberath M, Bauer D, Chen W, Salinas M, Mohabbat AB, Yang J, et al. Effects of COVID-19 pandemic on mental health of children and adolescents: A systematic review of survey studies. SAGE Open Medicine. 2022;**10**:20503121221086712

[18] Voy S, Robinson C, Blue S. A comparison of the number of referrals for psychiatric assessment and prescribing rates of psychotropic medication in the year leading up to the COVID-19 pandemic and the first year of the pandemic in a child and adolescent mental health service (CAMHS) in South Edinburgh. BJPsych Open. 2023;**9**(S1):S145

[19] O'Keeffe S, Martin P, Target M, Midgley N. 'I just stopped going': A mixed methods investigation into types of therapy dropout in adolescents with depression. Frontiers in Psychology. 2019;**10**:75

[20] Nock MK, Ferriter C. Parent management of attendance and adherence in child and adolescent therapy: A conceptual and empirical review. Clinical Child and Family Psychology Review. 2005;**8**:149-166

[21] Berg EL, Causey A. The life-changing power of the horse: Equine-assisted activities and therapies in the US. Animal Frontiers. 2014;**4**(3):72-75

[22] Bartels KP. Experiential learning: A relational approach to sustaining community-led social innovation. Innovation: The European Journal of Social Science Research. 2023;**36**(3):434-452

[23] Cagle-Holtcamp K, Nicodemus MC, Parker J, Dunlap MH. Does equine assisted learning create emotionally safe learning environments for At-risk youth? Journal of Youth Development. 2019;**14**(4):232-252

[24] Achterbergh L, Pitman A, Birken M, Pearce E, Sno H, Johnson S. The experience of loneliness among young people with depression: A qualitative meta-synthesis of the literature. BMC Psychiatry. 2020;**20**(1):1-23

[25] Rentko V, Warner A, Timlege E, Richman E. Equine-assisted learning–an experiential, facilitated learning model for development of professional skills and resiliency in veterinary students. Journal of Veterinary Medical Education. 22 Dec 2022:e20210165

[26] The Horse Course. 2023. Available from: https://www.thehorsecourse.org/method

[27] Inwood E, Ferrari M. Mechanisms of change in the relationship between self-compassion, emotion regulation, and mental health: A systematic review. Applied Psychology: Health and Well-Being. 2018;**10**(2):215-235

[28] Hamington M. Learning ethics from our relationships with animals: Moral

imagination. International Journal of Applied Philosophy. 2008;**22**(2):177-188

[29] Merleau-Ponty M. The visible and the invisible. In: Alphonso Lingis. Evanston, IL: Northwestern University Press; 1968. p. 145

[30] Chervonsky E, Hunt C. Emotion regulation, mental health, and social wellbeing in a young adolescent sample: A concurrent and longitudinal investigation. Emotion. 2019;**19**(2):270

[31] Kauten R, Barry CT. Externalizing behavior. Encyclopedia of Personality and Individual Differences. Jan 2020:1509-1512

[32] Bjork EL, Bjork RA. Making things hard on yourself, but in a good way: Creating desirable difficulties to enhance learning. Psychology and the Real World: Essays Illustrating Fundamental Contributions to Society. 2011;**2**:59-68

[33] Zepeda CD, Martin RS, Butler AC. Motivational strategies to engage learners in desirable difficulties. Journal of Applied Research in Memory and Cognition. 2020;**9**(4):468-474

[34] Rawana E, Brownlee K. Making the possible probable: A strength-based assessment and intervention framework for clinical work with parents, children, and adolescents. Families in Society. 2009;**90**(3):255-260

[35] Laursen EK. Frontiers in strength-based treatment. Reclaiming Children and Youth. 2003;**12**(1):12

[36] Christner N, Pletti C, Paulus M. Emotion understanding and the moral self-concept as motivators of prosocial behavior in middle childhood. Cognitive Development. 2020;**55**:100893

[37] Hards E, Ellis J, Fisk J, Reynolds S. Negative view of the self and symptoms of depression in adolescents. Journal of affective disorders. 2020;**262**:143-148

[38] Vallacher RR, Nowak A. Dynamical social psychology: Finding order in the flow of human experience. Social Psychology: Handbook of Basic Principles. 2007;**2**:734-758

[39] Li D, Deal B, Zhou X, Slavenas M, Sullivan WC. Moving beyond the neighborhood: Daily exposure to nature and adolescents' mood. Landscape and Urban Planning. 2018;**173**:33-43

[40] White MP, Alcock I, Wheeler BW, Depledge MH. Would you be happier living in a greener urban area? A fixed-effects analysis of panel data. Psychological Science. 2013;**24**(6):920-928

[41] Faber Taylor A, Kuo FE. Children with attention deficits concentrate better after walk in the park. Journal of Attention Disorders. 2009;**12**(5):402-409

[42] Amos GA, Byrne G, Chouinard PA, Godber T. Autism traits, sensory over-responsivity, anxiety, and stress: A test of explanatory models. Journal of Autism and Developmental Disorders. 2019;**49**:98-112

[43] Marques A, Marconcin P, Werneck AO, Ferrari G, Gouveia ÉR, Kliegel M, et al. Bidirectional association between physical activity and dopamine across adulthood—A systematic review. Brain Sciences. 2021;**11**(7):829

[44] Solinas M, Belujon P, Fernagut PO, Jaber M, Thiriet N. Dopamine and addiction: What have we learned from 40 years of research. Journal of Neural Transmission. 2019;**126**:481-516

[45] Waite C, Bourke L. "It's different with a horse": Horses as a tool for engagement in a horse therapy program

for marginalised young people. Youth Studies Australia. 2013;**32**(4):15-24

[46] Baier AL, Kline AC, Feeny NC. Therapeutic alliance as a mediator of change: A systematic review and evaluation of research. Clinical Psychology Review. 2020;**82**:101921

[47] Yorke J, Adams C, Coady N. Therapeutic value of equine-human bonding in recovery from trauma. Anthrozoös. 2008;**21**(1):17-30

[48] Dunlop K, Tsantefski M. A space of safety: Children's experience of equine-assisted group therapy. Child & Family Social Work. 2018;**23**(1):16-24

[49] Killian K, Hernandez-Wolfe P, Engstrom D, Gangsei D. Development of the vicarious resilience scale (VRS): A measure of positive effects of working with trauma survivors. Psychological Trauma: Theory, Research, Practice, and Policy. 2017;**9**(1):23

[50] Hemingway A, Carter S, Callaway A, Kavanagh E, Ellis S. An exploration of the mechanism of action of an equine-assisted intervention. Animals. 2019;**9**(6):303

[51] Smith SJ. Bringing up life with horses. Indo-Pacific Journal of Phenomenology. 1 Dec 2018;**18**(2):179-189

[52] Fuchs T. Intercorporeality and interaffectivity. Intercorporeality: Emerging Socialities in Interaction. 2017;**7853**:3-23

[53] HorseHeard. 2023. Available from: https://www.horseheard.com/project/being-friends/

[54] Fagan K et al. Successful Young Adults are asked 'In Your Experience, What Builds Confidence?': A Thesis Presented in Partial Fulfilment of the Requirements for the Degree of Master of Social Work at Massey University. Palmerston North, New Zealand (Doctoral dissertation): Massey University; 2012

[55] Parray WM, Kumar S. The effect of assertiveness training on behaviour, self esteem, stress, academic achievement and psychological well-being of students: A quasi-experimental study. Research & Development. 2022;**3**(2):83-90

[56] Wichers M. Critical slowing down as a personalized early warning signal for depression. Psychotherapy and Psychosomatics. 2016;**85**(2):114-116

[57] Schlote S. Security in connection and co-regulation: Safeguarding the horse from traumatic re-enactments in EQUUSOMA™. In: Parent I, editor. A Horse is a Horse, of Course: Compendium from the Third International Symposium for Equine Welfare and Wellness. Createspace Independent Publishing Platform; 2019. pp. 215-238

[58] Grandin T. Thinking in Pictures: My Life with Autism. 2nd ed. New York: Vintage; 2006. p. 84

[59] Maté G. When the Body Says No: The Cost of Hidden Stress. Toronto, Canada: Vintage Canada; 11 Feb 2011

[60] Smith SJ. Bringing up life with horses. Indo-Pacific Journal of Phenomenology. 1 Dec 2018;18(2):179-189

[61] Lebois LA, Li M, Baker JT, Wolff JD, Wang D, Lambros AM, et al. Large-scale functional brain network architecture changes associated with trauma-related dissociation. American Journal of Psychiatry. 2021;**178**(2):165-173

[62] Rousseau D, Long N, Jackson E, Jurgensen J. Empowering through

embodied awareness: Evaluation of a peer-facilitated trauma-informed mindfulness curriculum in a woman's prison. The Prison Journal. 2019;**99**(suppl. 4):14S-37S

[63] van der Kolk Laura BA, West J, Rhodes A, Emerson D, Suvak M, Spinazzola J. Yoga as an adjunctive treatment for posttraumatic stress disorder: A randomized controlled trial. The Journal of Clinical Psychiatry. 2014;**75**(6):22573

[64] Johnson EA, Portillo A, Bennett NE, Gray PB. Exploring women's oxytocin responses to interactions with their pet cats. PeerJ. 2021;**9**:e12393

[65] Lane A, Luminet O, Rimé B, Gross JJ, de Timary P, Mikolajczak M. Oxytocin increases willingness to socially share one's emotions. International Journal of Psychology. 2013;**48**(4):676-681

[66] Rector BK. Adventures in Awareness: Learning with the Help of Horses. Indiana, USA: Authorhouse; 2005

[67] Rashid M. Whole Heart, Whole Horse: Building Trust Between Horse and Rider. Delaware, USA: Simon and Schuster; 2009

[68] Sahdra BK, Shaver PR, Brown KW. A scale to measure nonattachment: A Buddhist complement to Western research on attachment and adaptive functioning. Journal of Personality Assessment. 2010;**92**(2):116-127

[69] Roseman L, Haijen E, Idialu-Ikato K, Kaelen M, Watts R, Carhart-Harris R. Emotional breakthrough and psychedelics: Validation of the emotional breakthrough inventory. Journal of Psychopharmacology. 2019;**33**(9):1076-1087

[70] Goodman R. The strengths and difficulties questionnaire: A research note. Journal of Child Psychology and Psychiatry. 1997;**38**(5):581-586

[71] Davis KL, Panksepp J, Normansell L. The affective neuroscience personality scales: Normative data and implications. Neuropsychoanalysis. 2003;**5**(1):57-69

[72] Beck JS, Fleming S. A brief history of Aaron T. Beck, MD, and cognitive behavior therapy. Clinical Psychology in Europe. 2021;**3**(2):1-7

[73] Hemingway A. A study exploring the implementation of an equine assisted intervention for young people with mental health and behavioural issues. Multidisciplinary Scientific Journal. 2019;**2**(2):236-246

[74] Hemingway A, Meek R, Hill CE. An exploration of an equine-facilitated learning intervention with young offenders. Society & Animals. 2015;**23**(6):544-568

[75] Nelson C, Dossett K, Walker DL. Equine-assisted therapy for posttraumatic stress disorder among first responders. Psychological Reports. 21 Dec 2022:00332941221146707

[76] Matias AR, Santos GD, Almeida N. Equine-assisted therapeutic intervention in institutionalized children: Case studies. International Journal of Environmental Research and Public Health. 2023;**20**(4):2846

[77] Xiao N, Shinwari K, Kiselev S, Huang X, Li B, Qi J. Effects of equine-assisted activities and therapies for individuals with autism spectrum disorder: Systematic review and meta-analysis. International Journal of Environmental Research and Public Health. 2023;**20**(3):2630

[78] Pendry P, Roeter S. Experimental trial demonstrates positive effects of

equine facilitated learning on child social competence. Human-Animal Interaction Bulletin; 2013;**1**(1):1-19

[79] Safran JD, Muran JC, Eubanks-Carter C. Repairing alliance ruptures. Psychotherapy. 2011;**48**(1):80

[80] Roemer L, Williston SK, Rollins LG. Mindfulness and emotion regulation. Current Opinion in Psychology. 2015;**3**:52-57

[81] Schutte NS, Malouff JM, Bobik C, Coston TD, Greeson C, Jedlicka C, et al. Emotional intelligence and interpersonal relations. The Journal of Social Psychology. 2001;**141**(4):523-536

[82] Smart D, Sanson AN. Social competence in young adulthood, its nature and antecedents. Family Matters. 2003;**64**:4-9

[83] Grandgeorge M, Tordjman S, Lazartigues A, Lemonnier E, Deleau M, Hausberger M. Does pet arrival trigger prosocial behaviors in individuals with autism? PloS One. 2012;**7**(8):e41739. DOI: 10.1371/journal.pone.0041739

[84] Pelyva IZ, Kresák R, Szovák E, Tóth ÁL. How equine-assisted activities affect the prosocial behavior of adolescents. International Journal of Environmental Research and Public Health. 2020;**17**(8):2967

[85] Hauge H, Kvalem IL, Berget B, Enders-Slegers MJ, Braastad BO. Equine-assisted activities and the impact on perceived social support, self-esteem and self-efficacy among adolescents – An intervention study. International Journal of Adolescence and Youth. 2014;**19**(1):1-21

[86] Burgon HL. 'Queen of the world': Experiences of 'at-risk'young people participating in equine-assisted learning/therapy. Journal of Social Work Practice. 2011;**25**(02):165-183

[87] Cochrane. 2017. Available from: https://rehabilitation.cochrane.org/sites/rehabilitation.cochrane.org/files/uploads/sosort_dubrovnik_-_cochrane_reviews.pdf

[88] Damasio AR. Descartes Error: Emotion, Reason and the Human Brain. New York, NY, USA: Grosset/Putman; 1994

[89] Cook N. Horses See Us as We Are. USA: Nova's Books; 2022. pp. 77-79

Chapter 12

Psychological Recovery Camps: Intensive Integrative Group Psychotherapy

Susana Roque López

Abstract

This one-week Group Psychotherapy Program is a multicomponent treatment for the resolution of traumatic memories (e.g., rape, sexual abuse, physical and emotional violence, etc.) for children and adolescents. It was designed and developed to support those children and adolescents who in general have not been able to develop the basic neural networks of feeling loved, cared for, and who often have attachment disorders. Children suffering from Adverse Child Experience (ACE), and also from Post-Traumatic Stress Disorder (PTSD), may find their confidence in themselves and in humanity, disturbed, preventing them from pursuing their development with joy. In a recent controlled study, it was shown that this program significantly decreased symptoms related to PTSD and improved attention-related outcomes. Furthermore, the program leads to changes in deoxyribonucleic acid (DNA) methylation at the genome level, and these modifications have been seen in genes whose biological processes are related to early childhood adversity-neural pathways. Data confirms the results of our previous uncontrolled studies using this multimodal program in children and adolescents with a history of sexual and physical abuse. In this chapter, we present the methodology of the program, the therapies, and techniques we use, as well as some authors who have inspired the intervention elements.

Keywords: intensive integrative group psychotherapy (IIG-psychotherapy), EMDR (eyes movement desensitization reprocessing), EMDR integrative group treatment protocol (EMDR-IGTP), adverse child experience (ACE), post-traumatic stress disorder (PTSD), deoxyribonucleic acid (DNA) methylation, mindfulness, art

1. Introduction

These Psychological Recovery Camps with the Intensive Integrative Group Psychotherapy (IIG-Psychotherapy) program have been conceived and developed within the framework of the Association Innocence In Danger Colombia (IID Colombia), a branch of Innocence In Danger International (IID), whose main office is in Paris. Since 2008, IID Colombia has been operating in Cali, a city in the southwest part of Colombia S.A. The humanitarian mission of IID Colombia is to provide psychological support and prevention of violence to children and adolescents.

Psychological treatment is provided for children and adolescents who are victims of violence in all its forms.

Children access their traumatic memories without plunging into despair. We practice an approach with several psycho-neurobiological means. This approach consists of artistic and playful activities, meditation practice, and emotional regulation, with the aim of treating children in their human wholeness, in their mental, cerebral, and interpersonal relationships, following D. Siegel's model of integration [1]. Several auteurs recommend working "top to down and down to top." For R. Lanius, in trauma, the lower brain structures function independently of the cortex, and this upper part of the brain can actually engage in top-down modulation; working both bottom-up and top-down helps the persons to regulate their feelings and connect intense feelings with what may have happened in the past and make sense of them [2]. For Bessel van der Kolk, by activating interoception, we help patients to find calm [3].

All activities in this protocol are organized so that children find external and internal safety conditions necessary to enable them to approach the sessions of the therapy EMDR (Eyes Movement Desensitization Reprocessing) [4].

- Artistic activities are practiced: the artists involved during the stays, as well as the other stakeholders in the treatment, accompany the children in a creative process in such a way that this path leads them to a transformation. On the first day of trauma treatment, children must come into intimate contact with their body and their sensations, and as they move forward, they must connect to their emotions, their own thoughts, and their own being. Playful practices aim to harmonize brain activity and motor skills. Discussions take place between the children so that they can express themselves and also respect the temporal presence and subjectivity of the other when the latter expresses himself. Also is taken into account the "awakening" of rhythm (walking, dancing), the original movement of the human being, a rhythm that was most likely interrupted by the violence to which children were subjected. According to A. Schore, early trauma affects the right side of the brain, the more emotional side of the brain. It can have an impact on our ability to form social connections and relationships [5]. It is important, though, to activate the right brain of patients who have had early adverse experiences. We postulate that through art, communication between the right brain of the children and the right brain of the caregivers is possible throughout the treatment.

- The practice of "Mindfulness" enables the direct experiencing of the body, the formation of new positive neural circuits, and the development of an attitude of self-compassion. Children are trained in the Mindfulness program, according to the Academy for Mindful Teaching (AMT) [6]. Also included is Thich Nhat Hanh's practice of compassion meditation [7].

- Concerning Emotional Regulation: practices such as contacting one's inner child [8], the butterfly hug [9, 10], dance, therapeutic massages [11, 12], heart coherence (Heart Math Institute) [13], working with the polyvagal perspective [14], integrating archaic reflexes [15], releasing bodily stress, installing internal resources like the protective self, the maternal self and the essential self of the therapy Developmental Needs Meeting Strategy (DNMS) [16], yoga, strengthen the organic security of children [17]. All this helps not only in the resolution of traumatic memories but also in reducing the risk of new trauma and making it possible for them to accept that these experiences were really lived but they belong to the past. Even preverbal memories, this means information stored in implicit memory, can cause symptoms; they can be retrieved and reprocessed. It is important to remain within the window of tolerance; otherwise, the patient is in the time of the trauma, does not feel safe, and is not present.

2. EMDR integrative group treatment protocol

In the EMDR Integrative Group Treatment Protocol (EMDR-IGTP), the group environment, allows for group administration of individual treatment, ensuring that many people can be treated simultaneously. During therapy, there is no interaction between people in the group, which guarantees confidentiality. Studies have used a number of terms to describe EMDR-IGTP, such as the EMDR group protocol, the EMDR group protocol for children, and the butterfly hug protocol [18]. These authors report that EMDR-IGTP has been used in its original format or with modifications to adapt to cultural circumstances, in many places around the world for thousands of survivors of natural or man-made disasters: anecdotal reports, nine pilot field studies with children and adults following massive natural disasters in Mexico, Nicaragua, El Salvador, Colombia and Venezuela, reports and field studies, have documented its effectiveness on children, adolescents and adults following natural or man-made disasters, during ongoing war trauma, during ongoing geopolitical crises, with women who have been sexually assaulted in Congo, with war refugee children in Germany, with children victims of severe interpersonal violence, with non-governmental organization staff caring for children suffering from severe interpersonal trauma, with caregivers of dementia patients, with Latin American survivors of domestic violence, with refugee children in the United Kingdom, Turkey, Ethiopia, and as emergency treatment for child survivors of the 13 November 2015 terrorist attacks in Paris.

3. Adverse child experience, post-traumatic stress disorder, and childhood

The ACE parameter (Adverse Child Experience) is used to describe the types of adversity experienced during the early years (sexual abuse, physical and emotional maltreatment, parental separation, parental abandonment, etc.). ACEs increase the risk of morbidity and mortality and can have a negative impact on life opportunities and lifelong social behavior. As soon as an adverse event occurs in a child's life, its normal development is further threatened [19]. Violence may threaten the optimum development of over a billion brains in children, every year [20]. There is evidence that extremely high exposure to early life stress in children is associated with changes in deoxyribonucleic acid (DNA) methylation levels in saliva, and that DNA methylation can modulate the binding of transcription factors on developmentally important genes in the brain [21].

4. Intensive integrative group psychotherapy

4.1 Trauma resolution and epigenetic progress

Designed and developed since 2008, this intensive multimodal group program has produced very encouraging results in a randomized controlled intervention with adolescent girls reporting an average ACE score > 5: the program significantly reduced symptoms linked to PTSD and improved results linked to attention [22]. These data confirm the results of our previous uncontrolled studies using this multimodal program in children and adolescents with a history of sexual and physical abuse [23]. For this study, a total of 14 adolescents (all male) aged between 14 and 18 took part in this trauma recovery program. All had been victims of interpersonal violence (sexual abuse, rape, maltreatment, prostitution). All the adolescents came from an institution accredited by the Colombian Family Welfare Institute. The results on the severity of PTSD showed that there was a statistically significant improvement in the participants' symptoms between the start and end of the study. In the study mentioned above, a statistical analysis of the effects of the psychological recovery intervention was carried out in all the groups who took part in the treatments from 2011 to 2013. Six groups of pre-adolescent children were treated. All groups followed a similar pattern between pre- and post-treatment in Short PTSD Rating Interview (SPRINT) scores. These results indicate that before EMDR therapy, participants had significant differences in their SPRINT scores. After EMDR therapy, participants had no significant differences in their SPRINT scores, meaning that the therapy had the same effect on all participants. There was an increase in the feeling of confidence with which they were able to cope with the terrifying memories. It is important to note that the treatment effects were widespread across the network of similar incidents (e.g., rape, sexual abuse, physical and emotional abuse, neglect, and abandonment).

In addition, this program has been studied for its epigenetic impact on adolescents who have had several negative childhood experiences, and the results show that it leads to genome-wide changes in DNA methylation, and these changes have been annotated to genes whose biological processes are linked to early childhood adversity - neuronal, immune and endocrine pathways, cancer and cardiovascular disease [24].

This IIG-Psychotherapy program is also designed and developed for young children with their guardians and also for adults. Both programs are currently the subject of studies looking toward publication.

4.2 IIG-psychotherapy, multicomponent treatment strategy

The treatment has been designed taking into account aspects such as:

- Empathy and the integration process (awareness, bilateral integration, vertical integration, memory integration, narrative integration, state integration, interpersonal integration, and temporal integration) as a fundamental mechanism of well-being [1]. Then, in the different treatment axes, practices are carried out to achieve integration of the brain with the rest of the body, integration of the three brains, integration of their life stories, etc.

- Teaching children methods of emotional regulation and promoting their integration as self-care practices, which are linked to close relationships and social life, and the ecosystem [25].

- Providing safe conditions in the place where the stay takes place, and follow the ventral vagal approach [14] in all activities to promote states of calm and self-regulation. In this way, avoidance (flight), anger (fight), and collapse (freeze or shut down) behaviors are not mobilized, and children can perceive the place as safe. This is the only way they can effectively receive treatment.

DOI: http://dx.doi.org/10.5772/intechopen.1003718

- Practicing mindfulness and other meditations: Research in neuroscience and molecular biology demonstrates the transgenerational transmission of behaviors and the positive changes generated by meditative practices [26].

- Providing states of calm, tranquility, and pleasure and strengthening the neural networks of the prefrontal cortex. Deep breathing, conscious walking, soft music, dance movements, reducing emotional tension during EMDR, etc., strongly stimulate acetylcholine production, which generates enriched and diversified thinking.

IIG-Psychotherapy treatment for children uses appropriate techniques to strengthen internal resources and create positive neural networks that can generate progress in self-esteem. We believe this can help children with complex trauma: Since they affect an entire personality state, we need to strengthen the associative links between emotional experiences and their meaning. This means enabling a semantic flow between a lived experience and its meaning. The cognitive system is antagonistic to the emotional system. When the latter is too intense, it takes over. Emotion dominates. But conversely, cognitive memory networks enable us to control our fears [27].

4.3 The eight-phase program

Phase 1. History

Meet individually with the children and a family member to establish each child's clinical history and determine which children can benefit from IIG-Psychotherapy. During this meeting, the number of ACEs is established. Children receive comprehensive information about the intervention. Assessments of the severity of PTSD are administered to the children on the first day of the stay.

Phase 2. Preparation

This phase focuses on the children's safety (internal and external), emotional regulation, and improvement of fundamental life skills. These are the activities prior to group EMDR. Phase 2 lasts 3 days (the first 3 days of the stay).

Each day

We start the day very early. The children have a shower and a hot drink (panela water with cinnamon), and at 6.45 am, we meet in "The Hall of Dreams" for arts, yoga, and meditation:

We start the day with some Brain Gym® exercises, which are the result of numerous applied neuroscience studies on learning and brain function [28]. It enhances the deep integration of brain and body, supporting the sense of balance and spatial awareness and orientation: sequential movements starting with spinal movements, passing through lateral, homolateral, and contralateral movements involving the vestibular system, etc. We continue with yoga, which is a practice based on postures and breathing techniques to create a sense of connection with oneself, cultivate skills for staying present by observing and accepting sensations and emotions during postures, and breath control. Trauma victims can improve their mental and physical problems by modifying their breathing. The yoga chosen is Ashtanga Yoga [29]. It is an intense, athletic, and dynamic practice that develops a perception of body and mind and warms the body in depth. Regular practice tones and strengthens muscles, cleanse the body of toxins, calms the mind, and enhances concentration. We recommend that children maintain full attention during practice to experience breathing and movement safely and effectively without risk of injury. Children are then guided through meditation exercises geared toward empathy and compassion.

After the previous session, the children have breakfast, and before starting the other activities, they have a mindfulness practice, AMT method for children and teenagers by Eline Snel [4]. Experience has shown us that meditation practices are a valuable aid for children to avoid emotional decompensation when in contact with their painful memories. Mindfulness practices help children to be more focused, calm, and relaxed during their stay. Taking advantage of the brain's calmer state after mindfulness, children are invited to recall the specific traumatic memory they will be reprocessing on the day of trauma therapy and are guided through the exercise of the Flash Technique (FT) [30] to make the trauma more accessible to therapy. This is a new technique used during the preparation phase of EMDR therapy as a quick and relatively painless way of reducing the intensity of extremely disturbing memories. Every day and before lunch, the children are directed to practice of Rhythmic Movement Training (RMT) [15]. In the RMT, children are led through exercises to integrate the Moro and Fear Paralysis reflexes, which play a very important role in the development of connections from the limbic system and brain stem to other parts of the brain, in particular the prefrontal cortex. These connections have an important effect on our behavior and emotions. When the paralysis reflex is active, it causes the person to become mute, overwhelmed by their emotions, and unable to express them. When the Moro reflex is active, the person can be highly reactive and excitable. If both reflexes are active, the person feels insecure in all interactions with others. They may then establish inappropriate behaviors to feel safe: withdrawing, acting violently, and feeling the need to control or manipulate others. The aim of these practices in IIG-Psychotherapy is the integration of these two reflexes, which can certainly help improve the ability to connect effectively with others. Children are also guided to practice Trauma Releasing Exercises (TRE). This is a series of exercises that release deep body tensions by evoking a process of self-controlled muscle tremor called neurogenic muscle tremor [31]. The originality of this technique lies in the fact that these tremors originate in the deep center of the body, in the psoas muscle. These tremors reverberate outwards along the spine, releasing tension from the sacrum to the skull. The TRE touches the unconscious part of the brain, revealing patterns of tension and contraction lodged deep within the body. The contractions release the tensions at this deep level. When this happens, the body becomes more flexible and resilient. The result is greater self-awareness and a greater sense of self. Biodynamic psychotherapeutic massages and Ayurvedic head and hand massages [11, 12] are offered to the children to promote relaxation, recovery and/or the installation of pleasant sensations, beautiful feelings, and emotions. The children attend the puppet show of the EMDR story of Buddy the Dog [32] so that they can understand the usefulness of alternating stimuli. The puppet show is performed the day before the EMDR group therapy.

Phases 3 to 7 (assessment, desensitization, future vision, body scan, closure)

Group therapy is administered to all children in a group in four sessions over a two-day period (days four and five). In the first session, children complete phases 3–4 (assessment and desensitization) of the Protocol EMDR-IGTP, the first measure of Subjective Disturbance Units (SUD); then, in phase 5, the children are asked to draw how they see themselves in the future and to write a word or sentence explaining what they have drawn (vision of the future). After this, in phase 6, children are asked to recall the event, close their eyes, scan their body, and then do the butterfly hug for

3 minutes. In phase 7, children are asked to go to their "safe place" and, after 1 minute, to breathe deeply and open their eyes.

In sessions 2, 3, and 4, children repeat phases 3 and 7 of the same group EMDR protocol (second, third, and fourth or last SUD measure) individually.

Phase 8. Reassessment and use of EMDR-IGTP protocol or standard EMDR protocol. Day six

Identify children who need individual EMDR sessions. These are children whose SUD for the chosen trauma has not reached 0 during the group intervention. Team members who are properly trained as psychotherapists in EMDR therapy can continue to work with participants who need more care: either by using this protocol again, in small groups, or by treating them with the individual EMDR therapy protocol. Individual EMDR: The target of the session is the same memory that was the focus of the group therapy. Children are also asked to identify a negative cognition. The session follows standard EMDR procedures. The treatment ends in this phase. Two or three months after the end of the stay, the follow-up measurement, self-descriptions, parent descriptions, and teacher descriptions are collected.

5. Pre-adolescent program: Happy children

At the pre-adolescent age, children find themselves in a world between dream and reality. That is why we have included the figure of a "fairy godmother" (playing the flute) who invites the children into the "room of dreams". Here, the children find everything they need for their art (the little stones, the treasure box, the leaves to draw their butterfly, the flutes, etc.), and they begin to enter into deep contact with the artists and with themselves. The artists are free to design and create their work with the children. They are asked to follow a line that leads to the proposed objectives. It is proposed to work on beautiful tales or stories, creating characters, costumes, and scenarios, as in Commedia dell'arte. The aim of theater for pre-teens is to work on presence, voice, the rhythm of their steps, and light; in short, the integration of life, the body, and emotions. The children, in addition to using musical and vocal instruments, become sensitive to the flute (wind instrument, internal safety, toning of the infra-diaphragmatic vague nerve). The general objectives are that children get in touch with their emotions, learn to differentiate between them, and experience happiness. The specific objective is that children free themselves from post-traumatic stress due to violence (rape, abuse, etc.).

6. Teen program: The hero's journey

During adolescence, limits are pushed, which can be a challenge but can also create disasters; adolescents tend to move away from what is known and safe, and at the same time, they feel they need protection; they also need immediate pleasures. Adolescents are trained in Eline Snel's comprehensive AMT protocol for adolescents. Adolescents find internal strengths and heal at least one negative belief about themselves through DNMS. Guided by the artists, the teenagers invent and stage The Hero's Journey. This program runs throughout the intervention. Also, during the stay, 1 day is devoted to the construction of polyhedral and mandala designs, to help them understand the structure of the universe. The general objectives of this teen program are: to sow the seeds of the essential desire to seek inspiration for themselves, so that it can appear at every moment of their lives; that young people find their place of balance between their own interiority and their place within the other beings of the world; that young people learn to take responsibility for their own physical, mental and spiritual health; that young people reflect on and integrate the following essential aspects: What are you looking for in life? Find your personal legend! The world of the earth - What are your fears? Transform them! And acquire pure willpower! The world of air and fire - What are your qualities for success? Listen to your inner voice! The world of water - Commit to yourself and to the world. Transcendental and spiritual world: Let young people rediscover the power of wonder. And the specific objective is That young people free themselves from post-traumatic stress due to violence (rape, abuse, etc.).

7. Conclusions

Intensive Integrative Group Psychotherapy is a week-long treatment program that provides significant mental health benefits associated with epigenetic changes in adolescents with a history of multiple ACEs and trauma. Children and adolescents create positive and peaceful relationships through group reconnections, find ways to focus on the present, and accept reality, which is key to recovering from trauma.

Acknowledgements

Our thanks to Dr. Ignacio Jarero for his constant guidance in the application and practice of his EMDR group protocols in our programs. Our thanks to Mrs. Homayra Sellier, president of IED International and creator of resilience camps in Switzerland, for having trusted us to create the IID Colombia branch and for having inspired us in the creation of camps. We would like to thanks Dr Richard Davidson for having this program as object of epigenetic study at the Center for Healthy Minds, University of Wisconsin-Madison. We thank Dr Perla Kaliman for her scientific support and for having provided us with a large part of the funding for this epigenetic study. Likewise, to Dr Elkin Llanes for his appreciation of the program since he first met it and for having made it possible for the University of Santander (UDES) to provide all the scientific, academic and ethical support and financial backing for this program to be the subject of the epigenetic study mentioned above. Our thanks to Mr. Alberto López, Master in Management, member of the administrative board of the Association IID Colombia for his moral and administrative support.

Conflict of interest

The authors declare no conflict of interest.

Thanks

We express our deep gratitude to the therapeutic team of the IID Colombia Association for having made possible the development of the Intensive Integrative Group Psychotherapy program: Dhelmis Guzman, physiotherapist; Megan Everts,

Psychologist; Laura Villa, artist; Vanessa Pahola Llano Cometa artist - psychologist; Fabian Bedoya Luna, artist; Danny Javier Poso Moreno, artist; Esperanza Alegria, Social worker; Dr Hugo Erazo, psychologist.

Declaration of competing interest

The program described in this chapter was designed by Susana Roque López, founder and director of the Association Innocence In Danger Colombia (IIDC). Email address: susanaied@orange.fr.

Author details

Susana Roque López
Association Innocence In Danger Colombia, Cali, Colombia

*Address all correspondence to: susanaied@orange.fr

References

[1] Siegel D. Il terapeuta consapevole. Sassari: Istituto di Scienze Cognitive Editore; 2013. 245 p. ISBN: 978-88-97386-10-0

[2] Lanius R. How to Help Clients Tolerate Dysregulation and Come Back from Hypoarousal Main Session #4. National Institute for the Clinical Application of Behavioral Medicine [Internet]; 2023. Available from: https://www.nicabm.com/confirm/treating-trauma-master-earlybird/?l=1 [Accessed: October 18, 2023]

[3] van der Kolk B. How to Help Clients Tolerate Dysregulation and Come Back from Hypoarousal Main Session #4. National Institute for the Clinical Application of Behavioral Medicine [Internet]; 2023. Available from: https://www.nicabm.com/confirm/treating-trauma-master-earlybird/?l=1 [Accessed: October 18, 2023]

[4] Shapiro F, Manueld' EMDR. Principes, Protocoles, Procedures. Paris: Dunod-Inter Editions; 2007. 567 p. ISBN: 978-2-10-050136-6

[5] Schore A. The Neurobiology of Attachment. Treating Trauma Master Series. Session #2. National Institute for the Clinical Application of Behavioral Medicine [Internet]; 2023. Available from: https://www.nicabm.com/confirm/treating-trauma-master-earlybird/?l=1 [Accessed: October 19, 2023]

[6] Snel E. Academy for Mindful Teaching, AMT [Internet]. Available from: https://www.elinesnel.com/en [Accessed: October 18, 2023]

[7] Nhat Han T. The Blooming of a Lotus. Essential Guided Meditations for Mindfulness, Healing, and Transformation. A Revised and Expanded Edition. Boston: Bacon Press; 2009. 152 p. ISBN: 978-080701787-6

[8] Nhat-Hanh T. Reconciliation, Healing the Inner Child. Berkeley: Parallax Press; 2006. 184 p. ISBN: 1935209647, 9781935209645

[9] Artigas L, Jarero I. The Butterfly Hug [Internet]. 2005. Available from: https://psycnet.apa.org/record/2009-16776-001 [Accessed: October 19, 2023]

[10] Artigas L, Jarero I. The Butterfly Hug [Internet]. 2010. Available from: https://psycnet.apa.org/record/2009-16776-001 [Accessed: October 19, 2023]

[11] Boysen G. Entre Psyche et Soma. Paris V: Editions Payot; 1997. 212 p. ISBN: 2-228-89064-2

[12] Johari H. Massage Tradionnel Ayurvedique. Le courrier du Livre. 1997. 180 p. ISBN: 2-7029-0356-8

[13] The Science of Coherence [Internet]. Available from: https://www.heartmath.org/resources/downloads/science-of-the-heart/ [Accessed: October 19, 2023]

[14] Porges S. Clinical Applications of the Polyvagal Theory: The Transformative Power of Feeling Safe [BtL Workshop]. Milan: Centro Moses; 2014

[15] Blomberg H, Dempsey M. Movements That Heal. Rhythmic Movement Training and Primitive Reflex Integration. Sunnybank Hills LPO: BookPal; 2011. 244 p. ISBN: 9781791985127(pbk.)

[16] Schmidt SJ. Ego State Therapy. Interventions to Prepare Attachment - Wounded Adults for EMDR. Gresham,

Oregon: DNMS Institute, LLC; 2020. 285 p. ISBN: 9798691660283

[17] Deb D. Polyvagal Exercises for Safety and Connection. 1st ed. New York: Norton; 2020. 1331 p. ISBN: 978-0-393-71385-5

[18] Molero RJ, Jarero I, Givaudan M. Longitudinal multisite randomized controlled trial on the provision of the EMDR integrative group treatment protocol for ongoing traumatic stress to refugee minors in Valencia Spain. American Journal of Applied Psychology. 2019;**8**(4):77-88. DOI: 10.11648/j.ajap.20190804.12

[19] Vega-Arce M, Núñez-Ulloa G. Experiencias Adversas en la Infancia: Revisión de su impacto en niños de 0 a 5 años. Enfermería Universitaria. 2017;**14**(2):4-5. DOI: 10.1016/j.reu.2017.02.004

[20] Hillis S, Mercy J, Amobi A, Kress H. Global prevalence of past-year violence against children: A systematic review and minimum estimates. Pediatrics. 2016;**137**(3):5-8. DOI: 10.1542/peds.2015-4079

[21] Papale LA, Seltzer LJ, Madrid A, Pollak SD, Alisch RS. Differentially methylated genes in saliva are linked to childhood stress. Scientific Reports. 2018;**8**(1):1-8. DOI: 10.1038/s41598-018-29107-0

[22] Roque Lopez S, Llanez Anaya E, Alvarez Lopez M, Everts M, Fernandez D, Davidson R, et al. Mental health benefits of a 1-week intensive multimodal group program for adolescents with multiple adverse childhood experiences. Child Abuse and Neglect. 2021;**22**(September):1-11. DOI: 10.1016/j.chiabu.2021.105349

[23] Jarero I, Roque Lopez S, Gomez J. The provision of an EMDR-based multicomponent trauma treatment with child victims of severe interpersonal trauma. Journal of EMDR Practice and Research. 2013;7(1):17-28. DOI: 10.1891/1933-3196.7.1.17

[24] Kaliman P, Cosín Tomás M, Madrid A, Roque López S, Llanez Anaya E, Papale L, et al. Epigenetic impact of a 1-week intensive multimodal group program for adolescents with multiple adverse childhood experiences. Scientific Reports. 2022;**12**:17177. DOI: 10.1038/s41598-022-21246-9

[25] Contamin E. Prenons Soin de Nous: Guide pratique d'auto-thérapie. Paris: Ed. BOD; 2018. 160 p. ISBN: 9782322164004

[26] Kaliman P. La Ciencia de la Meditación. De la mente a los genes. Barcelona: Ed. Kairos; 2018. 144 p. ISBN: 8499889220, 978849988922

[27] Roques J. Abrégé de Psychoneurobiologie au-delà de L'EMDR. Paris: Edit. BOD; 2018. 188 p. ISBN: 9782322089314

[28] Easy Brain Gym Exercises to Improve Focus and Memory [Internet]. Available from: https://www.stylecraze.com/.pdf [Accessed: October 05, 2023]

[29] Raisanen P. Ashtanga Yoga. Traditionnel. Le yoga selon l'enseignement de Sri K. Pattabhi. Jois. Paris: Ed. Almora; 2013. 189 p. ISBN: 978-2-35118-169-0

[30] The Flash Technique–Making Intense Trauma Memories more Accessible for EMDR Processing [Internet]. Available from: https://guerirdestraumaspsychologiques.comquest-ce-que-la-flash-technique/ [Accessed: October 10, 2023]

[31] TRE: A Condensed Explanation [Internet]. Available from: https://www.

bing.com/videos/riverview/relatedvideo?&q=David+Berceli&&mid=3CE601C9D895FB98BA113CE601C9D895FB98BA11&&FORM=VRDGAR

[32] Meignant I, Meignant C. L'EMDR de Bouba le chien. Paris: Ed. Meignant; 2007. 35 p. ASIN: B07YRS4CNY